Fix Your Gut

A Book Dedicated to "Fixing" All Your Digestive Ailments and Concerns

3rd Edition

By:
John Brisson

Edited By:
Jason Hooper
and
Paul Sweany

3rd Edition, 2017

info@fixyourgut.com

http://www.fixyourgut.com

DISCLAIMER

The author of this book is not a doctor, physician assistant, nurse practitioner, nurse, or in the health profession period. Information in this book cannot be used to diagnose, cure, or treat any disease. Do not follow any recommendations in this book without first discussing it with your medical professional. The research within this book is intended to provide options that were successful in the cited trials and could work for the reader as well. I hope this book improves your gut health and your life!

This book is a dedication to my beloved son Abel Scott Brisson. My inspiration for researching ways to improve our health often came because of me trying to give him and myself a better life. Even though you are gone, you will continue to touch lives both in your story and through me. I will love you always my son.

Table of Contents

Limonene

L-glutamine

Manuka Honey

Melatonin

Mitochondrial Support Supplements (Ubiquinol [CoQ10,] PQQ, and L-carnitine)

NAC

N-Acetylglucosamine

Nu-Nefarious

Ox bile

Oxaloacetate

R-lipoic Acid

Seacure

Undecylenic Acid

Zeaxanthin

Zinc Carnosine

Chapter 18

Herbs / Foods That Are Helpful for Digestive Ailments

Aloe Vera

Astragalus

Black Cumin Seed Oil

Black Raspberry Powder

Black Walnut Hulls

Boswellia

Butcher's Broom

Cardamom

Carnivora

Cayenne

Cinnamon

Chamomile

Echinacea

Fennel

Ginger

Goldenseal

Chapter 19

ANTIBIOTIC INFORMATION GUIDE

Chapter 24

Appendix / Sources

Gastroparesis
Cyclic Vomiting Syndrome
Barrett's Esophagus
Esophageal Spasms
Nutcracker Esophagus
SIBO
IBS
Chronic Functional Abdominal Pain
Intestinal Renewal
Celiac Disease
IBD
Appendix
Hemorrhoid
Colon Cleansing
Colon Cleansing Protocols

Chapter 1

My Story

For twenty-two years of my life, I thought natural medicine was a sham. My grandfather, who was a pharmacist, taught me that standard medicine was the only way to go and that the FDA (and drug companies) could do no evil. I laugh to myself now when I think of how foolish I was back then. Do not get me wrong; I still think conventional medicine has its place in healthcare, but I believe that we should consider all available options and make reasonable choices that are supported by the data.

I suffered from different medical conditions including being born extremely premature (twenty-two weeks) in 1985. I suffered from asthma, reduced lung capacity, and a poorly functioning immune system until I successfully healed myself a few years ago. Conventional medicine was just "treating" the symptoms of my asthma. It never addressed the actual causes of the disease, which were a deficiency in vitamin C, magnesium, omega 3 fatty acids, vitamin D, and chronic dehydration. Supplementation changed my life. My asthma symptoms disappeared within six months, and all tests showed my lung function was now completely normal. I asked my doctor how this was possible, and he was completely mystified and refused to consider the changes to my nutrition as a factor. It took conquering asthma and taking my life back to evaluate the relationship that I had with my doctor and the entire healthcare industry.

My mother passed away from systemic Lupus when I was five. She believed fully that conventional medicine would save her. My father was one of the first Americans in the early 90's to be diagnosed with hepatitis C. He participated in the first clinical trials of pegylated interferon with ribavirin. I remember taking care of my father throughout high school and listening to him vomit and sob for hours at a time after taking his medicine. When I was a senior in high school, the medication had left my father with cognitive deficits including memory loss, trouble focusing, and paranoid schizophrenia. He left this Earth when I was eighteen years old and about to leave home to go to college. He also believed that conventional medicine would have cured him, or at the very least, kept him alive to see me start my adult life, get married, or give him grandchildren.

I believe nutritional medicine would have saved both my parents. I believe that we should have opened our minds to other possibilities. What about people who have heart disease, cancer, diabetes, asthma, and autoimmune diagnoses? Are they aware of the treatment options that nutritional medicine has to offer? Conventional medicine does not always address the root cause of these illnesses. In many cases, only the symptoms are addressed.

I am not completely discounting the effectiveness of conventional medicine. The data shows that there is a high success rate of using certain treatments including antimicrobials to fight life-threatening infections, surgeries, and stabilizing someone during a medical emergency (like a heart attack, or stroke). One Christmas morning, I accidentally cut my artery in my left arm. I would have bled to death without emergency arterial repair surgery. I took antibiotics, and I followed my doctor's post-surgical recommendations and drug regimen for a month afterward. I have no problem admitting conventional medicine saved my life. The acceptance of both forms of healthcare is needed in the United States. We need to have access to a complete healthcare system.

I became interested in natural health when I learned about nutritional healing after listening to Dr. Joel Wallach on the Alex Jones Radio Show. He brought up many good topics like several key nutrients that are lacking in the Western diet. He addressed copper and magnesium deficiencies, which explain why we have an epidemic of heart disease in the United States. Although I do not completely agree with Dr. Wallach's entire body of work, I appreciate the fact that he encourages us to think about nutrition and the human body in different non-conventional ways. Discovering his work inspired me to dig deeper into natural health studies that served me well when I fell ill.

Ever hear of the "butterfly effect?" According to Edward Lorenz, it is theoretically possible for a butterfly to flap its wings and create a puff of air that will eventually cause a tornado somewhere. Looking back, I can point to a single cause to the deterioration of my health for years to come, but instead of a butterfly, it was a blood pressure cuff. The nurse took my blood pressure one day at the doctor's office and wrote down a number on the chart. The doctor reviewed the number later and wrote down a prescription for medicine on a pad. The pharmacist gave me an ACE inhibitor that I would later take a few years. The ACE inhibitor taxed my angiotensin-renin-aldosterone system. I eventually developed adrenal fatigue and LERD. You see how one simple medical decision can lead to something severe and unintended?

I remember the day when I first became sick like it was yesterday. I was at my grandmother-in-law's house eating a delicious catfish dinner. My stomach later burned for the first time in my life and ached badly. I tried to lie down, but after an hour, the pain was so overwhelming that I could barely move. I went to the emergency room, and they could not find anything wrong with me. They told me I was perfectly healthy.

Over the next month, I developed OCD, had significant anxiety, LERD symptoms, gastritis, stomach pain, and my resting heart rate increased thirty beats per minute. During this stressful period, I thought that I was going to die, or at the very least, I was concerned that I might be slipping into madness. For the first time in my life, my health was rapidly deteriorating. I visited several doctors, and their tests showed nothing significant except for an elevated heart rate. The only treatment my doctors offered me was a drug test in the hospital to see if I was a user. Once I passed the drug test, all they wanted to do was admit me into the hospital, and monitor my condition. My primary doctor planned to prescribe a series of prescription medicines, including some powerful heart and anti-anxiety medications to calm me down because he thought anxiety had caused all my problems. My grandfather told me to stop the ACE inhibitor and to wait a few days to see if I would improve. He said that any medicine, at any given time, might cause side effects in anyone. The next day, I discontinued my ACE inhibitor, checked my resting heart rate, and it relieved me to find that it had returned to normal.

Unfortunately, the damage had been done. The ACE inhibitor left me with horrible side effects, and I almost fell into an adrenal crisis. It took me over a year to recover from the severe adrenal fatigue that I had developed.

During my recovery, I noticed that my local supplement store needed employment. I asked the manager at the vitamin retailer if he had any job openings. He had seen me in the store frequently and knew I had some knowledge. He saw potential in me because of my willingness to help people and hired me immediately. I loved the work, learned everything that I could, and helped as many people as possible with their health problems. I had to resign when my youngest son was born with health problems, and I dedicated my life to take care of him.

My youngest son, Abel, was born with an extremely rare medical condition known as congenital myopathy with excess muscle spindles. He is only one of six children in the world to be given this diagnosis. The medical explanation of this condition is complex, but the simplest explanation that I can describe is that the gene that produces muscle fibers was stuck in the "off" position, while the gene that produces muscle spindles was stuck in the "on" position for some time in the womb. When he was born, we noticed that he was extremely fragile, and he could hardly move. His fragility was due to the higher concentration of muscle spindles, rather than muscle fibers, throughout his body.

Doctors told my wife and me that my son would continue to get weaker until he died. He was on a ventilator for the first three months of his life. My wife and I made a difficult choice, and his doctors removed the ventilator to end his suffering. Even though I consider myself a Theist, I often struggle with faith. There is no reasonable scientific answer for why Abel is still alive. Even though he was completely paralyzed, he coughed up the ventilator tube and began to breathe without the assistance. His spontaneous ability to breathe naturally on his own appeared to be medically impossible because his lungs were supposed to have atrophied. We took our son home the same month.

I am grateful for conventional medicine. They stabilized my son’s life. He lived in the ICU for a total of six months. I am grateful to all the doctors, nurses, and hospital staff that took care of my son. Conventional medicine stabilized my son. Supplementation extended and improved his quality of life.

There is very little information about Abel’s condition, and only one case study of five children has been presented for reference. He has surpassed his life expectancy of two years old, and I believe supplementation has made all the difference. He does not have any of the heart problems or conditions that any of the other children developed. His muscle tone is also increasing, and he can move his hands, feet, and make noises from his mouth. Neurologically, my son has above normal intelligence. The doctors were baffled at how well my son was doing. Abel sadly passed away right before the publishing of the first edition of Fix Your Gut from a sudden pulmonary embolism.

I do not suffer from LERD any longer. I tackled it as *H. pylori* overgrowth, even though all tests were negative. I had all the symptoms throughout my health journey of upper gut growth, and through taking the steps I did, I recovered. They say it takes becoming sick to take one's health in their own hands, and the same can be said for me. I wrote this book about digestive health and coached many clients with digestive problems and concerns because no one should have to suffer. I believe proper digestion is one of the most important components of health for everyone. Eating healthy food and having proper digestion is one of the things that make us human. Since my health is under control, my OCD and anxiety have disappeared, and I feel better than ever!

I want everyone who reads this book with digestion problems to know that they are not alone.

Chapter 2

Mechanisms of the Human Digestive System

The Importance of Digestive Health

There is an average of seventy million Americans diagnosed with digestive disorders every year. More Americans are rushing to their doctors to treat conditions like heartburn, gas, GERD, SIBO, IBS, ulcerative colitis and Crohn's disease. More digestive diseases and problems are also being discovered every year. The most concerning aspect of all these conditions is that science and natural medicine are way ahead of the curve in relieving all of these problems. Most people only rely on conventional medicine, which is ideal for emergency procedures, and life-threatening conditions, but does not always offer what is needed for the prevention of disease.

In every medical community, there should be a balance of natural and conventional medicine. All adults need to be given the information required to make their personal decisions not only for treatment options but to develop habits that will keep them healthy. One of the best ways to improve your health is to change your diet and optimize your digestive system to enhance total body function. An ideal digestive system eliminates toxins, governs the immune system, absorbs nutrients, provides peak mental health, and ultimately makes it possible to get the most out of life.

The Mouth and Esophagus

The most overlooked body part of digestion is the mouth. Your mouth is the starting point for all digestion. Do you remember when your parents used to yell at you for chewing your food too fast? They were right. Chewing your food thoroughly is critical for optimal digestion. Chewing your food well helps break down your food mechanically and makes it easier for your stomach to digest. Saliva helps lubricate your food and begins peristalsis. Saliva also contains the digestive enzyme amylase, which starts to break down carbohydrates from the moment you taste your food.

The next stage of the digestive system is the esophagus. The cilia and muscles of the esophagus push food downward (peristalsis) towards the stomach and through the LES. The lower esophageal sphincter relaxes and allows food to enter the stomach before closing tightly to keep stomach acid and pepsin from entering the esophagus.

Stomach

The stomach is the only digestive organ that mechanically, chemically, and enzymatically digests food in the human body. Through a complex system, the stomach works very hard to break down most of the meals that we consume. The food we eat is then absorbed and eliminated through our intestinal system.

Mechanically

The stomach has muscles that help churn food contents and mix it with stomach acid and pepsin. The sphincter at the lower part of the stomach opens and closes to propel food into the duodenum. These contractions can also squirt the food chyme upward back into the stomach if more digestion is required.

Chemically

The stomach produces hydrochloric acid that helps with the digestion process. Contrary to popular belief, this "stomach acid" does not directly digest food. The gastric acid instead maintains the proper pH balance in the stomach, allowing gastrin to be able to break down food, as well as eliminate any excess bacteria that were ingested. Gastric acid can help denature proteins, but pepsin does the majority of this form of digestion. The stomach also produces mucus, which coats and protects the stomach wall so that the stomach will not be harmed by gastric acid.

Enzymatically / Hormonal

Once the stomach distends from the ingestion of food, it releases gastrin. Gastrin can also be released through stimulation of the vagus nerve, undigested proteins in the stomach, and elevated levels of calcium in the blood. Gastrin has many different uses in the stomach. Gastrin stimulates stomach cells to release HCL, activates stomach cell growth, initiates the secretion of pepsinogen (which later becomes protein enzyme pepsin), induces pancreatic secretions, gallbladder emptying, and causes the LES to tighten and begin digestion. An excess of stomach acid inhibits gastrin production. This feedback loop causes the stomach to stop the digestion process over time.

Pepsin is the primary enzyme used by the stomach to digest protein. Pepsinogen activates and converts into the enzyme pepsin in the presence of stomach acid. Pepsin helps break down protein into amino acids the body can absorb and then becomes inactivated, by turning back into pepsinogen when it is mixed with bicarbonate released from the pancreas in the small intestine. This transformation protects the rest of the intestinal system from the pepsin and stomach acid.

The stomach produces other enzymes, as well. Gastric lipase helps break down different fats and digests fats like SCT's and MCT's that do not require bile to be broken down. Finally, mucin is an enzyme that the stomach produces to protect the mucosal lining of the stomach.

On Gastrin

Hormones control a lot of our digestion, and one of the most important hormones for the proper functionality of upper gut is gastrin. Gastrin is a hormone that is released into our bloodstream by our stomach to help control digestion. Gastrin is produced by the G cells in the antrum of the stomach.

Gastrin release occurs because:

- The stomach body expands from consumption.
- Vagus nerve stimulation.
- Partially digested protein or amino acid supplements in the stomach.
- Hypercalcemia.
- Ingestion of coffee and alcohol.
- H. pylori colonization of the antrum (stomach body).
- Using medications including adrenergic stimulating drugs, cholinergic agents, and H2 antagonists / PPI's (negative feedback loop, reduction in stomach acid and increased stomach pH leads to increased gastrin levels in some people).
- The hormone bombesin, epinephrine, and gastrin-releasing peptide.
- Gastrin-producing tumors (gastrinoma).
- Zollinger-Ellison Syndrome.

Gastrin, when it reaches the parietal cells of the antrum, signals the stomach to secrete gastric acid and release histamine. Gastrin does a lot to improve our digestion including:

- Causes the chief cells in the stomach to produce pepsinogen, which later becomes pepsin and helps to digest protein.
- Decreases upper stomach contractions and motility to help improve digestion by increasing stomach relaxation to allow ingestion of more food and further digestion by stomach acid and pepsin.
- Opens the pyloric sphincter and increases the rate of gastric emptying.

- Increases small intestine MMC function and helps relax the ileocecal valve.
- Induces pancreatic enzyme secretion.
- Stimulates bile release from the gallbladder.
- Helps regulate the production of gastric epithelial cells, tissue repair, and blood vessel growth in the stomach.

The body also has mechanisms to shut off gastrin production when stomach digestion is completed. When the stomach pH is below three, gastrin production by the stomach is limited. Fasting also decreases gastrin levels. The pancreas releases somatostatin to inhibit gastrin and histamine in the intestinal tract to stop digestion in the stomach. Other hormones that slow down or stop gastrin production include a gastric inhibitory peptide, secretin, glucagon, and calcitonin. Finally, when most of the ingested food has gone from the stomach into the duodenum or has passed into the jejunum, the enterogastric reflex occurs to reduce gastric motility, gastrin release, and gastric acid production.

Having a less acidic stomach over time, like when you consume PPI's or H2 antagonists might explain the increase in serum gastrin levels and rebound acid reflux if you are on these medications long term or if you discontinue them abruptly. An increase of gastrin causes more stomach acid to be produced in a less acidic stomach for a short period, as a way for the body to try to correct digestion and compensate for the less acidic stomach. People with lower stomach acidity are more prone to upper gut overgrowth and combined with increased gastrin, and stomach acid production can lead to stomach distension, weakened LES, increased gastric pressure, and worsen reflux symptoms. Most of the time the doses of medication are increased, which further hinders stomach acid production, which increases gastrin production further, and the cycle repeats itself. In addition, people with bile reflux see even worsening symptoms with up-regulation of gastrin because it also increases bile production and the opening of the pyloric sphincter, causing a mixture of bile and acid reflux, which irritates the stomach and esophagus when fluxed, causing issues.

The body to ensure proper digestion in the upper gut should tightly regulate gastrin levels. To produce appropriate gastrin levels, you need to make sure that your calcium levels are balanced, reduction of upper gut overgrowth like *H. pylori* if you have it, and maintain proper stomach pH for digestion. When you are consuming food, you want to make sure that the pH of your stomach is less than three after you finish your meal. You can achieve proper stomach pH by ingesting betaine HCL, acidic foods, or digestive bitters towards the end of a meal if you can tolerate them to help accurately control gastrin production and aid with digestion.

Intrinsic Factor

The intrinsic factor is also secreted by the stomach and is present in gastric juice and the mucous membrane of the stomach. The intrinsic factor helps absorb vitamin B12 further along in the intestines. Production of intrinsic factor in the stomach can be hindered by having low stomach acid or by taking certain medications that lower stomach acid like H2 antagonists and proton pump inhibitors.

Metformin, which is used in the treatment of diabetes, can also cause a loss of the intrinsic factor in the stomach. People with gastric bypass surgery might also lose their production of the intrinsic factor, as well. If you are dealing with any of these issues, have your doctor check your B12 plasma levels every few months. The supplementation of sublingual B12 or B12 injections might be needed for maintaining optimal health.

Liver, Gallbladder, and Pancreas

Aside from the stomach, the liver, gallbladder, and pancreas must function normally so that complete digestion can occur. These organs further regulate the enzymatic and chemical side of digestion. The Liver produces bile and releases it to the small intestine directly, or the gallbladder, where it is stored until needed. Bile helps break down fats so that the digestive enzymes can fully break down the food that you eat. The pancreas produces acinar cells, which are responsible for releasing most of these digestive enzymes into the intestines. The pancreas also makes ductal cells. Ductal cells release sodium bicarbonate into the small intestine to neutralize the stomach acid mixed with the food chyme that is released from the stomach into the duodenum.

Small Intestine

There are three parts of the small intestine, the duodenum, the jejunum, and the ileum. Most of the digestion that takes place in these three sections is accomplished enzymatically. Cilia and muscle contractions move chyme through the intestines (peristalsis).

Major Nutrients That Are Digested in the Small Intestine:

- Proteins break down into peptides and amino acids in the small intestine. Pepsin begins the process in the stomach, and enzymes secreted by the pancreas, including trypsin and chymotrypsin; cleave proteins into smaller peptides and amino acids in the small intestine.
- Lipids degrade into fatty acids and glycerol. Pancreatic lipase breaks down triglycerides into free fatty acids and monoglycerides. Pancreatic lipase accomplishes this task with the help of bile acid salts. The bile salts emulsify the triglycerides until the lipase can break them into smaller components. Then the broken down lipids can enter the villi for absorption.
- Pancreatic amylase breaks down some carbohydrates into oligosaccharides. Some simple carbohydrates can be converted quickly into glucose and are absorbed into the bloodstream. Other carbohydrates pass undigested into the large intestine where they ferment before they are broken down completely via bacteria. Dextrinase, glucoamylase, maltase, sucrase, and lactase are all digestive enzymes that are involved in these processes.

Some adults lack proper amounts of lactase, causing the digestive disorder known as lactose intolerance. Cellulose, cannot be broken down by humans and passes through the intestines undigested.

Nutrients That Are Absorbed in the Small Intestine:

- Iron is absorbed in the duodenum.
- Water, fat, and fructose are also absorbed.
- Vitamin B12 and bile salts are absorbed in the ileum.
- Sodium bicarbonate is also absorbed back into the body in the small intestines.

The duodenum releases secretin and cholecystokinin, which relaxes the stomach pylorus so that chyme can be released into the duodenum. It is primarily responsible for the breakdown of food in the small intestine, using other digestive enzymes. The hormones secretin and cholecystokinin also cause the liver or gallbladder to release bile, and the pancreas to release bicarbonate and digestive enzymes such as trypsin, lipase, and amylase into the duodenum as they are needed. Finally, secretin helps regulate the pH in the duodenum by inactivating gastric acid secretion by the parietal cells of the stomach.

The lining of the jejunum specializes in the absorption of small nutrient particles by enterocytes. Once absorbed, nutrients pass from the enterocytes into the enterohepatic circulation and enter the liver via the hepatic portal vein, where the blood is filtered. The jejunum is the end of chemical digestion, and most of the byproducts of chemical digestion (bile, bicarb) are absorbed back into the body in the ileum.

The ileum is the final section of the small intestine, which absorbs both nutrients and the byproducts of digestion. The main function of the ileum is to absorb nutrients, including vitamin B12. Byproducts of digestion like bile, fatty acids, and glycerol are absorbed, as well. The cells in the ileum also release protease to break down the remaining proteins. The remaining chyme deposits itself into the large intestine through the ileocecal valve to be turned into feces.

Large Intestine

Chyme moves from the small intestine into the large intestine through the ileocecal valve. The chyme is then made into feces and moves through the large intestine to the anus. Peristalsis in the large intestine slows to allow probiotic bacteria to ferment the chyme, so the final part of digestion occurs. The large intestine converts chyme into feces so that it can be eliminated from the body, a process that takes about sixteen hours. The large intestine removes excess water and any remaining absorbable nutrients from the chyme, before sending the indigestible matter to the rectum.

The large intestine houses over seven hundred species of bacteria that perform a variety of functions for the human body. The colon absorbs vitamins that are produced by the colonic bacterial metabolism from fermenting food. Those vitamins include vitamin K, vitamin B12, thiamine, riboflavin, and biotin. Undigested fiber other than cellulose is also metabolized into short-chain fatty acids and is then absorbed back into the bloodstream. Flatulence, caused by bacterial fermentation, is also formed and expelled through the large intestine during digestion. Probiotic gut flora is essential in developing large intestine epithelial cells, lymphatic cells, cross-reactive antibodies (that eliminate foreign bacteria), and help maintain the natural mucus barrier of the large intestine.

Feces travel further down the large intestine by peristalsis, pass through the colon, and are expelled out of the body through the anal sphincter.

Immune System and the Gut / GALT

The intestinal system is one of the most important components of one's immune system. The intestines are made up of both probiotics and gut-associated lymphoid tissue that helps regulate a significant part of the human immune system. If you have a poorly functioning immune system, one of the first areas the practitioner should begin to examine is your digestive health.

The gut contains the largest mass of lymphoid tissue in the body. The lymphoid tissue in the gut stores immune cells (T and B-lymphocytes) that help destroy pathogens. About fifty to eighty percent of your immune system is stored in the GALT. The GALT lies behind the mucosal lining of your gut and is only one cell wall thick. Your probiotic bacteria live in symbiosis with your GALT and partially compose your entire immune system.

Probiotics are both yeast and bacteria that live in your digestive tract, helping to maintain your intestinal integrity. Probiotic bacteria in the gut help maintain proper gastrointestinal function, break down lactose, manufacture and absorb vitamin K, vitamin B12, thiamine, riboflavin, biotin, destroy opportunistic bacteria, and help ferment carbohydrates for digestion in the large intestine.

The Gut: The Second Brain

If your gastrointestinal system is having problems functioning normally, it can create depression and increase anxiety levels in your life. The gut has a nervous system known as the enteric nervous system. The ENS influences your mental health function because of the large network of neurons, nerves, and neurotransmitters present. IBS has been theorized as a cause of some people developing anxiety and depression in people afflicted with the disease. Most medical professionals, on the other hand, believe that these mental health issues are the cause of IBS instead of being issues stemming from poor digestion.

The ENS communicates with the CNS using the vagus nerve and the prevertebral ganglia. Some studies explore the theory that the ENS can communicate directly with the CNS through neurotransmitters in the gut. This theory arose because the gut has been known to work properly even if a vertebrate's vagus nerve has been severed. The neurons in the ENS can also control the peristalsis of food, and what digestive enzymes are released. The ENS makes use of more than thirty neurotransmitters identical to the ones used in the CNS. Serotonin is used in large amounts in the gut for the muscle contractions needed in the peristalsis of food. More than ninety percent of anyone's serotonin and fifty percent of their total dopamine concentrations are found in the gut at any given time.

In the not too distant future, a link between depression, anxiety, and leaky gut syndrome may finally occur. Bacteria in the gut can influence what hormones and neurotransmitters are used and released into the gut. If you have a leaky gut, it may affect your brain by excessive amounts of neurotransmitters, pathogens, and toxins being able to cross the blood-brain barrier. If you have a spastic gut, like most people suffering from IBS, the spasms could create additional anxiety in your life because of increased vagal nerve function, increased epinephrine release, and heart palpitations. Misfiring of nerve signals can create anxiety as well as a neurotransmitter imbalance which will further mental anguish. Always remember if your gut is always in a panic, you will start to feel anxious as well.

What Is Melatonin?

Melatonin is a neurotransmitter that was originally believed only to be produced by our pineal gland within the brain. It is very important to the overall function of the human body acting as an antioxidant, regulating circadian rhythm (our internal clock) to help us sleep, reduces blood pressure, and leptin levels (the hormone that inhibits hunger) during sleep. Melatonin has also recently been discovered in large quantities in other organs as well.

Recent studies have shown that melatonin is also synthesized by our gut flora and rates at least 400 times greater than our pineal gland. Large quantities of melatonin have been located in the vermiform appendix, which appears to be a safe house for probiotic flora during gastrointestinal infection. Bacteria, like other life forms on Earth, have a circadian rhythm, so they also produce melatonin in the dark and possibly as a signaling hormone.

Melatonin and the Gut

There currently is not a lot of information about melatonin and its relation to the gut, because it is a recent discovery. Nevertheless, the information that we have from studies and proposed theories about a neurotransmitter that we believed was only important for healthy sleep is jaw dropping.

Here are some theories on the importance of melatonin and our gastrointestinal health:

- Melatonin protects the gastric mucosa from free radicals, medications (NSAIDS), and gastrotoxic agents.
- Reduces production of HCL and pepsin production when sleeping. Reduces the chance of esophageal, peptic, and duodenal ulcers.
- Reduction of reflux while sleeping and surprisingly also when awake.
- Improves LES and UES pressure regulation.
- Reduces the risk of developing Barrett's esophagus by increasing blood flow to the esophagus and reducing inflammation.
- Reduction of bowel spasms and improving MMC function in people with SIBO-D.
- Reinforces proper MMC function during sleep by regulating the interstitial cells of Cajal. A majority of MMC function occurs while we sleep; it is the longest period of fasting for our body.

Sleep Hygiene and Melatonin

We are supersaturated with blue light during the night. Blue light (part of the light spectrum or the color spectrum) reduces melatonin production and increases serotonin that helps us to be awake. The light from our cell phone screens and LED monitors. Even the light pollution that creeps in through our blinds at night is interfering with our sleep.

So what do we do to ensure that we have proper melatonin production?

First, before we even discuss reducing blue light to increase melatonin production, we have to make sure our gut flora is happy and well fed and remember diversity is key! We should avoid sugar and polyols as much as possible and focus on a diverse seasonal diet. We should eat prebiotic fiber (limit supplemental prebiotics, except for GOS occasionally) from time to time and fermented foods including organic grass-fed sour cream, kimchi, fermented cabbage, and fermented pickles. Remember, the flora in our gut produce a lot of melatonin, so we have to make sure that it is happy to assist us with proper digestion.

Second, this is what everyone writes about; we need to limit blue light at night.

Here are some tips:

- Wearing blue light blocking glasses at night to increase melatonin. I do not recommend doing this if you are driving, however, since you need to be awake while you drive, and some people including Dr. Jack Kruse believe that blue light hitting the retina is important for global positioning (this does weirdly make sense, I felt weird while going to the store a few times wearing the glasses).
- Install programs like F.lux on your PC or Mac to reduce blue light or Twilight on your Android phone.

- Do not fall asleep with the television or any electronic device on if possible that emits blue light. If you have any emitting LED light in your room, try to block it or cover it with electrical tape.
- If your child requires a night light while they sleep, get one that emits low levels of blue light.
- If you cannot limit blue light while you sleep, try to wear an eye mask if possible.
- If you live in an area with heavy light pollution, you might need to put up blackout curtains (caution, it is talked about in the health blogosphere that most are heavily treated and contain VOC's so you want them to out gas awhile before hanging) and try to make your room as dark as possible. If you live out in the country, it might be best to make your room as dark as possible since the proper reflection of moonlight when the moon is fuller might tie into a proper circadian rhythm. Even though the light reflected from the moon is of course sunlight that has plenty of blue light, the light is not bright enough to reduce melatonin production.

Finally, here are some tips to improve your sleep hygiene:

- Do not sleep in a frigid or sweltering bedroom. It is optimal for you to keep the room temperature between 60 – 70 degrees at night.
- Do not go to sleep on a full stomach. Melatonin production at night hinders the stomach's capacity to digest food. It tightens the sphincters and reduces HCL and pepsin production.
- Sleep on your left side or back with only one pillow for greatest oxygen saturation during sleep. Sleeping on your left side puts more pressure on the LES keeping it closed and prevents reflux.
- Do however take in a small amount of carbohydrates before bed. One to two teaspoons of raw honey or twenty grams of trehalose before bed mixed with spring water can help improve sleep by stabilizing your blood glucose during the night.
- Turning off non-native EMF (while experimental) may help improve sleep quality. I turn off my wifi at night and place my phone as far away from the bed as possible.

What Is CCK and What Does It Do?

CCK stands for cholecystokinin, and it is synthesized in the mucosal epithelium of the small intestine and secreted into the duodenum. The release of CCK is stimulated by a peptide released by pancreatic acinar cells and, CCK-releasing protein secreted by enterocytes in the mucosa. In addition, vagus nerve stimulation by acetylcholine may trigger its release. Finally, the greatest stimulator of CCK is the presence of fatty / amino acids in chyme when it enters the duodenum for further digestion.

The hormone does a lot in our body including:

- Stimulating the release of bile from the gallbladder and digestive enzymes from the pancreas.
- Increases bile production by the liver.
- Increases sodium bicarbonate production by the pancreas to neutralize stomach acid.
- Slows down gastric emptying and decreases stomach acid secretion.
- Induces satiety.
- Increases opioid tolerance.
- Plays a role in increasing sensitivity to pain.
- Reduces inflammatory markers including TNF and Il-6.
- Increases aldosterone (a hormone that increases retention of sodium and increases blood pressure) and cortisol.
- Helps to regulate MMC function in conjunction with the hypothalamus.
- Overproduction can lead to postprandial fatigue and sleepiness (the ITIS!)

As the chyme, digestive enzymes, and bile pass further into the small intestine, CCK release diminishes. In addition, more digestive enzymes produced by the pancreas to aid in digestion like trypsin and somatostatin further inactivate CCK.

So What Does All This Have to Do With Anxiety?

A single CCK peptide known as CCK-4 is to blame. In someone that is healthy, most CCK peptides are broken down effectively in the digestive tract or do not cross the BBB easily. When someone is having fat digestion issues, upper gut infections, SIBO, or leaky gut, CCK peptides are more likely to cross the BBB (specifically CCK-4). What does CCK-4 do when it gets into the brain? It overstimulates the vagus nerve for one and induces panic. Studies show that CCK-4, injected into the bloodstream, causes panic attacks. It is quickly metabolized in the brain, so the duration of its effects are short unless the act of panicking releases excess catecholamines, which cause some people to have panic attacks for an extended amount of time.

CCK production, inactivation, and leaky gut issues can also cause rapid dumping syndrome in consuming foods that stimulate its release (mainly fat), which can also overstimulate the vagus nerve and create anxiety. Capsaicin has been shown to blunt some of the effects CCK-4 has on the vagus nerve by desensitizing it and reducing anxiety. Digestive enzyme supplements that include amylase and trypsin might also reduce CCK overproduction in the intestines by activating feedback loops within the body.

So CCK Is Not to Blame for Digestive Caused Anxiety, Right?

Correct.

The issue is not CCK but instead either an overproduction of CCK from digestive issues or leaky gut. Most of the time too much CCK will be produced when you either eat a high fat meal (if you are not "fat adapted") or have some type of issue with your organs that help with fat digestion (liver, gallbladder, stomach, and pancreas). Fat malabsorption can also cause diarrhea and in doing so overstimulates the vagus nerve, which exacerbates anxiety. In addition, if you are suffering from leaky gut (more than likely from overgrowth) CCK peptides (including CCK-4) might be more likely to cross the BBB and induce anxiety. Try to reduce overgrowth and work to improve the lining of your intestinal barrier and restore your microbiome to good health.

When it comes to anxiety and digestion, do not blame the hormone CCK, which provides many important functions within our body. Instead, work to improve your digestion so that CCK production maintains homeostasis to improve your overall health.

Chapter 3

The True Cause of Heartburn / GERD

Heartburn is a result of too much pressure in the gastrointestinal system. Excessive pressure causes stomach acid to push through the LES and up through the esophagus where it is then stopped by the UES and sent back down into the stomach. The constant increase in pressure, weakening of the LES, and reflux causes the symptoms of GERD.

Reflux Can Be Caused By:

- Bacterial / archaeal overgrowth in the intestines causes excessive hydrogen / methane gas production, increasing gastrointestinal pressure.
- Upper gut overgrowth in the stomach upregulates protein fermentation and increases pressure, weakening the LES.
- Over ingestion of fermenting food and beverages (carbonated water, FODMAPS, and protein).
- Ingestion of GMO's.
- Tight fitting clothing (bras, belt, shirts, pants) putting excessive pressure on the gastrointestinal tract.
- Having incorrect posture increases gastrointestinal pressure.
- A weakened LES that is due to increased pressure causing more stomach contents to be forced up through the esophagus.
- Lack of digestive enzymes, resulting in poor digestion of food that can lead to excessive fermentation.
- Yeast overgrowth causes excessive fermentation and increases gastrointestinal pressure.
- Constipation leading to toxin retention, leaky gut, downregulation of MMC function, increased fermentation, and dysbiosis.
- The decrease of stomach acid productions leads to microbiome dysbiosis and poor protein digestion.
- Poorly functional gallbladder, liver, or pancreas resulting in either digestive enzyme or bile production problems.
- Having a hiatal hernia.
- Improper defecation posture.
- Parasites.

To eliminate heartburn, you have to identify its cause. Some digestive issues may overlap so tackle each problem accordingly.

GERD

Gastroesophageal Reflux Disease is a condition in which mucosal damage is done to the esophagus from chronic stomach acid and pepsin being trapped between the stomach and the upper esophageal sphincter. This "trapping" gives the afflicted person the characteristic feeling of heartburn. Having GERD can eventually lead to esophagitis, strictures, or even cancer from chronic inflammation if left untreated.

The most common symptoms of GERD are heartburn and dysphagia (trouble swallowing). Anyone with GERD can also display symptoms like regurgitating acid and food, sore throat, chest pain, increased salivation, and nausea. If GERD is left untreated, it can cause a reversible condition called Barrett's esophagus. When you have Barrett's esophagus, the epithelial lining of your esophagus turns into squamous or intestinal mucous epithelium, and it may cause you to have a greater risk of esophageal cancer.

Diagnosis of GERD is usually made by acknowledgment of symptoms by a doctor. An endoscopy may also be performed to get an idea of how damaged your esophagus is and the general function of your LES and stomach. During an endoscopy, a flexible wire with a camera positioned at the end of the wire is swallowed. The camera takes pictures down the esophagus and into the stomach. Traditional endoscopes are known to have issues associated with the procedure including potential injury or death from sedation, increased risk of aspiration, and infections from improperly sterilized scopes. I recommend you talk to your doctor about the safer, transnasal esophagoscopy procedure that does not require sedation. Pros, cons, and information about each procedure are located in chapter 21 to help you make an informed decision about what procedure is best for you.

One of the best assessments utilized in the diagnosing of GERD is an esophageal pH monitoring test. A flexible catheter with a pH monitor on the end is placed through the nose down into the esophagus for at least 24 hours. It is uncomfortable to have a tube down your nose and throat, but it is very useful in establishing a GERD diagnosis.

Conventional Medicine's Failed Treatments for GERD / The Average GERD "Cycle"

GERD Medicine Treatment

Conventional medicine tries to treat GERD with acid-reducing medications, and if all else fails surgery. Acid-reducing medications like H2 antagonists or the dreaded Proton Pump Inhibitors work by blocking natural stomach acid production. In theory, this works by limiting the stomach acid that can get into the esophagus from the stomach, creating less damage and overall inflammation.

H2 Antagonists – (Ex. Pepcid AC, Zantac) H2 antagonists are the safest of the stomach acid reducing medications because they only suppress acid for about six hours. H2 antagonists work by lowering histamine levels in the stomach that lower stomach acid production. H2 antagonists may still cause the same issues of reduced levels of stomach acid, seen in long-term PPI use, even if the medications have a smaller side effect profile.

Proton Pump Inhibitors – (Ex. Prilosec, Prevacid) if you take a PPI longer than a month then some extra issues might develop from a lack of stomach acid. People who take PPIs long-term start to have a whole host of problems including B12 deficiency, bone fractures, increased risk of *C. Diff* Infection, magnesium deficiency, food allergies, and SIBO. These drugs inhibit the hydrogen/potassium ATPase enzyme system in the gastric cells that secrete stomach acid. PPI's last longer than H2 antagonists and usually block acid for 1-2 days.

Both of these routes fail to correct any of the above causes of GERD. They only mask the symptoms. This can lead eventually to the loss of the intrinsic factor of the stomach (becoming deficient in B12), the weakening of the LES, causing a greater chance of developing a magnesium deficiency, developing food allergies from improper digestion, and the acquisition of SIBO once the lack of stomach acid disrupts the bacterial biome present in the gut. Taking any of these medications long term creates a whole host of new problems while the original cause of GERD remains.

PPI's are but a crude patch and do not directly treat the causes of GERD; this explains the general worsening of one's GERD after discontinuing the PPI. The body upregulates stomach acid production to recover from the numerous digestion issues that occur during extended PPI use. This upregulation causes worse GERD than previously experienced because the higher acid and pepsin output result in higher abdominal pressure and esophageal issues. The average person goes back on their PPI, and the dreaded cycle continues until the doctor recommends Nissen fundoplication surgery.

Nissen Fundoplication

A Nissen fundoplication is a useless and harmful surgery for the average GERD suffer. The procedure involves stapling the top part of the stomach (gastric fundus) around the LES or known as the bottom part of the esophagus so that it is strengthened. This procedure is done so that reflux into the esophagus is eliminated. Studies show that 90% of patients are cured of their GERD, which is great, right?

The problem lies in side effects from the procedure including "gas" bloat syndrome, dysphagia, and gastric dumping syndrome. A fundoplication may also come undone over time, which occurs in about 10% of people that have the procedure. "Gas" bloat syndrome is a condition disrupting the proper expelling of gas. In extreme cases, you will not be able to burp or vomit at all, which may cause severe pain. "Gas" Bloat Syndrome has about a 41% occurrence rate in people who have had a Nissen done and though it can go away in about two months; occasionally for some people they will suffer from it until the surgery is either redone or reversed. This surgery should be avoided at all costs!

Chapter 4

Protocols for Elimination of Heartburn / GERD

Protocol 1 - SIBO Protocols

See Chapter 9, *Disorders of the Intestines, SIBO*

Protocol 2 – Possible Eradication or Reduction of Opportunistic *H. pylori*

There is a lot of ongoing research being done to determine H. pylori's coexistence with humans.

Is it commensal, or severely opportunistic? Is it normal flora?

H. pylori, like an evil mastermind, knows when the "shields are down" in the stomach (reduced acid and pepsin production), and proliferates in the stomach and upper gut to cause numerous digestive woes.

But what about when it coexists with our commensal flora? Can it improve our health?

H. pylori and Humans

H. pylori have coexisted with humans for a very long time. At least 60,000 years of coexistence. Our mouth and stomach are a perfect environment for *H. pylori* to thrive, easily spread from both organs.

H. pylori are believed to be spread through saliva exchange, gastric juice exchange, and fecal contact. It is the true "kissing disease." *H. pylori* are believed to have evolved the ability to penetrate the mucosal barrier of the stomach. It loves us so much it evolved to coexist with us.

H. pylori colonization at this time is at least half the world's population. It has however seen a decline in virulence in first world countries, since the dawn of proper hygiene and sanitation.

What health conditions have also increased during modernization?

The Esophagus / Lungs Paradox

When you think of someone with a *H. pylori* infection, you think of gastritis and GERD.

You would expect to see people with *H. pylori* to show issues associated with GERD, including Barrett's Esophagus and even asthma.

The studies mostly show the exact opposite.

Barrett's esophagus is an abnormal mutation to the cells in the lower part of the esophagus. Long-term GERD, LERD, bile acid reflux, or vomiting may cause the stratified squamous epithelium cells to be replaced by simple columnar epithelium with goblet cells. The reasoning behind this replacement of cells is that over time pepsin and stomach acid degrade the cells in the esophagus (chronic inflammation) to the point where the body tries to replace them with cells that secrete more mucus to protect the esophagus from further damage. Even though the body is trying to adapt to protect itself from further damage, it comes at a cost.

This change in the cells of the esophagus greatly increases the risk of esophageal cancer formation that has a high mortality rate. The tissue change in Barrett's esophagus will reverse itself usually after the causes of the disease are remedied, and the risk of cancer then becomes reduced over time.

So in people with an *H. pylori* infection, you would believe they would have higher rates of Barrett's esophagus.

"The effect of *H. pylori* on Barrett's esophagus varied by geographic location and in the presence of selection and information biases. Only four studies were found without obvious selection and information bias, and these showed a protective effect of *H. pylori* on Barrett's esophagus (Relative risk = 0.46 [95% CI: 0.35, 0.60])."

In other words, if you have *H. pylori* colonization you may have a lot less risk of developing Barrett's esophagus. But the type of *H. pylori* infection may play a role in the reduced risk of Barrett's esophagus, those include:

Strain of *H. pylori* is CagA positive.

Location of infection. If you have a duodenal *H. pylori* infection, bile acid reflux may occur, and the risk of Barrett's esophagus may increase. You also have an increased risk if the antral part of the stomach (bottom of the stomach) is infected or have atrophic gastritis from the infection.

What About Asthma?

There are numerous studies linking *H. pylori* and developing asthma and allergies, but studies have shown its proposed benefits rather than drawbacks.

One study states:

"The loss of this ancient, dominant, and persistent member of the normal biota of humans would be predicted to have consequences, and now there is much information about the beneficial and deleterious aspects of this change on the health and disease of the gastrointestinal tract. However, increasing evidence is pointing to extra-intestinal manifestations of the disappearance of *H. pylori*, including asthma. An inverse association of *H. pylori* and childhood asthma, allergic rhinitis, and atopy is becoming increasingly obvious."

But what does *H. pylori* colonization in early childhood do to prevent the development of allergies and asthma?

"Indeed, its absence is associated with the loss of a metabolically active lymphoid compartment in the stomach. This compartment, with both activator and regulatory T cells, could be involved in setting the age-dependent threshold for allergic sensitization to environmental allergens"

It would appear that a diffuse *H. pylori* colonization in the stomach helps to create robust low-grade mucosa-associated lymphoid tissue (MALT) which is the first line of defense against allergic proteins that we consume.

There is one study, however, that does attempt to shed some doubt on *H. pylori's* protection against asthma and allergies. The study is a meta-analysis based on 770 cases and 785 controls. The study did not find a huge link between *H. pylori* and asthma and allergies.

There were issues with the study because they used serological ELISA tests for *H. pylori* that would show the body's reaction to a prior infection but not if the *H. pylori* were flora.

"In this present study, the included studies used a stable serological method, ELISA, as a unique approach for detecting the presence of *H. pylori* infection. Nevertheless, the serology of *H. pylori* is not a reliable criteria for detecting its effect on asthma. The serologic tests could not give us any information on current *H. pylori* infection. Therefore, a number of further investigations using multi-approaches such as immunhistochemistry, polymerase chain reaction and smears for exploring the presence of *H. pylori* are required.

The study even brings up more limitations:

"The present study has several limitations. Firstly, the papers identified in our study were limited to those openly published up to Jul 2012; it is possible that some related published or unpublished studies that might meet the inclusion criteria were missed, resulting in any inevitable bias, though the funnel plots and the Egger's tests failed to show any significant publication bias. Secondly, the results may be interpreted with care because of the limited number and small sample sizes of each included studies. Thirdly, subgroup analyses regarding other confounding factors such as smoking status, age and gender have not been conducted in the present study because sufficient information could not be extracted from the primary literature."

It appears that colonization may be beneficial when it is a part of normal flora.

H. pylori the Hobo Bacteria

H. pylori can become normal or opportunistic flora in three or more different parts of the human body. The mouth, the stomach, and the duodenum are known as the big three parts of the body that it colonizes. *H. pylori* is a transient bacteria; that can move freely in different parts of the body if kept unchecked.

So what do *H. pylori* being transient have to do with whether or not it is friend or foe? Well, studies have indicated that depending on what area of the stomach and duodenum *H. pylori* is currently colonized at the time, the greater the chance it is normal flora or the cause of your digestive woes.

There are four main areas in the stomach; they include from the LES down to the duodenum:

- **Cardia** – the part of the stomach where the esophagus empties into the stomach. The LES is located here.
- **Fundus** – the top part of the stomach.
- **Body** – the largest part of the stomach, the middle.
- **Pylorus** – the lower part of the stomach that is attached to the duodenum by the pyloric sphincter. The pylorus is broken up into two parts the pyloric antrum and the pyloric canal.

Now depending on where *H. pylori* are colonized within the stomach determines if it is either normal or opportunistic flora.

H. pylori opportunistic colonization of the mouth has been linked to possibly being the cause of the auto-immune conditions Sjogren's syndrome and burning mouth syndrome. There are mixed studies about it being the cause, but that being said concerns have been raised in the studies finding none or small amounts of correlation between the two, that the bacteria is transient and can be very difficult to biopsy. It has also been theorized that *H. pylori* can colonize the esophagus, depending on the cell structure of one's esophagus.

Cardia dominant colonization of *H. pylori* is associated with increased risk of developing cancer in that region of the stomach. Paradoxically, *H. pylori* dominant cardia colonization is not linked to increased GERD symptoms, which makes less sense to me because I believe that gastritis in that area should weaken the LES and increased pressure in the stomach because of the overgrowth should cause more reflux symptoms. Furthermore, it would appear that *H. pylori* colonization of the cardia also coincides with the colonization of the pyloric area of the stomach, which should further increase one's chances of suffering from GERD. The theory of dual colonization is based on the fact that in cardia colonization, inflammation and gastritis increase in the pyloric areas and does not occur within the body of the stomach. It is possible that this could occur however from unknown hormonal changes of the gastrointestinal system (modifying digestive hormones) by cardia overgrowth instead of dual colonization.

Body dominant colonization of *H. pylori* reduces your chances of having GERD (esophageal inflammation) by reducing stomach acid production. That being said it appears that a body dominant *H. pylori* colonization is greater linked to the development of gastric ulcers and stomach cancer. It is truly a catch-22, you might have a less chance of having acid reflux, but greater chances of developing gastritis, gastric atrophy, ulcers, and stomach cancer.

Pyloric dominant colonization of *H. pylori* has a set of different symptoms. Pyloric colonization seems to spread to the duodenum and seems to cause pre-pyloric and duodenal ulcers. GERD may develop as well from increased gastrin production (impairment of local somatostatin release), causing up-regulation of stomach acid and increased localized pressure from *H. pylori* overgrowth.

It does, however, appear that an equal colonization of both parts of the stomach by the bacteria appear to be asymptomatic, coincide with no reduction in stomach acid, and are believed to be linked to *H. pylori* being considered "normal" flora. It also appears that single colonization of one strain, like *H. pylori* cagA+, for example, might lead to it being normal flora, instead of multiple co-colonization or co-infections of multiple strains. *H. pylori* may be one instance where microbiome diversity of a specific strain might be a bad thing for your gastrointestinal health.

The transient nature of the bacteria and being able to embed itself deeply within the mucosal barrier and avoid immune system detection is why it can be so hard to biopsy accurately. This causes issues for accurate studies and diagnosis of opportunistic bacteria to help further understand the nature of *H. pylori* and in being able to help people who are made ill by an overgrowth of this Gram-negative bacteria.

There is so much we do not know about *H. pylori* or our microbiome as a whole. We will continue learning about this fascinating bacteria together in part three, which will be on the perils of opportunistic *H. pylori*.

When H. pylori Goes Rogue

H. pylori is a nasty bacteria when it becomes opportunistic. It has multiple factors to its advantage to promote its survival:

- *H. pylori* can bury itself deep into the stomach mucosa, protecting itself from stomach acid, pepsin, and our immune system.
- The bacteria are able to colonize multiple parts of the digestive system: the oral cavity, esophagus, the LES, the stomach, and the duodenum.
- *H. pylori* are transient bacterium and move freely throughout the different areas they colonize if given the chance.
- Manipulate and infect the brain-gut axis to increase survival by completely modulating digestion. *H. pylori* are able to reduce stomach acid and pepsin production to proliferate further the stomach and duodenum. It can regulate esophageal and gastric motility, change hypersensitivity to chemical and mechanical digestive stimulants, manipulate gastric blood

flow, and influence what we eat (increased cravings or decrease food intake). It can modulate digestive neurotransmitters including acetylcholine, noradrenaline, adrenaline, and dopamine. Finally, it is also able to modulate leptin, ghrelin, calcitonin gene-related peptide (CGRP), nitric oxide, neuropeptide Y, substance P (SP), somatostatin (STS) and cholecystokinin (CCK).

- *H. pylori* are able to avoid easily immune system detection by modulating inflammatory pathways, avoiding immune pattern recognition receptors by using endotoxins and flagellin, produce biofilms, reduce phagocyte potential, reduce endogenous nitric oxide production (increases blood pressure and promotes vasoconstriction), and by reducing T cell response.

H. pylori also cause many different medical conditions and health issues, those include:

- *H. pylori* can shed potent endotoxins that can leak into the bloodstream and increase inflammatory markers. Because of this, it is a known increased risk for heart and liver disease.
- *H pylori* have been implicated as the cause of the following autoimmune conditions: immune thrombocytopenic purpura, co-infection *with K. pneumoniae* as the cause of rheumatoid arthritis, co-infection with *Staph* as the cause of Lupus, Sjogren's syndrome. Behcet's disease, Wegner's granulomatosis, burning mouth syndrome, and scleroderma.
- *H. pylori* are the main cause of gastrointestinal ulcers.
- *H. pylori* overgrowth increases the risk of developing duodenal, esophageal, stomach cancer, and MALT lymphoma.
- *H. pylori* can reduce esophageal motility, gastric emptying, and small intestine emptying (third wave of the MMC).
- *H. pylori* can elevate cortisol and adrenaline production over time causing adrenal fatigue.
- *H. pylori* may be a clear cause of histamine intolerance and eosinophilic esophagitis because of its ability to modulate histamine and mast cell function.
- *H. pylori* may infect the brain-gut axis, which would lead to, vagus nerve issues, anxiety, depression, brain fog, dementia, reduced memory capacity (lower BDNF), fluctuations in appetite, lower HRV, and digestive issues.

So what does this all mean? Here is a great conclusion from a recent study on *H. pylori's* ability to avoid our immune system and cause infections:

"*H. pylori* has been co-existing with human host for at least 30000 years. During this long time of co-existence the bacteria has undergone evolutionary adaptation and established a comfortable niche in the human host. Unlike most other pathogenic bacteria which are cleared by the host adaptive immune response, *H. pylori* successfully establishes a persistent infection in its host in spite of the presence of vigorous innate and adaptive immune response. *H. pylori* evolved an array of mechanisms to evade both innate and adaptive immune responses. Host mediated immune response not only fails to clear the bacteria but also helps the bacteria for colonization by proving increased availability of adhesion places such as MHC II and CD74, both of these components are induced by IFN-γ and IL-8 during *H. pylori* infection. *H. pylori* virulence factors VacA, HP-NAP, Cag T4SS have been shown to cause damage in the gastric epithelium which results in peptic ulcer or even gastric cancer, if left untreated. Bacterial virulence factors together with host factors determine the severity of disease. Though multiple studies have examined how the bacteria interact with its host there is still a lack of clear knowledge about how it avoids host mediated immune responses. Furthermore little is currently known about the role of T cell subsets in controlling *H. pylori* infection and associated immunopathogenesis, particularly in humans."

I could not write the explanation of why we need a greater understanding of *H. pylori* better myself. *Pylori* have colonized humans for centuries and because of our association it knows us inside out, we are the preferred host.

So is *H. pylori* an evil mastermind that can control our body or an ally that can help us better our health? It depends on if our immune system can keep it in check and not let it overgrow and infect different parts of the body, the state of our digestive health, when we became infected, and what strain.

If *H. pylori* do become a James Bond super-villain with his monocle, mustache, and a fluffy white cat, what can be done to knock it back into submission, so it becomes a tamer Dr. Evil?

Supplementation Protocol to Reduce H. pylori Colonization

Certain supplements are more localized to the upper gut, others affect the intestinal or systemic microbiome.

Supplements that would reduce intestinal microbiota diversity and should not be used in a first round protocol unless necessary include:

- Allicin-C
- Berberine
- Lactoferrin
- Interphase plus
- NAC
- Oil of oregano

Supplements that work systemically and may reduce systemic microbiome diversity and should not be used unless necessary include:

- NAC
- Oil of oregano

Part 1: Antimicrobial Supplements

Depending on the infection load of *H. pylori*, multiple agents may be needed to achieve remission.

Supplements to Reduce Overgrowth In the Mouth:

- Colloidal silver (Mesosilver) – take one tablespoon and swish for a few minutes, spit out silver after swishing and wash your mouth out.
- Zane Hellas Oil of Oregano – swish with two drops for a minute, spit out the oil of oregano and wash your mouth out.
- Ceylon cinnamon oil – swish with one drop, diluted in 2 oz of water for a minute, spit out cinnamon oil and wash your mouth out.
- Oil pulling with either organic extra virgin coconut oil or Californian extra virgin olive oil. Take a tablespoon of either oil and swish in your mouth for fifteen to twenty minutes daily. Spit out oil after swishing. Then brush your teeth and swish your mouth out.

Supplements to Reduce Overgrowth In the Stomach and Duodenum:

- Colloidal silver (Mesosilver) – follow supplement bottle recommendations.
- Zane Hellas Oil of Oregano – follow supplement bottle recommendations.
- Berberine – take two capsules, twice daily. Use with caution if you have ulcers, gastritis, or hypoglycemia.
- Allicin-C – two to eight capsules daily in divided doses with food.
- Bismuth – Kaopectate Vanilla (No dyes, but contains some questionable additives including caramel, flavor, sucrose [possible GMO source,] and xanthan gum), do not use if you have bleeding ulcers.
- Manuka honey – one tablespoon, twice daily with food.
- Ceylon cinnamon oil – take one drop in one tsp. of extra virgin coconut oil or extra virgin olive oil, twice daily. Use with caution if you have hypoglycemia.

A Supplement Only to Be Used in Severe Cases of Overgrowth:

- Sodium butyrate – WARNING, Butyrate lysis's *H. pylori* on contact, therefore, it may cause severe gastritis in some people from massive die off and endotoxin release. Might be best to be used with zinc carnosine to help protect the mucosal lining and only taken with food.

Allicin-C, berberine, oregano oil, and silver are strongly antibacterial.

Coconut oil is composed of MCT's that have antimicrobial properties.

Manuka honey has antimicrobial properties.

Olive oil has polyphenols that boost the immune system and have antimicrobial properties.

Part 2: Supplements That Reduce Biofilm Formation

- Symbiotics lactoferrin – one to two grams daily, in divided doses with food.
- Interphase plus – one to two capsules, on an empty stomach, twice daily.
- NAC – (Should only be used in systemic overgrowth of *H. pylori*), 600 mg, twice daily with food.

Biofilm agents break down biofilm and weaken the *H. pylori* so that the antibacterial agents can eliminate it.

Part 3: Supplements That Boost Immune Function

- Liposomial Colostrum – one tbsp. mixed in filtered water, consumed at breakfast.
- Olive leaf extract – one – two capsules, twice daily with food.
- S. bouardii – one – two capsules before bed. Use filtered or bottled water when ingesting. Use with caution if you suffer from histamine intolerance and/or Th2 dominance.
- GutPro Capsules – one – two capsules before bed. Use filtered or bottled water when ingesting.
- GOS prebiotic – one – two scoops, mixed well with water, consume during breakfast.
- Immunoglobulin Y – follow supplement instructions.

Immunoglobulin Y helps the immune system recognize and reduce *H. pylori* overgrowth.

Olive leaf contains polyphenols that upregulate immune function and reduce *H. pylori* overgrowth.

Probiotics compete with *H. pylori* to reduce their concentrations.

Part 4: Supplements That Impede H. pylori Growth

- Betaine HCL – in some people increasing stomach acid production may cause severe inflammation from increased endotoxin production from *H. pylori* and increased burrowing of the bacteria into the mucosal barrier. Use with caution in systemic stomach overgrowth, or if you have ulcers / gastritis. Supplementation with zinc carnosine, l-carnitine, and activated charcoal may reduce these issues.
- Broccoli seed extract – one – two capsules, twice daily with food.
- Organic concentrated cranberry juice - drink a cup of straight cranberry juice daily.
- D-limonene – one softgel, twice daily with food.
- EGCG – one – two capsules, twice daily with food.
- Mastic gum – two capsules, twice daily with food.
- Zinc carnosine – two capsules, three times daily with food. If you are using another brand 40 – 50 mg of zinc from zinc carnosine total, daily in divided doses.

Mastic gum has proven in multiple studies to eliminate *H. pylori* by binding with it. Mastic gum also has strong antimicrobial properties.

Cranberry juice inhibits *H. pylori* by keeping it from adhering to the stomach wall.

Zinc carnosine repairs and heals the stomach lining.

Zinc also binds with the stomach wall to increasing white blood cell activity and help with eliminating *H. pylori*.

Betaine HCL increases stomach acid, deactivating *H. pylori*. Stomach acid also keeps *H. pylori* infections at bay if an infection is present.

H. pylori Harm Reduction Medication List:

Here is a list of believed safer medications that can be used to tackle *H. pylori* overgrowth or issues; ask your doctor about developing a regimen from this list:

- Amoxicillin.
- Bismuth.
- H2 antagonist (may increase growth in the stomach by reducing stomach acid production, but, decreases histamine and may be needed to help recover from gastritis or ulcers, better than PPI, Pepcid is the best one to use).
- Tetracycline.
- Third generation cephalosporin.

Other antibiotics that have more issues associated with their use:

- Flagyl.
- Macrolide antibiotics (clarithromycin for example) – supplementing with magnesium, ubiquinol, and pqq, may help prevent mitochondrial toxicity issues.
- Rifabutin.

Medications to definitely avoid if possible:

- Fluoroquinolones – supplementing with magnesium, ubiquinol, and pqq, may help prevent mitochondrial toxicity issues.
- PPI's.

Ulcers

Peptic ulcers are mostly caused by an *H. pylori* opportunistic infection. Ulcers can be caused by NSAID's and other certain medication overuse, infection, chronic gastritis, and cancer. Ulcers can occur in the duodenum, esophagus, stomach, and the diverticulum.

The most common symptoms of an ulcer are abdominal pain (stomach ulcer during eating, a duodenal ulcer pain is usually felt three hours after a meal), bloating or a sense of fullness, rush of saliva during pain, nausea, vomiting, vomiting of blood, and melena (tarry, dark stools). If an ulcer is left untreated, a perforation can occur (hole in the stomach). Perforations are a medical emergency and must be surgically treated immediately because of the chance of massive infection and inflammation from opportunistic bacteria and gastric juice outside the stomach. The main symptoms of perforation are an extreme stabbing pain in the abdomen and high fever.

Most ulcers are diagnosed through clinical symptoms. However, endoscopies and barium X-rays can also be used. I recommend instead of an endoscopy have a transnasal esophagoscopy performed if needed.

Healing a Ulcer (Supplementation)

- Pure Encapsulations zinc carnosine – take one capsule with a meal, twice daily.
- DGL licorice chewable – follow supplement recommendations on the bottle (take thirty minutes before a meal; chew very well and mix with saliva for effectiveness).
- L - glutamine - take 4,000 - 10,000 mg daily with food (use with caution if you have a sensitivity to glutamic acid, deficiency in GABA, or severe leaky gut and brain).

Zinc carnosine and L-glutamine repairs the stomach and gut lining in multiple studies.

DGL extract heals and protects the stomach lining according to multiple studies.

Zinc carnosine is prescribed in Japan to remedy ulcers, and DGL is prescribed in Germany to remedy ulcers.

Healing a Ulcer (Herbal)

- Solaray marshmallow extract – follow supplement bottle recommendations.
- DGL licorice chewable – follow supplement recommendations on the bottle (take thirty minutes before a meal; chew very well and mix with saliva for effectiveness).
- Now slippery elm extract - follow supplement bottle recommendations.
- Organic chamomile tea – drink a cup twice daily.
- Follow cayenne pepper protocol (Ch. 18).
- Georges Always Active aloe vera – follow supplement bottle recommendations.

Marshmallow, DGL extract, slippery elm, aloe vera, helps coat and protect the stomach lining.

Cayenne and chamomile help heal inflammation and stimulate the immune system.

Protocol 3 - Ditch the Standard American Diet

The standard American diet is rife with foods that hinder optimal functioning of the human intestinal system. The standard American diet is full of wheat, GMO's, dairy, carrageenan, artificial sweeteners, and excessive fructose. All of these food items wear down or even destroy the integrity of the intestinal system over a period of time in differing populations. A proper diet is necessary for most people with digestion problems to improve their symptoms.

Following a high fat / medium animal protein / low carbohydrate diets like the Primal® Diet or Bulletproof® Diet improves digestion (or a vegetarian diet using eggs and whey protein). Following a right fat / medium plant protein (no soy protein) / high carbohydrate diet that excludes wheat and whole grains and emphasizes carb intake from low fructose fruits, white rice, wild rice, cassava, and taro, improves digestion. Sometimes short-term specialty diets like the GAPS diet, SIBO diet, or elemental diet, might be needed for people with specific digestive needs. Not every diet is perfect for everyone. The best approach is to look for a diet tailored to your specific health needs by experimenting with different diets until digestion perfection occurs.

Protocol 4 - GMO Reduction / Elimination

Discussion about GMO food is everywhere lately in the alternative media, but what exactly are GMO's? GMO stands for genetically modified organism. A GMO is an organism with its genes modified artificially by humans. Some people believe that modern wheat, seedless cucumbers, purple potatoes, and other common examples of modifications to plants are GMO's, but this is not the case. These are examples of natural mutations. Granted, even though humans (as a form of selected breeding) caused some of the mutations they are still natural and are not considered GMO's.

A GMO food product is a product that has had a gene deleted, mutated, or inserted through artificial means. An example of a GMO food product would be genetically modified BT Corn. GMO BT corn has genes from a common bacterium *Bacillus thuringiensis* directly inserted into the corn so it can produce a natural insecticide called BT Toxin. Some early studies showed that BT Toxin was originally thought to be harmless in mammals. More recent studies, however, indicate that the rogue genetic material from the corn can embed in your gut and begin producing a significant amount of BT Toxin in your colon that can destabilize your gut bacteria and health.

This is why you must attempt to buy as much organic food as you can or purchase items labeled non-GMO by the non-GMO Project. Here is a list of food items that are GMO in the United States, Mexico, and Canada.

Common Crops and Animal Products that Are GMO:

- Corn
- Soybean
- Papaya
- Zucchini
- Canola
- Cotton
- Alfalfa
- Sugar beet
- RBGH dairy
- Animal meat where the animal was fed GMO feed

Common Ingredients that are GMO:

- Aspartame
- Maltodextrin
- Soy lecithin

- Corn or soy protein
- Corn, cottonseed, soy, or canola oil
- Sugar that is not listed as non-GMO or cane sugar
- High fructose corn syrup
- RBGH milk
- Citric acid
- Modified food starch
- Cornstarch
- Vegetable protein (that is not labeled non-GMO)

After eliminating GMO's for one month, you should follow my rebuild the gut protocol (Ch. 9) and continue limiting exposure if all possible.

Protocol 5 – Clothing

Wear loose fitting clothing and do not tighten your belt to the very last notch. Also, do not wear tight pants if possible. Tight clothing including bras, can put pressure on the stomach and LES, which will aggravate GERD symptoms.

Protocol 6 - Proper Posture

Sit straight as much as you can. See a chiropractor to get your spine aligned if needed. The excess curvature of the spine increases pressure on the stomach and LES. If you have GERD, elevate the top of your bed by putting cinder blocks under the front support of the bed. This change in elevation puts less pressure on the stomach, but more pressure on the LES keeping it closed.

Protocol 7 - Strengthen Your LES!

The lower esophageal sphincter is a sphincter that connects the top of the stomach with the bottom of the esophagus. The LES first relaxes to allow food to enter the stomach. The LES then closes tightly after food enters the stomach to keep stomach acid and pepsin from traveling up the esophagus from the equalization of pressure. The LES also relaxes to allow air to travel out of the stomach in the form of a burp. Finally, the LES will also typically relax to allow the vomit to travel out of the stomach when one is vomiting.

The lower esophageal sphincter may become weakened over a period of time if you consistently ingest certain foods (peppermint, chocolate, uncooked onions), frequently use nicotine or caffeine, take certain medications (SSRI antidepressants, anticholinergic medicines, uniphyl, sedatives, and estrogen replacements), if you have had nerve damage done to the vagus nerve, or have a stomach infection like *H. pylori*. The LES might also become damaged if you are suffering from SIBO, if you have a hiatal hernia, or if you were born with a malfunctioning LES. If one's LES is weakened, excess gastrointestinal pressure can easily push gastric contents into the esophagus, causing reflux symptoms to occur. In addition, if the LES is weakened heartburn can occur easily during sleep because of the lack of necessary LES pressure, which normally hold gastric contents in the stomach in place.

Strengthening the LES is hard because no known exercise can be used to strengthen the sphincter. You can relieve excessive pressure off the LES and stomach physically by wearing loose clothing and losing excess weight. You should also limit foods that weaken the LES, cause SIBO, and attempt to switch medications to avoid those that may weaken the LES.

Some supplements can help by strengthening the LES, lowering gastric pressure, and repairing nerve damage. All of these suggestions should help your LES heal and function better.

LES Protocol

- Now calcium citrate powder – consume 500 mg, twice a day mixed with filtered water.
- L-glutamine shake – take 4,000 mg of L-glutamine mixed well with one scoop of grass-fed whey in filtered water, consume twice daily (use with caution if you have a sensitivity to glutamic acid, deficiency in GABA, or severe leaky gut and brain).
- Jarrow R-lipoic acid – take one capsule, twice daily with meals.
- Enzymedica Digestive Enzyme Gold – take one capsule with every meal daily.
- Thorne Research B complex– take one capsule daily, do not use if you are an overmethylator.
- Pure Encapsulations zinc carnosine – take one capsule with a meal, twice daily.
- Do not wear tight clothing or tight belts.
- Melatonin Life Extension extended release – take 3-10 mg before bed daily.

If all else fails to relieve LES issues:

- Jarrow 5-HTP – follow supplement bottle recommendations, and supplement no longer than two weeks.

Calcium citrate, in theory, should strengthen the LES when it encounters it if you drink it in powder form mixed with water. One of calcium's roles in the body is to be used as a strengthener in muscle contractions; this is just a theory, though; no In Vivo studies have been done.

R-lipoic acid ensures that the LES has little nerve damage and strengthens the vagus nerve.

Digestive enzymes help break down the food in the stomach, reducing gas, and pressure on the LES.

L-glutamine and grass-fed whey help rebuild the integrity of the gastrointestinal system and the LES, as well.

Melatonin and 5-HTP have been shown to increase LES strength.

Protocol 8 - Digestive Enzymes!

Take one - two capsules of Enzymedica Digest Gold at the start of a meal to help with digestion and food breakdown if you have frequent indigestion. Digestive enzymes should not be taken indefinitely unless needed (an example of this would be if you had a poorly functioning pancreas or gallbladder). It is better for you to train your body to make digestive enzymes by helping your gallbladder and pancreas to work optimally. You can do this by using Swedish bitters.

Swedish Bitters (Gentian):

- **Uses**: helps stimulate digestion, improves gallbladder issues, and increases digestive enzyme production.
- **Brand**: Urban Moonshine Digestive Bitters
- **Side effects**: RARE: hypersensitive allergic reaction

Swedish bitters are a mixture of herbs that vary depending on the brand. Swedish bitter supplements can be used to help stimulate digestion and help the body make natural digestive enzymes. Swedish bitter herbs help stimulate digestion and improve gallbladder function and gastric emptying.

Gentian is a bitter herb from a plant native to China and is used in most digestive bitter formulas. Gentian has been shown to help ease gallbladder issues and indigestion. The herb helps increase appetite, stimulates the production of digestive juices, increases pancreatic activity, and boosts blood supply to the digestive organs. Gentian is also known to stimulate the flow of bile.

Protocol 9 – *Candida*

Candida albicans is usually found in the gut and vaginal flora of most humans, and most of the time is relatively harmless. *Candida* may become an opportunistic yeast that can cause many digestive problems. If you have taken too many antibiotics and eliminated the beneficial bacteria and yeast that keep *Candida* in check in your intestines, *Candida* will flourish. Is it also impossible to know if you have an active *Candida* infection, unless the *Candida* becomes fungal, or you develop thrush. If you have thrush, the *Candida* will be visible as white patches usually inside one's mouth, throat, or vagina. An active thrush infection may be found in any part of the body that has a mucous membrane, but it may be found on the skin, as well.

Candida spit tests that you have read about on the Internet that can help diagnose active *Candida* infections are a scam. An alcohol fasting challenge might be useful in the diagnosis of an active yeast infection. During an alcohol challenge test, sugar is consumed, and a few hours later, alcohol and acetaldehyde blood levels are measured to determine *Candida* intestinal overgrowth. Yeast converts sugar into alcohol and acetaldehyde as a source of energy during digestion. Testing D-arabinitol in a urine culture may also be an accurate diagnostic marker of yeast overgrowth. Finally, stool *Candida* tests including Genova GI Effects test might be accurate in determining and active gastrointestinal *Candida* infection, as well.

Since *Candida* can be opportunistic, being overrun with it is usually a sign of poor health instead of being a direct cause of poor health. *Candida* only becomes opportunistic if you give it a chance! Therefore, unless you have thrush or digestive issues that point to an active *Candida* infection (white tongue, heartburn that is not relieved by any of the other protocols, brain fog, or allergic reactions), then the average person can take extra virgin coconut oil and occasional probiotics, to keep *Candida* at bay.

Herx Reaction

A herx reaction can be a sign of the body's natural healing process. The herx reaction occurs from the body's overreaction to inflammatory products that are released by lysised bacteria, mycobacteria, archaea, viral infected cells, and yeast. It takes a while for the body to filter out these toxins and reduce inflammation; a herx reaction can mimic symptoms of the flu.

General symptoms of a herx reaction are a headache, body aches, rashes, brain fog, extreme fatigue, light sensitivity, irritability, tachycardia, low blood pressure, nightmares and a low-grade fever. If you have a fever higher than 102.5 F then you need to see a doctor; you might not be suffering from a herx reaction and instead are either sick or septic. Lab work during a herx reaction may show elevated creatinine levels, blood urea nitrogen levels, liver enzymes, sedimentation rate, gamma globulin (a decrease in white blood cells), hemoglobin, and an elevated CRP test.

Supplements to Stop a Yeast Herx Reaction (Must Be Taken All Together):

- Thorne Naturals molybdenum glycinate - take one capsule daily.

- Clean Chlorella – consume ten tablets daily with food.
- Glutathione Force – ingest two ml, twice daily.
- Sodium ascorbate - take 3,000 mg, two to three times daily.
- Upgraded™ Activated Charcoal – follow supplement bottle recommendations.
- L-glutamine powder - consume 4,000 mg, daily, mixed in a glass of filtered water, with food (use with caution if you have a sensitivity to glutamic acid, deficiency in GABA, or severe leaky gut and brain).
- Black cumin seed oil – One tablespoon with a meal. Use with caution if you have gastritis.

Molybdenum is used in the body to produce two enzymes, aldehyde dehydrogenase, and aldehyde-oxidase. These enzymes allow the liver to neutralize a potent and otherwise relatively inert toxin (neurotoxin), aldehyde. Yeasts release aldehydes as a byproduct of their cellular respiration, causing the main side effects from yeast die off including brain fog.

Vitamin C helps reduce histamine and inflammation triggered from yeast die off.

Chlorella and charcoal help absorb the toxins released by the yeast.

Glutathione is reduced in yeast overgrowth and people with an elevated Th2 immune system.

Black cumin seed oil reduces an elevated Th2 system.

L-glutamine helps repair the digestive tract.

Maintenance Candida Protocol

- Organic extra virgin coconut oil – consume two tablespoons with meals, daily.
- Follow the Bulletproof® Diet.

Mild Candida Protocol - Taken for 2 - 3 Weeks

- Organic extra virgin coconut oil – consume two tablespoons, daily.
- Lactobacillus plantarum 299V Jarrow – take one capsule nightly with a glass of chlorine free water.
- Pure Encapsulations caprylic acid – follow supplement bottle recommendations.

Follow the Bulletproof® Diet and stay hydrated. Coconut oil contains many anti-yeast goodies like caprylic acid and lauric acid. Both caprylic acid and lauric acid are found in breast milk that is one of the reasons you can still breastfeed if you have an active yeast infection and the main reason breast milk cures thrush!

Lactobacillus plantarum is present in fermented foods and is one of the few probiotics that produces a barrier in the digestive tract blocking unwanted pathogens. It also reduces Th2 immune reactions.

Moderate Candida Protocol - Taken for 3 - 4 weeks

- Organic extra virgin coconut oil – consume two tablespoons, daily.
- Niacinamide – take 500 mg, daily.
- S. boulardii Jarrow Formulas AND Lactobacillus reuteri OR / AND Lactobacillus plantarum Jarrow - take one capsule nightly with a glass of chlorine free water, do not supplement with the *S. boulardii* probiotic if you have elevated histamine, yeast sensitivities, or severe Th2 issues.
- Pure Encapsulations caprylic acid – follow supplement bottle recommendations.
- Lauricidin – follow supplement bottle recommendations.
- SF722 – follow supplement bottle recommendations.
- Follow the Bulletproof® Diet and stay hydrated.

Niacinamide inhibits yeast growth within the body.

Lauricidin is a concentrated form of monolaurin, which has been shown in studies to inhibit yeast.

S. boulardii is a yeast found on lychee fruit that will compete with the *Candida* and eliminate it.

Lactobacillus reuteri is a probiotic found mostly in human breast milk that produces anti-yeast compounds and reduces Th2 reactions.

Undecylenic acid is a fatty acid derived from castor oil. Undecylenic acid inhibits *Candida's* ability to become virulent.

Advanced Candida Protocol - Taken for 1 - 3 Months

- S. boulardii Jarrow Formulas AND Lactobacillus reuteri AND Lactobacillus plantarum Jarrow - take one capsule nightly with a glass of chlorine free water. Do not supplement with the *S. boulardii* probiotic if you have elevated histamine, yeast sensitivities, or severe Th2 issues.
- Niacinamide – take 1,000 mg, daily.
- SF722 – follow supplement bottle recommendations.
- Lauricidin – follow supplement bottle recommendations.
- Pure Encapsulations caprylic acid – follow supplement bottle recommendations.
- Gymnema – follow supplement bottle recommendations, use with caution if you suffer from hypoglycemia.
- Follow the Bulletproof® Diet and stay well hydrated.

Gymnema sylvestre is a herb that has been found to inhibit yeast cell growth and reduce *Candida* virulence.

Herbal Candida Protocol

- Zane Hellas Oil of Oregano - take two drops under tongue, twice daily.
- Allicin C – follow supplement bottle recommendations.
- Dr. Hulda Clark's black walnut tincture – follow supplement bottle recommendations.
- Organic extra virgin coconut oil – consume two tablespoons, daily.
- Gymnema – follow supplement bottle recommendations, use with caution if you suffer from hypoglycemia.

Gymnema sylvestre is a herb that has been found to inhibit yeast cell growth and reduce *Candida* virulence.

The carvacrol in oregano oil has been found to be both antibacterial and anti-yeast. The Zane Hellas brand is one of the strongest and best brands of the oil and the capsules and oil are non-gmo!

The garlic in Allicin C has been shown to inhibit yeast.

Remember to rebuild your gut one week after all symptoms have subsided, or the protocols have stopped, whichever comes first.

I do not recommend the following method to reduce yeast overgrowth in the gut. Some people, however, have had great success in using it, so I believe it is worth mentioning.

- Turpentine

Protocol 10 – Constipation

See Chapter 9, *Disorders of the Intestines, Constipation*

Protocol 11 –Maintain Proper Chloride Levels in the Stomach

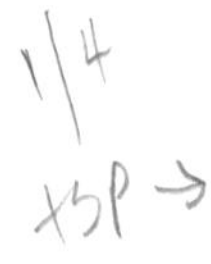

It is essential for optimal health that you intake the right amount of salt in your diet and that it is pure salt so that your body can properly make hydrochloric acid. Gastric acid is made up of hydrochloric acid, sodium chloride, and potassium chloride in the stomach. Take 1/4 tsp. of a good quality sea salt, Real Salt, or pink salt in a glass of filtered warm water upon waking to help adrenal function and to jump start digestion. If you have low stomach acid drink the saltwater formula in a small cup of warm filtered water twenty minutes before the start of every meal.

Protocol 12 - Proper Liver, Gallbladder, and Pancreas Function

There are a lot more organs associated with your digestion than just your stomach and intestines. The liver, gallbladder, and pancreas must function normally so that complete digestion can occur. These organs deal with the enzymatic and chemical side of digestion whereas the stomach and mouth are mixtures of enzymatic, mechanical, and chemical digestion.

The liver produces bile and releases the bile either directly into the small intestine or into the gallbladder. When the bile is released into the gallbladder, the bile is then stored in the gallbladder until it is needed. Bile helps digest fat and breaks down the fat into individual fatty acids for assimilation. It further breaks down the food chyme so that the other digestive enzymes can fully digest and assimilate the food that you eat. The pancreas produces cells that release most of these digestive enzymes into the intestines. The pancreas also releases sodium bicarbonate to neutralize the stomach acid mixed with chime, which has been released from the stomach into the duodenum for further digestion. The cells the pancreas produces to help with digestion are the ductal cells, which produce bicarbonate and the acinar cells, which in turn produce digestive enzymes. Medical issues with these organs can cause GERD, diarrhea, constipation, gastritis, SIBO, or even IBS. Occasionally, the health of these different organs can be determined by the color and quality of one's stool.

Liver – Poor liver function can be hard to identify in the early stages because the liver itself is one of the few organs that can regenerate easily. Early stages of poor liver function are diagnosed through random metabolic panel blood tests. Jaundice or yellowing of the skin and eyes is usually the only major physical manifestation of poor liver function. However, when it comes to digestive issues, signs of poor liver function include unrelenting GERD in combination with a very light-colored stool. These symptoms together can be a powerful indicator of potential liver disease.

Gallbladder – Poor gallbladder function can produce many symptoms of digestive discomfort. These include abdominal pain after eating fatty meals, GERD, greasy bowel movements ranging from pale to yellow in color, constipation, diarrhea, and bowel movements with a very strong odor. These signs are either caused by a lack of bile or too much bile being released into the small intestine. If too little bile is released, it tends to cause abdominal pain, constipation, GERD, and a yellow, greasy, foul-smelling stool. If too much bile is released, on the other hand, usually causes frequent diarrhea. Another sign of possible gallbladder attacks or failure is referred right shoulder pain. Most gallbladder symptoms and attacks usually occur right after eating a meal high in fat. The symptoms occur after eating a meal high in fat because of the large bile release required to digest the high amount of fat after a meal.

Pancreas – The digestive signs of poor pancreatic function are similar to indicators of disease in the gallbladder. Diarrhea can also occur when foods high in fat are eaten. Signs of poor pancreatic function outside of the digestive tract include the development of insulin resistance, elevated pancreatic enzyme blood levels, and diabetes.

General Liver Health Protocol

- Once daily upon waking – drink one glass of warm non-chlorinated water mixed with lemon squeezed in it, 1/4 tsp. of sea salt, and 1/4 tsp. of cayenne pepper added.
- Jarrow Formulas R-alpha lipoic acid – you must take supplement with meals, R-lipoic acid may lower blood glucose; take two capsules daily.
- Jarrow Formulas milk thistle – take two - four capsules daily.
- Nordic Naturals Ultimate Omega - follow supplement bottle recommendations.

A glass of warm water, cayenne, salt, and lemon in the morning stimulates bile production and eliminates toxins.

R-lipoic acid and milk thistle are hepatoprotective, and both supplements help regenerate liver cells.

The fish oil supplementation increases the overall health of the person, and the body to reduce overall inflammation uses extra omega-3 fatty acids.

Extensive Liver Detox and Health Protocol

- Once daily upon waking – drink one glass of warm non-chlorinated water mixed with a lemon squeezed in it, 1/4 tsp. of sea salt, and 1/4 tsp. of cayenne pepper added.

Herbal Support of Liver:

- Jarrow Formulas milk thistle - take two to four capsules daily.
- Gaia Herbs Astragalus Supreme – follow supplement bottle recommendations.

Liver Detoxifying Supplement:

- Thorne Research calcium D-glucarate – follow supplement bottle recommendations.

Increase Glutathione Naturally:

- Solaray Schizandra berry – follow supplement bottle recommendations.
- Jarrow Formulas R-alpha lipoic acid – you must take supplement with meals, R-lipoic acid may lower blood glucose; take two capsules daily.
- Sodium ascorbate – take 1,000 mg daily.
- Grass-fed whey protein (Upgraded™ Whey) – mix one scoop in water or milk, consume daily.

A glass of warm water, cayenne, salt, and lemon in the morning stimulates bile production and eliminates toxins.

R-lipoic acid, astragalus, and milk thistle are hepatoprotective, and both help regenerate liver cells.

Schizandra, Jarrow R-lipoic acid, Jarrow Formulas NAC, Ester C vitamin C, and grass-fed whey protein (Upgraded™ Whey) all support natural glutathione production.

Calcium D-glucarate is a natural whole-body detoxifier.

Fish oil is for increasing the overall health of the person.

Gallbladder Protocol (Poor Gallbladder Health)

This protocol should only be used if you have poor gallbladder function, but only if your gallbladder has not completely failed. If at any time, you have a sharp stabbing pain in the abdomen for a considerable period of time and are vomiting; your bile duct might have become blocked with a gallstone. If this happens, go to the hospital immediately. It is considered a medical emergency.

- Once daily upon waking – drink a glass of warm non-chlorinated water mixed with lemon squeezed in it, 1/4 tsp. of sea salt, and 1/8 tsp. organic cayenne pepper.
- Jarrow Formulas Bile Acid Factors – follow supplement bottle recommendations.
- Enzymedica Digest Gold – take one to two capsules with every meal daily.
- Magnesium chloride – take 400 mg, daily.
- Limit greasy fried food in the diet and use organic extra virgin coconut oil as the source of fat.

Might Help Remove Gallstones:

- Food-grade humic acid supplementation – follow supplement recommendations.

The glass of water stimulates the liver and gallbladder to release bile and toxins.

The ox bile and digestive enzymes help give the gallbladder a rest in releasing bile and help with fat digestion.

I do not believe in using gallbladder flushes personally because some scientific studies have shown that the combination of oils and juices ends up producing soap in the stomach, and what is passed through the bowels is a soap bezoar, not gallstones.

The humic acid, in theory, might help the body to eliminate excess gallstones.

Gallbladder Protocol (Health after Removal of Gallbladder)

- Jarrow Formulas Bile Acid Factors (discontinue if diarrhea and bile acid malabsorption occurs) – follow supplement bottle recommendations.
- Enzymedica Digest Gold – take one - two capsules with every meal daily.
- Limit greasy fried food in the diet and use organic extra virgin coconut oil as your primary source of fat.
- In addition, limit gallbladder stimulators like lemon juice, spicy food, and ginger.
- Follow the Perfect Health® Diet and eat small meals frequently during the day.

Rapid Dumping Syndrome

Rapid dumping syndrome is a condition that is usually caused by gastric surgery. Ingested foods rapidly enter the small intestine before being fully digested and can happen immediately after a meal or up to three hours later. Symptoms of "early" dumping are nausea, bloating, vomiting, stomach pain and cramping, diarrhea and dizziness. Signs of "late" dumping are weakness, sweating, and dizziness. Most people with this condition also suffer from hypoglycemia.

Rapid Dumping Protocol

- Jarrow ox bile supplement – follow supplement bottle recommendations. Discontinue if diarrhea worsens or develops.
- Enzymedica Digest Gold - take one – two capsules with every meal.
- Organic vanilla hemp protein powder or Unifiber– follow supplement recommendations.
- Magnesium glycinate - take 400 Mg, before bed.
- Jarrow Formulas R-lipoic acid – take one capsule daily with your largest meal. Lipoic acid supplementation may lower blood glucose levels.
- Optimal Start – take two capsules a meal, twice daily.
- Jarrow Formulas methyl B12 – take one sublingual tablet daily. Use another form like adenosylcobalamin if you are an overmethylator.
- Limit greasy, fried food in the diet. Use organic, extra virgin coconut oil, eggs, meat, and Brain Octane Oil as primary sources of fat. In addition, limit items that stimulate bile including citrus fruits, malate (apples) or citric acid, spicy food, foods high in oleic acid (extra virgin olive oil and avocados are good examples), and ginger.
- Follow the Perfect Health® Diet and eat small meals frequently during the day.
- Follow the advanced probiotic regimen (Ch. 13) for one month then discontinue.

If You Have Continuous Diarrhea:

- Upgraded™ Activated Charcoal – follow the general supplement bottle recommendations.
- Rainforest Pharmacy sangre de drago – follow the general supplement bottle recommendations.

The ox-bile and digestive enzymes will help digest food before it is dumped.

The fiber will help bulk up stools. Charcoal supplementation may help as well.

The magnesium and R-lipoic acid will help regulate blood sugar.

The multivitamin and B12 help with nutrients that are lost during rapid gastric dumping.

Bile Acid Malabsorption

Some people with poor gallbladder function or who have had their gallbladder removed might have diarrhea from bile acid malabsorption. Bile acids are produced in the liver for fat digestion and are stored in the gallbladder for future use. Large amounts of bile acids during digestion are reabsorbed in the terminal ileum of the small intestine and are recycled through the liver.

These bile acids are then stored in the gallbladder for future use. In people with poor or absent gallbladder function, bile acids may not be reabsorbed properly because too many bile acids were dumped in the small intestine for fat digestion. The excess bile acids travel further into the large intestine, where they stimulate extra water secretion and intestinal motility, creating chronic diarrhea. A SeHCAT test can be used to diagnose bile acid malabsorption if you or your doctor believes you are suffering from this condition.

Bile Acid Malabsorption Protocol

- Enzymedica Digest Gold – take one to two capsules with every meal daily.
- Organic vanilla hemp protein powder – ingest one scoop mixed with filtered water, daily.
- Unifiber – follow supplement recommendations.
- Optimal Start – take two capsules a meal, twice daily.
- Jarrow Formulas methyl B12 – take one sublingual tablet daily. Use another form like adenosylcobalamin if you are an overmethylator.
- Limit greasy, fried food in the diet. Use organic, extra virgin coconut oil, eggs, meat, and Brain Octane Oil as primary sources of fat. In addition, limit items that stimulate bile including citrus fruits, malate (apples) or citric acid, spicy food, foods high in oleic acid (extra virgin olive oil and avocados are good examples), and ginger.

If You Have Continuous Diarrhea:

- Upgraded™ Activated Charcoal – follow the general supplement bottle recommendations.
- Rainforest Pharmacy sangre de drago – follow the general supplement bottle recommendations.

Consider the daily use of a probiotic that mostly contains *Bifidobacteria longum.*

Possibly consider the medication cholestyramine – If you take this medicine for an extended period of time, supplement with the fat-soluble vitamins A, D, E, and K.

The digestive enzymes will help digest the food before it is dumped.

The extra fiber will help bulk up stools.

The multivitamin and B12 help with nutrients that are lost during rapid gastric dumping.

The activated charcoal will help bulk up the stools and eliminate excess bile.

Sangre de drago is a latex herb that might help bind the bile and bulk up the stools.

Cholestyramine binds to bile in the gastrointestinal tract.

Bifidobacteria longum has been shown in multiple studies to help the body reabsorb bile acids.

Pancreatic Health Protocol

This protocol should be used if you are suffering from mild pancreatic insufficiency.

- R-Lipoic acid (stabilized) – take 300 mg daily. Must take supplement with meals, lipoic acid may lower blood glucose levels.
- Enzymedica Digestive Enzyme Gold – one to two capsules with every meal. Take unless your amylase level from a blood test is elevated, if so discontinue the enzymes.
- Magnesium glycinate – take 400 mg daily, before bed.
- Limit or eliminate tobacco use.
- Follow the Bulletproof® Diet.
- Exercise at least three times a week for at least thirty minutes at a time.

The digestive enzymes and R-lipoic acid give the pancreas a break by decreasing insulin resistance and the need for digestive enzymes.

Tobacco puts excess stress on the pancreas.

Protocol 13 – Hiatal Hernia

A hiatal hernia is the protrusion of the upper part of the stomach into the thoracic cavity through a weakness in the diaphragm. There are two different types of hiatal hernias.

- **Sliding Hiatal Hernia** – A sliding hernia is the most common hiatal hernia and represents close to 99% of all cases of hiatal hernias. A sliding hernia occurs when the gastroesophageal junction slides back and forth above the diaphragm. When a sliding hernia occurs, some of the upper parts of the stomach is pulled through the opening, weakening the lower esophageal sphincter (LES). A sliding hiatal hernia rarely creates strangulation of the stomach or surrounding organs and, therefore, might not have to be surgically treated unless it is symptomatic.

- **Rolling Hiatal Hernia** – A rolling hernia occurs when a part of the upper stomach herniates through the esophageal hiatus that lies beside the esophagus. This form of a hiatal hernia is a lot more serious because the top part of the stomach may become twisted when the stomach occasionally moves to the side and behind the lower part of the esophagus. A rolling hiatal hernia needs to be immediately repaired upon diagnosis because of the risk of strangulation in the stomach and the medical emergency that may arise from it.

It has been theorized that developing a hiatal hernia might be a natural part of the aging process. Around 60% of individuals aged, fifty or older have been diagnosed as having a hiatal hernia. Hiatal hernias later in life might occur more frequently because as we age we tend to gain more weight and the structural integrity of our organs and muscles, including the LES, decreases.

Lack of proper dietary fiber intake and sitting while defecating can lead to developing a hiatal hernia. The reasoning behind this theory is that hiatal hernias are rare in rural African communities where they squat to use the bathroom compared to their first-world counterparts who sit. Finally, frequent increases in pressure within the abdomen (such as heavy lifting, coughing, sneezing, and violent vomiting), obesity, genetics, smoking, and stress can also be risk factors for developing a hiatal hernia.

Symptoms of a hiatal hernia are a dull pain in the chest, acid reflux, shortness of breath, heart palpitations, and pain in the esophagus after swallowing. Most hiatal hernias are asymptomatic, and often go undiagnosed. If you have been diagnosed with a hiatal hernia and at any time feel extreme pain or experience a large increase in vomiting, hernia strangulation may have occurred, and you need to go to the hospital immediately!

The most common way to diagnose a hiatal hernia is by an x-ray. Other ways to diagnose a hiatal hernia are by upper GI series or transnasal esophagoscopy.

Hiatal Hernia Protocol

- Follow the strengthening the LES protocol above.
- Magnesium glycinate – take 600 mg, before bed daily.
- Visit a chiropractor; they might be able to manipulate down a hiatal hernia into the correct position.
- Lose weight if you are overweight.
- Possibly try Nu Nefarious homeopathic supplement.

Protocol 14 – Develop Proper Defecation Posture

Even though this is technically an intestinal recommendation, proper defecation posture is important to lower intra-abdominal pressure. So what is proper defecation posture you might ask? Well, if you guessed that it was sitting straight up when using the toilet, guess again. Observe any toddler, dog, or cat using the bathroom to learn the proper posture for defecation. Squatting during defecation is the optimal posture.

The problems with sitting on the toilet instead of squatting are numerous. When you sit on the toilet, it makes a narrow anorectal angle. The narrow anorectal angle obstructs the anus and causes you not to empty your bowels completely when you use the bathroom. When you do not completely empty your bowels, some stool is pushed back up into the colon when you stand up. Theoretically, feces back up eventually leads to appendicitis, from the irritation of the appendix from toxins and opportunistic bacteria that were supposed to be eliminated.

Sitting while defecating causes you to perform repeatedly the Valsalva maneuver, which puts excessive stress on both the vagus nerve and the cardiovascular system, as well. Finally, sitting on the toilet increases the chances of developing diverticulosis and hemorrhoids from straining. The pressure buildup during defecation, if you are constipated, is up to three times greater than if they used the squatting technique to eliminate.

To squat on the toilet, stand with your knees and hips sharply bent and position yourself over the toilet opening. Some people who squat while defecating obtain complete relief from their constipation. Theoretically, it is easier to defecate when you squat because of the increase in the anorectal angle. You can purchase a squatty potty; a platform to stand on so one can successfully squat over the toilet very easily without having to balance.

Protocol 15 – Elimination of Parasites

Parasite infections are more common than most people would predict, even in the first world! Parasites cause digestive problems ranging from GERD to complete abdominal distress. A common myth is that more ingestion of parasites comes from eating meat, because of the grave horrors of factory farming. Accumulating a parasite load from eating meat is a myth because animals, even those whose meat comes from factory farms are regularly tested and treated for parasites. In addition, as long as the meat is properly cooked if it did contain parasites, all parasites would be eliminated from the heat of cooking. Most parasites in the human diet come from raw food, especially vegetables. According to the research, most vegans have a greater chance of having parasites than their meat eater counterparts.

Most intestinal parasite diagnoses come from stool samples taken by your doctor. A blood test can also be used in some cases to test for antibodies to parasites.

Is Piperine the Golden Bullet for Parasite Elimination?

Piperidine is used in both the treatment of parasites and worms in animals and the treatment of schizophrenia, in humans. Researchers propose that schizophrenia may result from a parasite infection like *T. gondii*.

The mechanism behind piperine is currently unknown. It may cause paralysis in parasites by increasing the permeability of schistosome cell membranes causing an influx of calcium ions. This reaction would dislodge the parasites from the site of action and eliminate them by phagocytosis (engulfment by white blood cells of the immune system). Piperine may also reduce adenosine uptake by the parasites creating mitochondrial disruption, causing them to tire to death.

If this correlation is based on truth, then a simple bio-piperine extract in supplement form could prove to be effective in eliminating parasitic infections. Piperine is a natural alkaloid of piperidine. Piperine has shown to eliminate parasite populations with fewer side effects than piperidine medications. Piperine can increase absorption of supplements and medications and should be taken two hours before, or after ingestion of medicines and supplements to reduce the chance of too much concentration of the medication or supplement in the blood.

Is Diatomaceous Earth the Silver Bullet for Parasite Elimination?

Diatomaceous earth is a naturally occurring rock made from the skeletons of fossilized algae. When food grade diatomaceous earth is grounded into a fine powder and ingested, it is used to eliminate parasites in the human body. When the razor-sharp edges of the diatoms encounter the parasites, it punctures their cellular walls. It is recommended that the earth is mixed with water when taken so that the risk of inhalation is very low. Diatomaceous earth is irritating to the lungs, try not to breathe in the dust when pouring or mixing.

Diatomaceous earth may degrade the mucous membrane in the stomach and intestines if used over a long period. People with ulcers may need to limit the amount of diatomaceous earth they consume until their ulcers have healed.

Diatomaceous Earth Protocol

I would suggest mixing a half-teaspoon in a glass of water twice a day (upon waking and before bed) for a week and slowly working up to one teaspoon twice a day. Do not use the diatomaceous earth drink more than three times daily. The diatomaceous earth should be taken for at least a month but no more than three months. Mix the diatomaceous earth well with purified water, and then consume.

Common Parasites and Elimination Protocols

Blastocystis hominis

Blastocystis is a genus of single-celled protozoan, which its colonization in most cases is asymptomatic. The intestinal colonization of *hominis* is somewhat common because of the low host specificity of the protozoan. Colonization rates differ between developed (10%) and less developed (50%) countries, and it seems to infect people more frequently who work and live with animals.

Most people with adequate immune systems are asymptomatic carriers. There is much debate in the scientific community if *Blastocystis hominis* even cause infections in humans or if it is a commensal protozoan. Blastocystosis is an opportunistic infection of the protozoan that can rarely occur. Symptoms of blastocystosis mimic other gastrointestinal illnesses and include:

- Abdominal pain
- Constipation
- Diarrhea
- Fatigue
- Flatulence
- Weight loss
- Food allergies
- Intestinal inflammation
- Skin rashes
- Headaches
- IBS
- IBD

Blastocystosis might occur because of an infection of a different more unknown opportunistic strain of *Blastocystis.* Researchers for the longest time might have mislabeled other infectious *Blastocystis* strains as being *Blastocystis hominis*. Therefore, we might not know which strains are truly causing the infection. *Blastocystis hominis* could be mostly harmless for all we know, and another strain could be causing all the opportunistic infections.

Diagnosis of infection requires an ova and parasite stool culture. If large numbers of organisms are present, and you show symptoms of blastocystosis, then I would consider trying to rid yourself of the protozoan. Blastocystosis is very difficult to eliminate, so a combination of medication and natural supplements may be needed. It can take months or even years to rid yourself of a *Blastocystis* opportunistic infection.

Blastocystis Protocol

- Ask your doctor about using Secnidazole / Diloxanide Furoate / Bactrim as a prescription combination to help eliminate the protozoan.
- Food grade diatomaceous earth – follow diatomaceous earth protocol above.
- Dr. Hula Clark's black walnut tincture – follow the general supplement bottle recommendations.
- Herb Pharm wormwood – follow the general supplement bottle recommendations.
- Sodium ascorbate – take 4,000 mg, twice daily.
- Upgraded™ Activated Charcoal – follow the general supplement bottle recommendations.
- Clean Chlorella – follow the general supplement bottle recommendations.
- Symbiotics lactoferrin - follow supplement bottle recommendations (can increase up to two grams daily if needed).
- MRM Cardio Chelate – follow general supplement recommendations.
- Colloidal silver (Mesosilver, Sovereign Silver) – follow supplement recommendations.

Lactoferrin, silver, and EDTA deprive the parasites of iron that they need to survive.

Vitamin C, activated charcoal, and chlorella, to limit the herx reactions from toxic exposure from eliminating parasites.

Black walnut and wormwood naturally remove parasites.

Cestoda Class (Tapeworms)

Cestoda is a class of flatworms that are commonly known as tapeworms. Tapeworm infections caused by ingestion of live larvae from consuming undercooked food (pork, beef, vegetables, or fish, for example), contaminated water or soil. Tapeworm infections are asymptomatic, but some people may have gastrointestinal symptoms like abdominal discomfort, diarrhea, and loss of appetite. Anemia can occur if fish tapeworms infect you. Live tapeworms can be seen in passed excrement; because of this diagnosis of tapeworms can be easily performed.

Taenia solium (pork tapeworm) cause a specific human disease known as cysticercosis. Cysticercosis can be asymptomatic for years, and later painless solid bumps appear on the skin, vision loss and muscle issues. After a few years, the body's innate immune system eventually can rid itself of the tapeworm and the bumps resolved themselves. The tapeworm may eventually cross the blood-brain barrier if it is not eliminated and cause neurological symptoms including seizures. Diagnostic methods of cysticercosis include stool samples, biopsies of affected areas, antibody blood tests, and radiological scans.

If you are suffering from cysticercosis, ask your doctor about the use of Praziquantel (steroids can be used to reduce the life-threatening CNS symptoms dealing with parasite die off if it is in the brain) with an enema to help remove the tapeworms.

Echinococcus tapeworms can cause a different disease known as echinococcosis. Humans are dead-end hosts for these parasites and ingestion can occur from eating contaminated undercooked food (sheep, goats, pigs), or infections that manifest from canine species. There are two different types of echinococcosis: cystic echinococcosis and alveolar echinococcosis.

Cystic echinococcosis (caused by *Echinococcus granulosus*), infections come from dogs, sheep, goats, or pigs. Symptoms are usually asymptomatic, but the parasite can cause lung and liver infections in people with compromised immune systems. Alveolar echinococcosis (caused by *Echinococcus multilocularis*), infections mainly come from canines. Symptoms are more severe than the cystic infection, and parasitic tumors may form in the liver, lungs, and brain.

Diagnostic methods of echinococcosis include stool samples, biopsies of affected areas, antibody blood tests, and radiological scans. If parasitic tumors and cysts occur then, surgery might be needed.

Self-limiting Cysticercosis / Echinococcosis Protocol

- Dr. Hula Clark's black walnut tincture – follow the general supplement bottle recommendations.
- Herb Pharm Wormwood – follow the general supplement bottle recommendations.
- Source Naturals Bioperine – take ten mg, twice daily, four hours away from any supplements or medications.
- Food grade diatomaceous earth – follow diatomaceous earth protocol above.
- Sodium ascorbate – take 4,000 mg, twice daily.
- Upgraded™ Activated Charcoal – follow the general supplement bottle recommendations.
- Clean Chlorella – follow the general supplement bottle recommendations.
- Symbiotics lactoferrin - follow supplement bottle recommendations (can increase up to two grams daily if needed).
- MRM Cardio Chelate – follow general supplement recommendations.
- Colloidal silver (Mesosilver, Sovereign Silver) – follow supplement recommendations.

Cryptosporidium Genus

Cryptosporidium is a genus of apicomplexan protozoans that causes the disease cryptosporidiosis. Infection of *Cryptosporidium* generally comes from ingestion of contaminated food or water. *Cryptosporidium* infection mainly occurs from contact with improperly treated water, the protozoan is highly resistant to chlorine, but may succumb to it over long periods or when combined with ozone. Swimmers that swim in improperly treated swimming pools or other contaminated water may be susceptible to getting this parasite. *Cryptosporidium* appears to be susceptible to UV radiation filtration exposure, which when used properly might eliminate the parasite.

Cryptosporidiosis is a self-limiting condition in healthy people. Symptoms of a self-limiting infection include diarrhea, stomach cramps, vomiting, and a low-grade fever. Self-limiting infections generally last a week but can rarely last up to a month. Diagnostic tests performed to determine an infection include detection of antibodies and microscoped stool sample testing.

In people with compromised immune systems, Cryptosporidiosis can become an emergency. The *Cryptosporidium* can spread beyond the intestines and infect the lungs, ears, stomach, biliary tract, and pancreas. Unrelenting severe diarrhea and dehydration are the main cause of death in people infected with *Cryptosporidium* that have poorly functioning immune systems. If you have a compromised immune system and your infection is severe, use of medication may be needed to treat the parasite. I recommend you ask your doctor about using only Nitazoxanide if possible. I would add black walnut, diatomaceous earth, and wormwood to help eliminate the parasite.

Self-limiting Cryptosporidiosis Protocol

- Dr. Hula Clark's black walnut tincture – follow the general supplement bottle recommendations.
- Herb Pharm Wormwood – follow the general supplement bottle recommendations.
- Source Naturals Bioperine – take ten mg, twice daily, four hours away from any supplements or medications.
- Food grade diatomaceous earth – follow diatomaceous earth protocol above.
- Sodium ascorbate – take 4,000 mg, twice daily.
- Upgraded™ Activated Charcoal – follow the general supplement bottle recommendations.
- Clean Chlorella – follow the general supplement bottle recommendations.
- Symbiotics lactoferrin - follow supplement bottle recommendations (can increase up to two grams daily if needed).
- MRM Cardio Chelate – follow general supplement recommendations.
- Colloidal silver (Mesosilver, Sovereign Silver) – follow supplement recommendations.

Black walnut and wormwood naturally remove parasites.

Cyclospora Genus

Cyclospora is a genus of protozoans which different strains cause an infection known as cyclosporiasis. *Cyclospora cayetanensis* is a recorded pathogenic strain in humans. Infection occurs because of ingestion of contaminated food (it has been linked to fruit like raspberries) or water. Symptoms include diarrhea, vomiting, abdominal pain, fatigue, and low-grade fever. Infection is self-limited unless you have a compromised immune system. If you have a compromised immune system, medication and hospitalization might be needed to treat the infection.

The incubation period is usually a week, and the illness can last at most six weeks. Diagnosis is made through microscoped stool sample (can be difficult to identify correct strain) and PCR testing. PCR testing is preferred because it has a high accuracy rate of at least 84% but it can be a costly diagnostic method. If medication is needed to treat infection, I recommend you ask your doctor about using TMP-SMX.

Cyclospora Protocol

- Dr. Hula Clark's black walnut tincture – follow the general supplement bottle recommendations.
- Herb Pharm Wormwood – follow the general supplement bottle recommendations.
- Source Naturals Bioperine – take ten mg, twice daily, four hours away from any supplements or medications.
- Food grade diatomaceous earth – follow diatomaceous earth protocol above.
- Sodium ascorbate – take 4,000 mg, twice daily.
- Upgraded™ Activated Charcoal – follow the general supplement bottle recommendations.
- Clean Chlorella – follow the general supplement bottle recommendations.
- Symbiotics lactoferrin - follow supplement bottle recommendations (can increase up to two grams daily if needed).
- MRM Cardio Chelate – follow general supplement recommendations.
- Colloidal silver (Mesosilver, Sovereign Silver) – follow supplement recommendations.

Dientamoeba fragilis

Dientamoeba fragilis is a single-celled amoeba that generally causes an infection known as dientamoebiasis. It was originally theorized that pinworms were once the main cause of infection, which they co-infected the host infected with the amoeba. Further research concludes that the only cause of transmission is contaminated water or food. Nevertheless, if you have been diagnosed with dientamoebiasis, you should also be tested for pinworms.

Symptoms of dientamoebiasis include diarrhea, abdominal pain, fatigue, fever, skin rashes, and IBS. Infection can range from being asymptomatic to severe and can last more than a couple of weeks if it is a chronic infection. Diagnostic tests used to determine an infection include a microscoped stool sample test and blood tests. Dientamoebiasis also appears to be a more severe condition for children than adults, and children might have to be treated more often with medication. Medication might be needed to help eliminate the parasite. If you have to use medication, I recommend asking your doctor about using only Doxycycline or Secnidazole if possible.

Dientamoebiasis Protocol

- Dr. Hula Clark's black walnut tincture – follow the general supplement bottle recommendations.
- Herb Pharm Wormwood – follow the general supplement bottle recommendations.
- Source Naturals Bioperine – take ten mg, twice daily, four hours away from any supplements or medications.
- Food grade diatomaceous earth – follow diatomaceous earth protocol above.
- Sodium ascorbate – take 4,000 mg, twice daily.
- Upgraded™ Activated Charcoal – follow the general supplement bottle recommendations.
- Clean Chlorella – follow the general supplement bottle recommendations.
- Symbiotics lactoferrin - follow supplement bottle recommendations (can increase up to two grams daily if needed).
- MRM Cardio Chelate – follow general supplement recommendations.
- Colloidal silver (Mesosilver, Sovereign Silver) – follow supplement recommendations.

Entamoeba histolytica

Entamoeba histolytica is an opportunistic protozoan. Infection of the parasite occurs from ingestion of contaminated food and water. The parasite usually remains in the colon and cecum but can cause invasive infections in immunocompromised individuals. *Histolytica* can spread to the liver, brain, and lungs through the bloodstream if you are immunocompromised and requires emergency treatment.

Symptoms of infection usually appear one to four weeks after ingestion. Symptoms include diarrhea, stomach pain, stomach cramps, and rarely fever and liver issues. Diagnosis of the parasite is made from a microscoped stool sample test. There is a possibility that false-positive results can occur due to confusion with other amoebas like *Entamoeba dispar.* Antibody tests might be needed if you test positive for the parasite to make sure you are suffering from an *Entamoeba histolytica* infection.

Entamoeba histolytica Protocol

If you require medication to rid yourself of the parasite, ask your doctor about using Diloxanide furoate, Iodoquinol, or Tindamax.

- Dr. Hula Clark's black walnut tincture – follow the general supplement bottle recommendations.
- Herb Pharm Wormwood – follow the general supplement bottle recommendations.
- Source Naturals Bioperine – take ten mg, twice daily, four hours away from any supplements or medications.
- Food grade diatomaceous earth – follow diatomaceous earth protocol above.
- Sodium ascorbate – take 4,000 mg, twice daily.
- Upgraded™ Activated Charcoal – follow the general supplement bottle recommendations.
- Clean Chlorella – follow the general supplement bottle recommendations.
- Symbiotics lactoferrin - follow supplement bottle recommendations (can increase up to two grams daily if needed).
- MRM Cardio Chelate – follow general supplement recommendations.
- Colloidal silver (Mesosilver, Sovereign Silver) – follow supplement recommendations.

Is the Magic Bullet for GERD, D-Limonene?

If there is one magic bullet that could eliminate most of the causes of Gerd at once, it is D-limonene. Texas scientist, Joe S. Wilkins, suffered from GERD for years and searched for alternative protocols. He was working with orange oil and noticed how D-limonene, a component of the oil acted as a cell rejuvenator. D-limonene is an extract from orange peel, which is non-toxic to humans and might have some anti-cancer properties. The daily intake of just one 1000 mg capsule of D-limonene every other day for twenty days, and has been shown to reduce or eliminate GERD symptoms in most people for six months or longer.

D-limonene is lighter than water, so it floats to the surface of gastric juices in the stomach. When someone has reflux, the D-limonene coats the esophagus, protects the esophagus from acid and gastrin, and helps heal erosions. D-limonene also increases gastric emptying and helps improve the flow of bile.

Joe S. Wilkins, the Houston-area scientist who developed this natural approach to heartburn relief, believes that the minor burping that occurs with D-limonene makes this orange peel extract to be directly carried into the esophagus. By coating the esophagus, D-limonene may protect the esophagus against caustic contents that would have otherwise been regurgitated from the stomach. D-limonene may promote quicker gastric emptying of food and gastric juices out of the stomach so that these esophageal irritants do not promote as much reflux. Finally, D-limonene might inhibit *H. pylori*, help the stomach produce extra mucus, and repair itself.

D-limonene Protocol

- Jarrow Formulas D-limonene or Enzymatic Therapy D-limonene - Take one softgel of D-limonene, during or with a meal, every other day for twenty days.

Chapter 5

Silent Reflux / Barrett's Esophagus

LERD: Laryngopharyngeal Reflux Disease

Laryngopharyngeal reflux disease is a newer, less understood cousin of GERD. LERD differs from GERD in that people with LERD suffer from more of the upper airway symptoms of reflux disease. Symptoms of LERD include coughing, hoarseness, tachycardia after eating, esophageal spasms, post-nasal drip, sore throat, lump in the throat feeling (globus pharyngis), hoarseness, dry mouth, bad taste in mouth, bad breath, loss of smell and nose function, ear infections, hearing problems, and asthma.

Most people who suffer from LERD do not have traditional heartburn, pain in the throat or chest, or any symptoms of GERD. LERD sufferers usually have their symptoms during the day, whether they eat or not, and symptoms usually arise when they are sitting. GERD sufferers typically have their symptoms in the evening, after they eat, and when they are lying down. Most LERD symptoms are instead felt upon waking from sleep in the morning. It is also harder for LERD to be diagnosed correctly because the symptoms are so universal for most people. LERD can disguise itself as being asthma, mouth, ear, or sinus issues.

Unlike GERD, the esophagus usually appears undamaged in people with LERD. The esophagus appears undamaged because the acid and pepsin that are refluxed are quickly swallowed downward. The stomach contents not being trapped in between the two sphincters creates a lot less damage to the esophagus itself and more damage to the upper airway and larynx because pepsin remains there and breaks down the tissue.

Pepsin is the main enzyme used by the stomach to digest protein. Pepsinogen activates and converts into the enzyme pepsin in the presence of stomach acid. Pepsin helps break down protein into amino acids the body can absorb and then becomes inactivated by turning back into pepsinogen when it is mixed with bicarbonate released from the pancreas in the small intestine. This transformation protects the rest of the intestinal system from the pepsin and stomach acid.

The inactivation of pepsin by sodium bicarbonate does not occur in the esophagus. Anytime you swallow anything with a low pH like vinegar, for example, pepsin is reactivated and begins to damage the tissue. I recommend drinking Alkaline water after meals, throughout the day, and before bed to inactivate pepsin. In addition, limiting acidic foods like citrus fruits or vinegar can also help relieve the symptoms of silent reflux.

An endoscopy may also be performed to get an idea of esophageal damage and the general function of your LES, UES, and stomach. During an endoscopy, a flexible wire with a camera positioned at the end of the wire is swallowed. The camera takes pictures down the esophagus and into the stomach. Traditional endoscopies are known to have issues associated with the procedure including potential injury or death from sedation, increased risk of aspiration, and infections from improperly sterilized scopes. I recommend you talk to your doctor about the safer transnasal esophagoscopy procedure that does not require sedation.

One of the best assessments utilized in the diagnosing of LERD is an esophageal pH monitoring test. A flexible catheter with a pH monitor on the end is placed through the nose down into the esophagus for at least 24 hours. It is uncomfortable to have the tube down your nose and throat, but it is very useful in establishing an LERD diagnosis.

In most people with LERD, the upper and lower esophageal sphincters are not functioning properly. The UES, known as the upper esophageal sphincter, closes off the oral cavity and the upper airways from the esophagus. In most people with GERD, the LES, known as the lower esophageal sphincter, is the only sphincter in the esophagus not functioning properly. The nonfunctioning LES causes acid to become stuck in-between the stomach and the UES. The UES is the sphincter at the top of the esophagus that open and closes when you swallow to protect the upper airways from aspiration; the trapped acid between the two sphincters is what causes the sensation of heartburn for most people.

The main problem with LERD is conventional medicine does not have an effective treatment for it. There is no proven diagnostic cause of LERD. My best hypothesis is that it is caused by any combination of any of these issues: SIBO, magnesium deficiency, adrenal fatigue, hypothyroid, vagus nerve issues, zinc deficiency, improper collagen production in the body, possible unknown infection, and / or nerve damage to both the LES and UES.

General Advice for LERD

- Ask a physical therapist about "shaker" neck exercises that can be used to strengthen neck muscles (and the UES) after someone has a stroke.
- Drink only room temperature water during meals, and do not overeat. Eat three meals daily only and try not to snack at night to help maintain proper MMC function.
- Chew your food well while you eat especially if you are eating anything with carbohydrates (to mix well with what little amylase we have in our saliva). The more you masticate your food, the less your stomach needs to work to digest properly your food.
- Drink two oz. of naturally alkaline water (Evamor, Icelandic Spring, and Mountain Valley Spring Water are good brands) two hours after a meal to deactivate pepsin in the larynx (from stomach contents reflux) that might cause irritation. Swish well with the alkaline water before swallowing. In addition, drink two oz. of naturally alkaline water before bed.
- Wash the nasal passages out with saline at least once a day. In addition, use saline drops in the nose daily and blow your nose afterwards. The saline is to deactivate excess pepsin that might be in your nose from the reflux caused by the LERD. Do not use a neti pot unless needed because it can wash away the beneficial mucus barrier in the nose.
- Sleep on your left side at night to prevent reflux. Sleeping on our left side or back prevents LES weakness and helps with maintaining proper anatomical position. Possibly consider using the Reza Band at night to prevent reflux. I cannot fully recommend it because it is

relatively new and more post-market studies need to be performed. Finally, practice good sleep hygiene. Melatonin production is important for proper digestive health and LES function.

- Reduce intake of acidic foods that can trigger silent reflux. I would try to limit what I ingest with a pH lower than 5.5.
- If you are suffering from bile reflux, combined with silent reflux, reduce your ingestion of foods high in omega 9, known as oleic acid. Avocados and extra virgin olive oil is an example of foods high in oleic acid.
- Increased endogenous production of vitamin D seems to help most people with silent reflux. I cannot stress the importance of this advice enough; it has made the biggest difference in my life and those I have coached that made the lifestyle changes. If you live in an area where it is hard to get sun or UVB, the use of a UVB producing tanning bed or supplementation might be needed. Get your 25-hydroxy and 1-25 hydroxy levels checked to see if your vitamin D levels are in range.
- Maintain proper amounts of Omega-3 fatty acids in your diet. Ingest leaner fish like cod, flounder, and salmon.

LERD Protocol

- Zinc carnosine – One to two capsules with each meal.
- Magnesium glycinate – 200 mg per 50 pounds of body weight, taken at bedtime.

Coat and Rebuild Your Esophagus and Larynx

- Supplement with collagen daily.
- Recipe to help coat and relieve your throat – In one cup of hot filtered water, mix in 1/2 teaspoon of slippery elm powder and 1/8 teaspoon of DGL powder, consume after each meal. Swish well, mixing with saliva before swallowing.
- Eat organic grass-fed beef liver once weekly for a good source of retinol and ceruloplasmin-bound copper.
- Consider using D-limonene to help coat and protect the esophagus and larynx. For some people, it helps immensely, but for others it may not be easily tolerated.
- Consider using liposomial colostrum to help invigorate your immune system and reduce inflammation.

Tackle Outstanding Medical Problems which may cause LERD

- Follow the strengthen LES protocol (Ch. 4).
- Relieve adrenal fatigue or/and hypothyroidism.
- Be tested by a doctor for SIBO; if positive or have a lot of the symptoms, follow SIBO protocol (Ch. 9).
- Follow *Candida* protocol (Ch. 4) if you are suffering from *Candida* overgrowth.

Barrett's Esophagus

Barrett's esophagus is an abnormal mutation to the cells in the lower part of the esophagus. Long-term GERD, LERD, bile acid reflux, or vomiting may cause the stratified squamous epithelium cells to be replaced by simple columnar epithelium with goblet cells. The reasoning behind this replacement of cells is that over time pepsin and stomach acid degrade the cells in the esophagus (chronic inflammation) to the point where the body tries to replace them with cells that secrete more mucus to protect the esophagus from further damage. Even though the body is trying to adapt to protect itself from further damage, it comes at a cost.

This change in the cells of the esophagus greatly increases the risk of esophageal cancer formation. Esophageal adenocarcinoma has a high mortality rate. The increased risk of cancer develops from the chronic inflammation damaging cells, increasing free radical damage from refluxed gastrointestinal contents, and from the cells mutating into abnormal cells outside of their normal body organs (stomach and intestines). The tissue change in Barrett's esophagus will reverse itself usually after the causes of the disease are remedied, and the risk of cancer then becomes reduced over time.

Signs of symptoms of Barrett's esophagus include frequent and long-term GERD / LERD, dysphagia, vomiting of blood, pain under the breastbone, and possible weight loss. If your Barrett's esophagus is caused by LERD, it may be asymptomatic. Barrett's esophagus is more common in overweight people and affects men more than women.

Diagnosis of Barrett's esophagus is usually made from an endoscopy. Biopsies from the endoscopy are examined under a microscope, and changes of esophageal tissue are seen in people suffering from the disease. I recommend that you get a transnasal esophagoscopy instead of an endoscopy. Someone with Barrett's esophagus is recommended to get a transnasal esophagoscopy three years after remission of the disease to make sure the condition is in remission.

Barrett's Esophagus Protocol

- Follow GERD protocol (Ch. 4), LERD protocol above, or gallbladder protocol (Ch. 4) to remedy underlying disease to reverse Barrett's esophagus.

Any supplement recommended below is to be taken if they are not in any of the above-mentioned protocols.

- Pure Encapsulations zinc carnosine – take one capsule with a meal, twice daily.
- DGL licorice chewable – follow supplement recommendations on the bottle (take thirty minutes before a meal; chew very well and mix with saliva for effectiveness).
- Georges Always Active aloe vera – follow bottle recommendations.
- Organic black raspberry powder – consume one teaspoon with a glass of filtered water mixed well, once daily.
- Magnesium glycinate – 600 mg, taken at bedtime.
- Drink a half cup of naturally, alkaline water (Evamor and Mountain Valley Spring Water are recommended brands) two hours after a meal to deactivate pepsin in the larynx (from stomach contents reflux) that might cause irritation. In addition, drink a half cup of naturally alkaline water before bed.
- Follow D-limonene protocol (Ch. 4) if no relief in ten days.

Zinc carnosine, D-limonene, DGL licorice, aloe vera, alkaline water, magnesium glycinate, and black raspberry powder may help to reduce inflammation and help protect the esophagus from further damage.

Chapter 6

Disorders of the Stomach

Gastritis

Gastritis is inflammation of the lining of the stomach. Gastritis can occur acutely or become chronic. Most causes of acute gastritis include excessive alcohol consumption, use of NSAIDS (ibuprofen, naproxen sodium, or aspirin as examples), food poisoning, traumatic injury to the stomach, and major intestinal surgery. Chronic causes of gastritis include *H. pylori* infection, bile reflux, stress, upper gut overgrowth, liver or kidney disease, stomach cancer, Zollinger-Ellison syndrome, and long-term use of certain medication like NSAIDS. Finally, the food additive carrageenan has been implicated in causing chronic gastritis and excessive intestinal inflammation.

The most common symptoms of gastritis are a burning feeling in your stomach, stomach gnawing sounds, abdominal pain, nausea, loss of appetite, vomiting, a feeling of fullness in the stomach, ulcers, indigestion, and bloating. Pernicious anemia, which is known as anemia that is caused by a B12 deficiency, is a symptom of chronic gastritis.

Diagnostic tests useful in the diagnosis of gastritis are X-rays, ECG, an endoscopy, blood cell count to determine pernicious anemia, *H. pylori* tests, liver, kidney, gallbladder, or pancreatic function tests (to determine possible bile reflux cause), and possible stomach biopsy. I recommend that you get a transnasal esophagoscopy instead of an endoscopy if possible.

Carrageenan

Carrageenan is a family of linearly sulfated polysaccharides that are extracted from red seaweed. The food industry uses carrageenan in meat and dairy (even in natural and organic products) for its gelling, thickening, and stabilizing properties. Multiple studies show that carrageenan causes gastrointestinal problems and immune responses. It has also been linked to gastrointestinal cancer. Anyone suffering from gastritis or inflammatory diseases should eliminate carrageenan until their gastrointestinal tract heals. People who are seeking optimal gut health should avoid carrageenan altogether.

Mild to Moderate Gastritis Protocol

- Pure Encapsulations zinc carnosine – take one capsule with a meal, twice daily.
- DGL licorice chewable – follow supplement recommendations on the bottle (take thirty minutes before a meal; chew very well and mix with saliva for effectiveness).
- L - glutamine – take 4,000 - 10,000 mg daily with food (use with caution if you have a sensitivity to glutamic acid, deficiency in GABA, or severe leaky gut and brain).
- D-limonene – one softgel daily with food.
- Nordic Naturals cod liver oil – follow the general supplement bottle recommendations.
- George's aloe vera – only use when the stomach is inflamed. Follow the general supplement bottle recommendations.
- Sodium Bicarbonate – follow box recommendations for consumption, only use when stomach inflammation is at its worst.
- I would reduce consumption of gluten (wheat), oats (avenin), spinach, and casein (dairy except for butter and ghee) to help improve digestion and reduce inflammation.

Lowering stomach PH might be a bad idea if an *H. pylori* infection is the cause of your gastritis; therefore, D-limonene may be used as an alternative to sodium bicarbonate if this is the case. Follow D-limonene protocol (Ch. 4) if bicarbonate causes issues.

Zinc carnosine, DGL, and L-glutamine will repair the mucus and stomach lining.

Fish oil will help reduce inflammation.

Aloe vera will help soothe the stomach.

Severe Gastritis Protocol

Follow protocol above and add:

- Proton Pump Inhibitor: Zegerid (All PPI use comes at a risk, use only with caution).

TAKE PPI NO LONGER THAN 1 MONTH.

Afterward, follow SIBO protocol (Ch. 9), *Candida* protocol (Ch. 4), and Betaine HCL protocol (Ch. 12).

I chose Zegerid because it contains Prilosec, the PPI that has been in use the longest. Therefore, its mechanism of action and side effects are well known. Zegerid is Prilosec mixed with sodium bicarbonate.

Herbal Gastritis Protocol

- George's aloe vera – only use the aloe vera when your stomach is inflamed. Follow the general supplement bottle recommendations.
- DGL licorice chewable – follow supplement bottle recommendations (take thirty minutes before a meal; chew very well and mix with saliva for effectiveness).
- Solaray marshmallow extract – follow the general supplement bottle recommendations.
- Now slippery elm extract - follow the general supplement bottle recommendations.
- Organic chamomile tea – drink twice daily.

Aloe vera will help soothe the stomach.

DGL, marshmallow, chamomile, and slippery elm will help soothe and repair the stomach's mucous lining.

Gastroparesis

Gastroparesis is also known as delayed gastric emptying. When someone has Gastroparesis, the pylorus at the bottom of the stomach has trouble pushing chime through the stomach into the small intestine. In a healthy person, the vagus nerve controls these contractions. The vagus nerve is a cranial nerve that begins at the brain and travels all the way down to the large intestine. One of its primary functions in the body is to control peristalsis throughout the digestive system. Gastroparesis is usually caused by nerve damage done to the vagus nerve.

When someone has gastroparesis, food moves slowly (or even not at all) through the digestive system because of nerve signaling problems from the brain to the vagus nerve. It can also be caused due to signaling problems from the vagus nerve to the digestive system. Symptoms of gastroparesis are GERD, chronic nausea, chronic diarrhea, vomiting, abdominal pain, heart palpitations, lack of appetite, bloating, SIBO, and blood glucose regulation issues. Morning nausea may be a warning sign that you might have, at the very least, mild Gastroparesis from the lack of stomach emptying during the night.

Gastroparesis can be diagnosed with stomach X-rays, manometry, and a gastric emptying scan. Some causes of gastroparesis are diabetic neuropathy, drug-induced neuropathy, anorexia or bulimia (damage to the vagus nerve from vomiting or extreme loss of weight), and lastly, even PPIs can cause mild gastroparesis (from lack of stomach acid to digest proteins that in turn slows stomach transit time).

Gastroparesis Supplementation Protocol

(The gastroparesis protocol is almost identical to the LES protocol [Ch. 4])

- Now Calcium citrate powder - 500 mg, twice daily mixed with water.
- L-glutamine "shake" - 4,000 mg of L-glutamine, mixed with a glass of water, with food (use with caution if you have a sensitivity to glutamic acid, deficiency in GABA, or severe leaky gut and brain).
- Jarrow R-lipoic acid - one capsule, twice a daily with meals.
- Magnesium malate - 600 mg total daily.
- Enzymedica Digestive Enzyme Gold - take one capsule with every meal.
- Thorne Research B complex - one capsule daily, do not use if you are an overmethylator.
- Pure Encapsulations zinc carnosine - one capsule with meals, twice daily.
- Melatonin Life Extension extended release - take three mg at night daily.

If all else fails to provide relief:

- Jarrow 5-HTP - follow supplement recommendations on the bottle. Only take for two weeks at most.
- Follow SIBO protocol (Ch. 9) if bacteria are present.
- Consider a low residue diet.
- Consider using spicy food or ginger to increase gastric emptying.
- Eat small meals and frequently. Large meals can further slow down stomach emptying.

Calcium citrate, in theory, should strengthen the pylorus in the body when it encounters it. Calcium strengthens muscle contractions. This is just a theory; no in vivo studies have been done.

R-lipoic acid has multiple benefits in the body, but in this role, it works by ensuring that the pylorus has little nerve damage as possible, and also strengthens the vagus nerve.

Digestive enzymes help break down the food in the stomach that reduces gas and pressure on the pylorus.

The L-glutamine and the grass-fed whey helps rebuild the integrity of the gastrointestinal system and the pylorus as well.

Melatonin and 5-HTP have been shown to increase LES strength.

Gastroparesis Herbal Protocol

- Follow the Cayenne Pepper Protocol (Ch. 18).
- New Chapter Ginger Force – take one softgel with your largest meal.

- Swedish bitters - follow the general supplement bottle recommendations.

Cayenne pepper, ginger, and Swedish bitters have been shown to increase gastric emptying time.

Zollinger – Ellison Syndrome

Zollinger – Ellison syndrome is a condition that is caused by a non-beta islet cell, a gastrin-secreting tumor of the pancreas that causes the stomach to overproduce gastrin. When gastrin is overproduced in the stomach, excess stomach acid is also produced. The tumor is usually discovered in the pancreas, duodenum, or abdominal lymph of the person. The tumor somehow manages to shut off the body's natural acid production feedback loop. This shutdown causes an extreme amount of gastrin, pepsin, and stomach acid to be produced, which creates massive digestive issues.

Most people with Zollinger - Ellison syndrome present with differing symptoms. The person usually suffers from intolerable GERD, chronic diarrhea (fatty yellow stools), pain in the esophagus after meals and at night, nausea, wheezing, and weight loss. It is usually diagnosed with blood work including a secretin stimulation test, gastrin level test, and a chromogranin A test. All tests are usually elevated in people with this syndrome. If the blood tests are positive, an MRI, Endoscopy, or CAT scan is usually performed to show the location of the tumor. I recommend that you get a transnasal esophagoscopy instead of an endoscopy.

General Advice for Zollinger - Ellison Syndrome

- Follow gastrointestinal cancer advice (Ch. 9) for possible reduction or elimination of tumors.
- Drink alkaline water two hours after meals and before bed to deactivate pepsin.
- Weigh surgery options.
- Zollinger – Ellison syndrome is one of the few conditions where PPI's might be needed on a long-term basis. If you need to use one, I recommend that you supplement with magnesium and B12 on a regular basis for optimal health.

After Surgery Stomach and Intestinal Recovery Protocol

For Two – Three Months:

- L-glutamine - 20,000 – 40,000 mg daily for one week after surgery. Then, take at least 10,000 mg daily for a month after surgery. Then, take 4,000 mg for the remainder of the protocol. Take with food (use with caution if you have a sensitivity to glutamic acid, deficiency in GABA, or severe leaky gut and brain).
- GOS – take one scoop daily mixed with filtered water. Use with caution if you have yeast overgrowth or Th2 elevated issues.
- Florastor probiotic - follow supplement-boxed instructions; take while on an antibiotic. Do not use if you have yeast or histamine sensitivities.
- Thorne Curcumin - follow the general supplement bottle recommendations
- N-acetylglucosamine - (do not use if allergic to shellfish or have yeast overgrowth) – follow the general supplement bottle recommendations.
- Pure Encapsulations zinc carnosine – take one capsule with a meal, twice daily.
- SeaCure white fish protein supplement (do not use if you are allergic to fish) – follow the general supplement bottle recommendations.
- For three months: magnesium glycinate – take 600 mg, before bed.
- Follow a gluten-free / GMO-free diet.

L-glutamine is the most abundant amino acid and helps rebuild both the stomach lining and the gut.

Probiotics help protect the gut from opportunistic bacteria.

Curcumin is to increase immune cells in the gut and heal inflammation.

The body makes N-acetylglucosamine to increase mucus production in the stomach and gut and to make a protective barrier.

The zinc carnosine should help repair the stomach lining.

SeaCure might help your intestines recover from the surgery faster.

Nausea / Vomiting

Nausea is a sensation of unease and discomfort in the upper stomach, which can lead to an urge to vomit. You may occasionally feel nauseated, but this does not always mean you will vomit. Some common causes of nausea are motion sickness, anxiety, dizziness, migraine, gastroenteritis, or food poisoning.

Vomiting is the forceful expulsion of the content of one's stomach, through the mouth or nose. Vomiting is different from regurgitation. Regurgitation is the return of undigested food back up through the esophagus into the mouth, without the dynamic action of vomiting, almost like a burp. Vomiting has many common causes like poisoning, overeating, ingestion of certain medications, gastroenteritis, gastritis, food poisoning, foodborne illness, anxiety, exposure to ionizing radiation, and increased intracranial pressure.

Vomiting for most people is harmless for an acute period, but it can lead to complications acutely and chronically. Aspiration occurs mainly in people that are incapacitated, under the influence of incapacitating medications, or people who have issues with or cannot swallow properly. Aspiration occurs when gastric contents enter the respiratory tract. Aspiration into the respiratory tract may cause someone to choke and asphyxiate, or suffer from aspiration pneumonia. Vomiting also causes dehydration, electrolyte imbalance, and causes hypochloremic metabolic acidosis (low chloride levels together with elevated CO2 levels that lead to increased blood PH) and hypokalemia (potassium depletion). Finally, excessive chronic vomiting causes small tears and erosions in the esophagus that are known as Mallory-Weiss tears.

The Pathophysiology of Vomiting

Receptors on the floor of the fourth ventricle of the brain represent a vomiting chemoreceptor trigger zone. When this receptor is triggered, you may become nauseated and vomit. The chemoreceptor trigger zone has numerous D2 receptors, 5-HT3 serotonin receptors, opioid receptors, acetylcholine receptors, and receptors for substance P. The D2, 5-HT3, opioid, and Substance P receptors are the receptors that trigger vomiting. It seems that these receptors exist in the brain to monitor these neurotransmitters, and an increase of these neurotransmitters can cause vomiting. Acetylcholine receptors signal the stomach, causing contractions that eventually lead to vomiting.

Before the act of vomiting, you will have increased salivation. The increase in saliva is the body's attempt to protect your teeth enamel. Then, the body signals a respiratory response causing you to take a deep breath to close off the lungs so that aspiration of vomit will not occur. Retroperistalsis starts from the middle of the small intestine and sweeps up digestive tract contents into the stomach. Intrathoracic pressure lowers coupled with an increase in abdominal pressure. The increase in abdominal pressure propels the stomach contents into the esophagus as the LES relaxes, and with great force, the vomit exits the body through the mouth. The person may also begin sweating and suffering from tachycardia during the action of vomiting.

Colors of Vomit

Bright red streaks in the vomit suggest bleeding from the esophagus.

Dark red vomit with clots suggests profuse bleeding in the stomach, such as an ulcer.

Dark brown vomit suggests lesser chronic bleeding in the stomach because gastric acid changes the composition of the blood over time to a browner color.

Yellow vomit suggests bile reflux.

Boerhaave Syndrome

Boerhaave syndrome also known as esophageal rupture is a medical emergency where there is a rupture of the esophageal wall. Most ruptures come from medical accidents during endoscopy or surgery, but it can occur from vomiting. Boerhaave syndrome occurring because of vomiting is thought to be the result of a sudden rise in internal esophageal pressure. The sudden change in pressure is a result of neuromuscular incoordination during vomiting causing failure of the cricopharyngeus muscle to relax properly. The cricopharyngeus muscle failing to relax properly and the sudden change in pressure leads to esophageal rupture. The rupture can also occur from ingestion of caustic materials, pill esophagitis (a pill is stuck in the throat), and long-term Barrett's esophagus.

Symptoms of Boerhaave syndrome include severe vomiting, severe chest, and upper abdominal pain. Trouble breathing, swallowing, fever, and shock also develop shortly after esophageal rupture. Most diagnosis of Boerhaave syndrome is performed by symptoms, chest X-ray, or CT scan.

Treatment requires immediate surgery to fix the rupture followed by antibiotic therapy. IV rehydration therapy is also needed since nothing can be taken by mouth for a while. Mortality without treatment is near 100% and even after surgery; the risk of mortality is 25%.

General Nausea Protocol

- Ingest ginger (ginger beer, ginger chews, or ginger tea) if you are suffering from nausea.
- Ingest fennel seeds if you are suffering from nausea.
- Thorne Research pyridoxal 5' phosphate – one to two capsules daily in divided doses.

Ginger, vitamin B6, and fennel help relieve nausea.

Boerhaave Syndrome after Surgery Protocol

Only follow the protocol after the doctor allows you to take anything by mouth.

For Two – Three Months:

- L-glutamine - 20,000 – 40,000 mg daily for one week after surgery. Then, take at least 10,000 mg daily for a month after surgery. Then, take 4,000 mg for the remainder of the protocol. Take with food (use with caution if you have a sensitivity to glutamic acid, deficiency in GABA, or severe leaky gut and brain).
- Florastor probiotic - follow supplement-boxed instructions; take while on an antibiotic. Do not use if you have yeast or histamine sensitivities.
- GOS – take one scoop daily mixed with filtered water. Use with caution if you have yeast overgrowth or Th2 elevated issues.
- Thorne Curcumin - follow the general supplement bottle recommendations.
- N-acetylglucosamine - (do not use if allergic to shellfish or have yeast overgrowth) – follow the general supplement bottle recommendations.
- Pure Encapsulations zinc carnosine – take one capsule with a meal, twice daily.
- SeaCure white fish protein supplement (do not use if you are allergic to fish) – follow the general supplement bottle recommendations.
- For three months: magnesium glycinate – take 600 mg, before bed.
- Follow a gluten-free / GMO-free diet.

L-glutamine is the most abundant amino acid and helps rebuild both the stomach lining and the esophagus.

Probiotics help protect the body from opportunistic bacteria.

Curcumin is to increase immune cells in the esophagus and heal inflammation.

The body produces N-acetylglucosamine to increase mucus production in the stomach and esophagus and to make a protective barrier.

The zinc carnosine should help repair the stomach lining.

SeaCure might help your esophagus recover from the surgery faster.

Cyclic Vomiting Syndrome

Cyclic vomiting syndrome is a condition in which someone has recurring attacks of intense nausea, vomiting, and abdominal pain. Cyclic vomiting syndrome typically develops during childhood and usually remits when the person becomes an adult.

Anyone who is affected with this disorder vomits in a pattern. The person usually vomits six to twelve times an hour, and each episode lasts a few hours to at most a month. During these periods of vomiting, the person might feel very tired and have migraine symptoms during an attack. Some people might even have warnings before the attack much like migraine sufferers; this is also known as a prodrome. During a prodrome, anyone with this disorder might have extreme nausea, sensitivity to light and sound, muscle pain, and fatigue. The disease has intermittent periods where you might function normally before you suddenly suffer from another vomiting fit.

The cause of CVS has been undetermined in conventional medicine, but some studies have linked it to mitochondrial dysfunction. Mitochondrial dysfunction is why people who have cyclic vomiting syndrome also suffer from migraine symptoms, as well. If this is the case, increasing mitochondrial function might help relieve cyclic vomiting syndrome symptoms. Research Dr. Richard Boles if you want more information on this correlation.

Cyclic Vomiting Syndrome Protocol for Children

- Now liquid CoQ10 – take 200 mg, once daily before noon.
- Magnesium malate – follow instruction dosage and recommendations for children.
- L-carnitine – follow instruction dosage and recommendations for children.
- Children's B vitamin supplement – purchase B vitamin supplement from these companies: Jarrow, Thorne Research, Pure Encapsulations.
- Drink pH balanced alkaline water after a vomiting attack to limit pepsin degradation of tissue in the esophagus.

CoQ10, magnesium, L-carnitine and B vitamins all help with mitochondrial support.

Cyclic Vomiting Syndrome Protocol for Adults

- Jarrow Formulas ubiquinol – 200 mg, taken once daily before noon.
- Magnesium malate – 600 mg total, take 200 mg with every meal daily.
- Jarrow L-carnitine supplement – 2,000 mg, take on an empty stomach, divide the dosage if you wish.
- Life Extension PQQ – take 10 mg, once daily.
- B vitamin complex Thorne Research – take once daily, do not use if you are an overmethylator.
- Black raspberry powder – follow the general supplement bottle recommendations.
- Drink pH balanced alkaline water after a vomiting attack to limit pepsin degradation of tissue in the esophagus.

If there is no improvement after a month of following the protocol:

- Jarrow Formulas R-lipoic acid – take twice daily with meals.

R-lipoic acid, PQQ, CoQ10, magnesium, L-carnitine, and the B vitamins all help with mitochondrial support.

Black raspberry powder helps protect the esophagus from free radical damage.

Roemheld Syndrome

Roemheld syndrome is also known as gastric-cardia syndrome and was discovered by Ludwig Roemheld in the 1930's. Simply put, it is a condition where poor digestive health leads to cardiac symptoms and issues. Ever felt a very low or very high heart rate during or after eating that was relieved by burping? You probably suffer from Roemheld syndrome.

Most of the following symptoms of Roemheld syndrome seem to occur after eating, especially a large meal. Some people have also reported their symptoms occur after strenuous activity, when excessive pressure is applied to their abdomen, or during sleep.

Here are the proposed symptoms of Roemheld syndrome:

- Sinus bradycardia followed by sinus tachycardia
- Hypotension followed by hypertension
- Abnormal amount of premature ventricular contractions (PVC's)
- Arrhythmia (heart palpitations)
- Chest pain (angina pectoris)
- Anxiety
- Syncope
- GERD, bile, and / or silent reflux symptoms
- Sleep disturbance
- Fatigue
- Weakness
- Muscle cramps
- Trouble breathing
- Tinnitus
- Hot flashes
- Facial flushing
- Vertigo
- Visual snow
- Atrial fibrillation
- Coughing and throat clearing
- Heart disease
- Sudden cardiac death

The syndrome consists of both mechanical and neurological triggers. Mechanical triggers of the illness occur when pressure is placed on the fundus of the stomach or the esophagus. When the increased epigastric pressure occurs, the diaphragm's position is elevated and puts pressure on the heart and vagus nerve. Hiatal hernias are known to be a significant mechanical trigger of Roemheld syndrome.

The neurological conditions of the syndrome occur from increased vagus nerve pressure and misfiring. When the vagus nerve is compressed your heart rate and blood pressure decrease and in doing so the body's autonomic nervous system is triggered creating a catecholamine dump into the bloodstream. The increased circulating catecholamines cause a massive increase in blood pressure and heart rate. Unless an underlying arrhythmia is triggered, the fluctuation from low to high cardiac pulses and pressure may be undetectable unless you are actively monitored during an attack and can be easily mistaken as anxiety. When an attack occurs, strong coronary reflexes happen, causing many of the cardiac symptoms associated with the syndrome and if the heart is stressed enough a heart attack may occur!

Over time, the syndrome can lead to a weakening of the heart. It can cause arrhythmias to develop including atrial fibrillation and may cause heart disease and eventually heart failure.

Causes of Roemheld syndrome include:

- Hiatal hernia
- Abdominal hernia
- Abdominal hernia repair (mesh)
- Excessive gas in the abdomen (SIBO, lactose intolerance, fructose intolerance, food intolerance, upper gut infection)
- Gas bloat syndrome (failure to burp)
- Gastric bypass
- Gallbladder issues
- Being overweight

What Can Be Done to Help Recover from Roemheld Syndrome?

Here are some tips to try to help reduce the issues from having Roemheld syndrome:

- If your Roemheld syndrome is caused by a hiatal hernia, try to work on reducing it.
- Reduce gas formation in the stomach and intestinal tract.

- Try to follow a low FODMAP diet throughout the week and a gluten-free diet on weekends to see if that helps reduce gas buildup.
- Treat SIBO or an upper gut infection if you have it.
- Taking activated charcoal may reduce gas formation in the stomach and intestines.
- Taking digestive enzymes may help reduce gas formation.
- Make sure your stomach acid production is optimal.
- Chew your food well and eat slowly. Do not over stuff yourself. If you need to burp, make yourself by swallowing a little bit of water and try to burp. Most of the time making yourself burp relieves the symptoms of Roemheld syndrome.
- Exercise regularly to strengthen your heart, supplement with magnesium, and maintain proper intake of dietary omega 3 fatty acids to help reduce chances of developing serious heart arrhythmia.
- Try to sleep on your back or side. Some people have fewer symptoms of Roemheld syndrome sleeping on their left or right side. Laying on the right or left side during an attack may provide instant relief. For most people laying on the right side seems to help more, even if that is counterproductive to sleeping recommendations individuals who have GERD.
- Strengthen your diaphragm!

Chapter 7

Motility Disorders of the Esophagus

Esophageal Spasms

Esophageal spasms cause many people a lot of pain and often lead to symptoms including dysphagia, food regurgitation, GERD, and chest pain. Feeling of food "stuck" in the throat, and tachycardia can be present in someone suffering from these spasms.

The causes of most esophageal spasms are unknown. It has been linked to GERD, weakness of the LES, restrictive LES disorders, and magnesium deficiency. The diagnosis of esophageal spasms is usually made by either a barium test or endoscopy. I recommend that you get a transnasal esophagoscopy instead of an endoscopy.

On the Importance of Capsaicin and TRPV1 Activation in People Suffering from Esophageal Spasms

Your body has receptors for capsaicin (this is what makes spicy foods taste hot) in the digestive tract and on the skin. The receptor it is associated with is named TRPV1. TRPV1 is also the receptor that deals with the detection and regulation of body temperature, and it provides a sensation of heat and pain. The upregulation of the TRPV1 receptors is why you sweat, and your body temperature rises after consuming spicy food; this is also why capsaicin has been proven to dull pain receptors.

The endocannabinoid anandamide binds with TRPV 1 receptors, which may be why marijuana can help relieve pain. Tylenol also weakly binds to TRPV1 receptors, and this is why it can be used as a pain reliever.

Stimulation of TRPV1 also greatly reduces anxiety, increases hippocampal function, and restores memory. Simulating the receptor also might mediate long-term depression and PTSD. Stimulation of TRPV1 is why spicy foods and marijuana have been shown to elevate mood and eliminate both depression and PTSD.

Now to the vagus nerve problem at hand, and the reason that most people experience heart palpitations with upper digestive problems. CCK is an important peptide hormone that helps with digestion and feelings of satiety. When too much CCK is present, people will suffer from stomach, gallbladder, or pancreas disorders. Elevated amounts of CCK cause the nervous system to be constantly overstimulated while eating. When the nervous system is overstimulated, the vagus nerve will also become overactive causing anxiety, a poor functioning LES, and heart palpitations. Capsaicin inhibits the effects of overproduction of CCK and increases gastric emptying. The increase in gastric emptying might also be why people report feeling hungry one hour after eating a spicy meal!

Esophagus Spasms Protocol

- Follow GERD protocol (Ch. 4) if GERD is present.
- If GERD is not present, follow LERD protocol (Ch. 5) for at least three months.
- Follow SIBO protocol (Ch. 9) if SIBO is present.
- Follow LES protocol (Ch. 4). Increase elemental magnesium to at least 600 mg daily for three months.
- Follow average probiotic protocol (Ch. 13) for a month.
- Do not drink hot liquids or extremely cold liquids when eating a meal.
- Optional: Follow cayenne pepper protocol (Ch. 18).
- Optional: Ingest liquid peppermint oil to relax muscles. Non-enteric coated peppermint oil may cause heartburn.
- Black raspberry capsule or powder – follow the general supplement bottle recommendations.

Nutcracker Esophagus

Nutcracker esophagus is another esophagus motility disorder in which peristalsis in the esophagus does not function properly. Issues with peristalsis in the esophagus cause spasms, abnormal pain when swallowing, and even food obstruction. Most people suffering from nutcracker esophagus are asymptomatic.

Signs of someone suffering from nutcracker esophagus are non-cardiac related chest pain and dysphagia. Chest pain often occurs in people suffering from nutcracker esophagus even when they are not swallowing because of random esophagus spasms associated with the disorder. If food obstruction happens in the esophagus, it becomes a medical emergency, and surgery is needed to remove the obstruction. Nutcracker esophagus has been linked to GERD, nerve damage, increased pressure of the LES, and magnesium deficiency.

Nutcracker esophagus is diagnosed with esophageal motility study. The person swallows pressure instruments that determine peristalsis of the esophagus. An endoscopy is also helpful in diagnosing nutcracker esophagus.

Nutcracker Esophagus Protocol

- Follow the GERD protocol (Ch. 4) if GERD is present.
- If GERD is not present, follow the LERD protocol (Ch. 4) for at least three months.
- Follow the SIBO protocol (Ch. 9) if SIBO is present.
- Black raspberry capsule or powder – follow supplement recommendations on bottle
- Follow the LES protocol (Ch. 4). Increase elemental magnesium to at least 600 mg daily for three months.
- Follow the average probiotic protocol (Ch. 13) for a month.
- Do not drink hot liquids or extremely cold liquids when eating a meal.
- Optional: Follow cayenne pepper protocol (Ch. 18).
- Optional: Ingest liquid peppermint oil to relax muscles. This may cause heartburn.

Achalasia

Achalasia is a condition where the smooth muscle of the esophagus and the LES are compromised, and they cease to function properly. In some people with achalasia, the LES will not relax limiting food from entering the stomach properly. Peristalsis is also lacking, and people often have trouble swallowing.

The main symptoms of achalasia are difficulty swallowing, food regurgitation, and chest pain. Dysphagia will worsen over time. Food and liquid sometimes become aspirated. The tests completed confirming the diagnosis of achalasia are barium swallow tests, endoscopy, and esophageal manometry. I recommend that you get a transnasal esophagoscopy instead of an endoscopy. Achalasia has been linked to the failure of distal esophageal inhibitory neurons that regulate LES function.

An esophageal manometry is the most commonly used diagnostic test for achalasia. When someone gets a manometry, a tube is inserted into the nose, and into his or her esophagus to record swallowing with pressure instruments. Common findings are that the LES fails to relax upon swallowing, the pressure of the LES is greater than 100 mm Hg, and peristalsis is observed during the test.

Achalasia Protocol

- Eat slowly, chew food very well, and drink water with meals.
- Raise the head of your bed, or sleep with a wedge pillow.
- Follow the GERD protocol (Ch. 4) if GERD is present.
- Black raspberry capsule or powder – follow instructions on the bottle.
- If GERD is not present, follow the LERD protocol (Ch. 5) for at least three months.
- Follow the SIBO protocol (Ch. 9) if SIBO is present.
- Do not drink hot liquids or extremely cold liquids when eating a meal.

- Optional: Follow the cayenne pepper protocol (Ch. 18).
- Optional: Ingest liquid peppermint oil to relax esophagus muscles. This may cause heartburn.
- L-glutamine shake – 4,000 mg of L-glutamine with a scoop of grass-fed whey, twice daily with food (use with caution if you have a sensitivity to glutamic acid, deficiency in GABA, or severe leaky gut and brain).
- Jarrow R-lipoic acid – take one capsule, twice daily with meals.
- Enzymedica Digestive Enzyme Gold – take one capsule with each meal.
- Thorne Research B complex– take one capsule daily, do not use if you are an overmethylator.
- Pure Encapsulations zinc carnosine – take one capsule with a meal, twice daily.
- Do not wear tight clothing or tight belts. Tight clothing and belts increases pressure on the LES.
- Pure Encapsulations magnesium glycinate – 600 mg, take before bed.
- Melatonin Life Extension extended release – three mg, take before bed.

If all else fails:

- Jarrow 5-HTP – Follow the supplement recommendations on bottle. Only take for two weeks at most.
- Optional: Achnical supplementation.

Calcium citrate strengthens the LES on contact. R-lipoic acid has multiple benefits in the body but in this role, it works by preventing nerve damage to the LES while strengthening the vagus nerve.

Digestive enzymes break down the food in the stomach reducing gas and pressure on the LES.

The L-glutamine and grass-fed whey help rebuild the integrity of the gastrointestinal system and the LES.

Chapter 8

Disorders of the Abdominal Area

Abdominal Hernia

An abdominal hernia is a weakness of abdominal muscles or the abdominal connective tissues that may cause many health issues in those affected. An abdominal hernia is the most common hernia. Hernias either can be congenital (from birth) or acquired (from injury or disease).

The risk factors for developing an abdominal hernia include being a male, old age, and congenital abdominal weakness. Other risk factors include if you frequently lift very heavy objects, have had invasive abdominal surgery, chronic cough or vomiting, constipation, or a sports injury / general accident.

Symptoms of an abdominal hernia include protruding or bulging hard skin / muscle mass in the abdomen, pain or occasional numbness in the abdominal area (rare because most hernias are asymptomatic for quite some time, more likely for strangulated hernias). Obstructive hernias may cause nausea, vomiting, and fever if the herniated tissue blocks the functioning of the intestines.

Strangulated hernias and obstructive hernias are medical emergencies in some cases because of the potential loss of blood supply to specific areas or bowel obstruction.

Abdominal hernias are treated with surgical repair by mesh repair method, older tension repair method, tension free repair method, and the Shouldice repair method.

As someone with a hernia abdominal mesh repair performed more than ten years ago, I would recommend the Shouldice repair procedure if all possible.

Abdominal Hernia Repair Methods

Tension Repair

Tension repair was the first hernia surgery method to be developed in the late 1800's. During a tension repair, parts of the herniated tissue are pushed back in their proper place. Layers of the herniated tissue are then sutured or stapled together to the surrounding muscle tissue. The abdominal muscles are then slid over the hernia hole and are sewn together to reinforce the area without the use of any mesh. All materials used in a standard tension repair stay in the body and are not absorbed. These materials are left to put “tension” on the hernia to keep the tissue in place.

This form of repair can be more painful and require longer recovery time than the other procedures because of the permanent tension in the herniated area.

Mesh Repair

There are many different types of mesh repairs. During a standard mesh repair, plastic mesh is placed over or inside the herniated tissue to reinforce and patch the affected area. Most plastic meshes are made from polyethylene, polypropylene, polyester, or a mixture. A proper plastic mesh repair depends on scar tissue to grow into the mesh properly, forming a large layer of scar tissue to help reinforce the repair. The scar tissue will eventually shrink, and sometimes creates a mass of fibrous tissue compressed together with a plastic mesh that may cause many complications including strangulation and chronic pain. Most mesh repairs are laparoscopic surgeries.

During a laparoscopic hernia mesh repair, three small openings are made in the abdomen. The abdomen is then filled with carbon dioxide gas so that the surgeon can see the abdominal organs through different tiny cameras that display the images on the screen. Other medical instruments are inserted through the openings and are used to insert dissolvable staples / screws to anchor the mesh to the herniated tissue in the repair of the hernia. Most of the staples or screws dissolve in a few weeks, but the mesh always remains. Although a laparoscopic repair is described as a minimally invasive surgical procedure, it does require three incisions and deep surgical intervention that may cause significant scar tissue and tissue trauma.

Mesh repairs are associated with many additional complications compared to other repair procedures. If an infection or chronic pain develops, the plastic mesh in most cases has to be removed. Plastic mesh has also been associated with chronic inflammation because of a foreign object being embedded in the body. In some cases, the body rejects the mesh, which leads to severe pain, obstruction or strangulation, and other health issues.

Organic meshes developed from pigs are new and appear to have less medical issues. The organic meshes seem to reinforce the herniated tissue so that it can heal with less scar tissue. The mesh also either partially dissolves or fully dissolves. The organic meshes have not been out on the market yet for me to make a full recommendation, though.

Shouldice Repair

The Shouldice repair is performed in a specialized hospital in Canada. Specially trained surgeons also perform the surgery. During the Shouldice repair, herniated tissue is repaired by overlapping and reinforcing each affected muscle layer. The reinforced herniated tissue is then stapled together with absorbable sutures for a short-term tension repair.

During the procedure, they also search for hernias in the localized area and repair them, as well. This procedure is known for faster recovery times, lower instances of hernia recurrence, and less postoperative pain and complications. Surgical recovery occurs within a week.

I also recommend following my surgical recovery protocols (Ch. 9) after any hernia surgery.

Abdominal Hernia Surgery Recovery Protocol

For Two – Three Months:

- L-glutamine - 20,000 – 40,000 mg daily for one week after surgery. Then, take at least 10,000 mg daily for a month after surgery. Then, take 4,000 mg for the remainder of the protocol. Take with food (use with caution if you have a sensitivity to glutamic acid, deficiency in GABA, or severe leaky gut and brain).
- Florastor probiotic - follow supplement-boxed instructions; take while on an antibiotic. Do not use if you have yeast or histamine sensitivities.
- GOS – take one scoop daily mixed with filtered water. Use with caution if you have yeast overgrowth or Th2 elevated issues.
- Thorne Curcumin - follow the general supplement bottle recommendations.
- N-acetylglucosamine - follow the general supplement bottle recommendations. Do not use if you have yeast issues.
- Pure Encapsulations zinc carnosine – take one capsule with a meal, twice daily.
- SeaCure white fish protein supplement (do not use if you are allergic to fish) – follow the general supplement bottle recommendations.
- For three months: magnesium glycinate – take 600 mg, before bed.
- Follow a gluten-free / GMO-free diet.

L-glutamine is the most abundant amino acid and helps rebuild both the stomach lining and the gut.

Probiotics help protect the gut from opportunistic bacteria.

Curcumin is to increase immune cells in the gut and heal inflammation.

The body makes N-acetylglucosamine to increase mucus production in the stomach and gut and to make a protective barrier.

The zinc carnosine should help repair the stomach lining.

SeaCure might help your intestines recover from the surgery faster.

Chapter 9

Disorders of the Intestines

SIBO / SIYO / Leaky Gut Syndrome

SIBO is a medical condition where you have an opportunistic bacterial infection in the small intestine. SIBO is usually caused by a combination of the poor American diet and long-term use of acid-reducing medications. Long-term use of acid-reducing medications causes opportunistic bacteria that would normally be eliminated by stomach acid to survive and flourish in the small intestine. A lack of stomach acid causes food proteins to become partially undigested. Allergies develop from the undigested proteins. Undigested proteins also cause excessive flatulence and increase inflammation. The standard American diet of FODMAP carbohydrates allows opportunistic bacteria to thrive, infect the small intestine, and produce excess gas.

Bacteria also produce protective biofilms (one of the most common examples of a biofilm is the “film” on your teeth that appears when you do not brush your teeth after a while) which make eradication with antibiotics very difficult. The biofilm protects the opportunistic bacteria from antibiotic treatment, bactericides, and probiotics. To eliminate the opportunistic bacteria you also have to disrupt the biofilm that protects the bacteria. Biofilm disruption can occur by either breaking down the biofilm itself using systemic enzymes or by chelating the iron out of the biofilm to dissolve it. To chelate the iron you can use either calcium disodium EDTA, lactoferrin, or NAC.

The main symptoms of a SIBO infection are indigestion, a sharp increase or decrease in flatulence, constipation or diarrhea, reflux, and bloating. Most people with IBS are walking around with SIBO, and SIBO is their main cause of their digestive problems. Other symptoms of SIBO include abdominal pain, diarrhea, food allergies, and low-grade fever. There is also a big correlation between rosacea and SIBO. In one study, the majority of patients with rosacea were in remission or cured for at least nine months after taking Rifaximin. Rifaximin at the time was being used to treat their SIBO.

How to Diagnose SIBO

The hydrogen / methane breath test is used to diagnose if you have SIBO. You still have a large amount of bloating, gas, and stomach discomfort, but your breath test results were negative.

Is it possible still to have SIBO, if your breath test results were negative?

The hydrogen / methane breath test is a non-invasive fasting test in which your doctor has you breathe into a machine that monitors excess hydrogen or methane that is released by the opportunistic bacteria in your small intestine. You are given glucose, dextrose, or lactulose, during the test to consume, and the test input is collected at twenty-minute intervals for at least three – five hours. If you produce at least twenty ppm of hydrogen or three ppm of methane during the test, you test positive for an active SIBO infection (but even a result of twelve ppm hydrogen should be treated at the very minimum). If your hydrogen and methane are flat lined or do not rise during the test, you may have the third type of SIBO, hydrogen sulfide producing bacterial overgrowth.

It is debatable about which test is better, lactulose or glucose? Bacteria have to ferment lactulose in the intestines for it to be absorbed by the body. Glucose is easily broken down by the microbiome or directly absorbed by the gastrointestinal system. The use of glucose as a test marker may give a false negative reading because at least seventeen feet of the small intestine may not be tested. Finally, in people with IBS-D, the glucose might reach the cecum and begin fermentation sooner creating a false positive SIBO result in people with strictly colonic overgrowth.

There are some issues with the use of lactulose that might produce some false negatives. Not all bacteria / archaea that would cause an overgrowth ferment lactulose, which may cause a false negative test result. Lactulose increases bowel transit time, which may skew the test results. It might be best to get both tests done (glucose and lactulose) to determine bacterial overgrowth. Finally, it may be best to have a bowel transit test done as well, like a sitz marker test to determine one's motility and how long it would take the test substances to reach the colon.

People can still have symptoms of SIBO, and both tests come back negative. How can that be?

Again, not every overgrowth of bacteria in the gut will contain bacteria that produce hydrogen, so these tests could be inaccurate in determining SIBO. There is also no unified medical interpretation of SIBO breath tests, therefore, a doctor might perceive it to be normal and it is not. If your values do not rise during the test, you may have hydrogen sulfide producing bacterial overgrowth in the small intestine. I recommend using the guidelines of hydrogen / methane breath interpretation by the leading SIBO expert, Dr. Allison Siebecker.

I recommend getting a GI Effects performed by Genova Diagnostics through your gastroenterologist. I can help interpret the results of your bacterial culture, lactoferrin levels, pH, and antibody levels to determine if you have SIBO. Contact me for coaching if you are interested.

It is best to tackle your SIBO if you have many of the symptoms of SIBO instead of relying on breath test results. If you are not any better within a month of following the FODMAP diet and SIBO protocols, then SIBO was either not your problem in the first place (might be a yeast issue instead or SIYO), or the protocol was not strong enough to eliminate some hardy bacteria like *MAP* or *Klebsiella*. There is no public test for *MAP* currently (outside of specific testing at a university or hospital pathology laboratory), but *Klebsiella* can be tested for by using the GI Effects.

Are Opportunistic Bacteria One of The Main Causes of Leaky Gut?

Opportunistic bacteria in the small intestine can wreak havoc on your health and lead your intestinal health into a vicious cycle of destruction. The more opportunistic bacteria in your small intestine, the more food they consume, and the more gas byproducts and toxins they will produce. This cycle can lead to nutrient deficiencies in vitamin B12 and iron, which further leads you to develop anemia. The opportunistic bacteria also consume more nutrients that are now unabsorbed by the gut that leads to both an increased flora of opportunistic bacteria and gas production. From the blooming of opportunistic bacteria in the small intestine, you might start having abdominal bloating, diarrhea, pain, and excessive flatulence.

The opportunistic bacteria then begin to decrease fat absorption in the intestines that lead to stool problems with color / fat content. The decrease in fat absorption leads to deficiencies in the fat-soluble vitamins A and D. The intestinal lining further degrades and eventually cannot digest larger food particles correctly. These larger food particles start to cause food allergies and sensitivities (gluten first, then usually followed by fructose malabsorption and lactose digestion problems).

The opportunistic bacteria begin to enter the bloodstream from the loss of integrity in the intestinal wall. Opportunistic bacteria in the bloodstream lead to an immune overreaction that causes fatigue, systemic joint pain, and elevated liver enzymes. Finally, the bacteria start to excrete acids that cause neurological and cognitive problems including brain fog and memory problems. The vicious cycle continues as the body's immune system tries to eliminate the opportunistic bacteria, which when reduced poison the body with acids, toxins, and different opportunistic bacteria then continue to flourish. The vicious cycle then repeats itself, and you become chronically ill.

The Migrating Motor Complex and SIBO

Your digestive system eliminates waste through a process known as the migrating motor complex. The cycle of the peristalsis of the gut occurs every two hours. The MMC cycle includes four phases:

1. The first phase is a period of intestinal smooth muscle calmness lasting 45 to 60 minutes, which only rare action potentials and contractions occur.
2. The second phase is a period of roughly thirty minutes in which peristaltic contractions occur and progressively increase in frequency. Peristalsis originates in the stomach and propagates throughout the small intestine.
3. The third phase lasts 5 to 15 minutes and consists of rapid, evenly spaced peristaltic contractions. In contrast to the digestive period, the pylorus remains open during these peristaltic contractions, allowing many indigestible materials to pass into the small intestine.

4. The fourth and final phase is a short period of transition between the strong contractions that occur in the third phase and the inactivity that occurs in the first phase.

During the migrating motor complex increased gastric, biliary, and pancreatic secretion occurs to help further digestion and decrease bacterial buildup in the proximal segments of the digestive tract. It is believed that the MMC is controlled by the enteric hormone motilin. Ingestion of food overrides the MMC. Therefore, fasting has to occur regularly to help complete the process. The typical "growling" sounds you hear when you are hungry might be the MMC doing its job, cleaning your bowels of waste and excessive bacteria through increased peristalsis.

As much as 70% of people afflicted with SIBO experience a disruption of MMC rhythm. Excessive methane / hydrogen gasses produced by overgrowth of bacteria in the gut has been linked to decreased MMC function. When the second and third phase of the MMC is reduced, bacteria remain in the small intestine instead of being pushed back into the large intestine. Bacteria are then able to adhere and propagate in the small intestine, which increases inflammation and intestinal permeability. Inhibition of MMC homeostasis drives the vicious SIBO cycle.

Reduction of stomach acid by using acid reducing medications or *H. pylori* infection can contribute to poor MMC function. Lack of exercise, grazing, and constipation can contribute to poor MMC homeostasis. Being over-stressed and anxious can also decrease the MMC. Finally, low thyroid function and adrenal fatigue can lower MMC function.

Fasting for at least four hours after meals during SIBO protocols might be beneficial in regulating the MMC. The increase in fasting time gives your body longer time to complete the MMC process. MMC also occurs during sleep, which is why proper sleep may be more helpful than fasting because of the longer total fasting time that normally occurs during sleep. Frequent exercise also helps to regulate the MMC properly.

Does SIYO (Small Intestinal Yeast Overgrowth) Exist?

In some people, *Candida* overgrowth can manifest itself in the small intestine and cause similar symptoms as if the person is infected with SIBO. SIYO is a rare condition, but systemic yeast infection of the intestines can happen in some people. The same vicious cycle that exists with SIBO occurs in people with SIYO. The yeast in SIYO will rob nutrients from the body, reduce vitamin absorption and fat digestion (by eliminating probiotic bacteria), causing food allergies and sensitivities, as well as of the excretion of toxic byproducts (antibodies, and aldehydes) that destroy the immune system. Often joint pain and cognitive issues occur in addition to the digestive issues you may be facing.

Other yeasts besides *Candida* can cause SIYO; an example of this would be the probiotic yeast *Saccharomyces boulardii. Boulardii* is a great probiotic yeast and is very useful in helping relieve certain medical conditions. Caution should be used when supplementing if someone has a severely compromised immune system. If you are suffering from an opportunistic *Boulardii* infection or any other yeast infection, follow my candida protocols (Ch. 4) for relief.

The two tests that are used to diagnose SIYO are an alcohol challenge test and a Genova GI Effects. During the alcohol challenge test, you will ingest a lot of sugar that feeds the yeast and then a blood measurement is taken to determine how much alcohol is produced from the fermentation. A stool sample test will test the stool for any excessive amounts of yeast colonies and antibodies that are cultured from a provided sample. If you read about a "spit" test online, it is unreliable and should not be used.

If someone is suffering from SIYO, then the person should try any of my *Candida* protocols. After completion of the protocol, they should rebuild their gut for a month.

Restore Proper MMC Function Protocol

SIBO-C:

- Wait at least four hours in between meals before eating another meal. No snacking!
- Exercise more and walk as much as possible.
- Use a squatty potty when you defecate.
- Supplement with triphala – one capsule, twice daily with food.
- Magnesium malate – supplement 200 mg per 50 pounds of body weight.

SIBO-D:

- Include ECPO as one of your antimicrobial agents.
- New Chapter Ginger Force – one softgel, twice daily with meals.
- Wait at least four hours in between meals before eating another meal. No snacking!
- Exercise more and walk as much as possible.
- Use a squatty potty when you defecate.
- Take Upgraded™ Activated Charcoal, two capsules two hours after every meal.
- Magnesium glycinate – supplement 200 mg per 50 pounds of body weight.

If you have low stomach acid:

- Follow Betaine HCL protocol (Ch. 12).

- Urban Moonshine Digestive Bitters – follow the general supplement instructions, do not use if you have histamine intolerance, ulcers, or gastritis.

If suffering from SIYO:

- Thorne Research molybdenum glycinate – one capsule every other day with meals.
- Pure Coenzyme A – follow the general supplement instructions.

General SIBO MMC Advice:

- Consider talking to your gastroenterologist about the use of erythromycin (fifty mg nightly) if your SIBO does not approve in a few months.
- Ginger, fasting between meals, exercising, using a squatty potty, magnesium, increasing stomach acid, and the use of the medications have been shown to help properly regulate the MMC.
- Aldehydes have been shown to interfere with the MMC and molybdenum can help your body detoxify them.
- SIYO reduces coenzyme A production which interferes with the MMC.
- ECPO helps to calm the MMC and can help reduce diarrhea by reducing intestinal spasms.

Mild SIBO-C Protocol

For two to four weeks:

Choose one strong antimicrobial agent:

- Colloidal silver (Mesosilver, Sovereign Silver) – follow supplement bottle recommendations.
- Thorne Research Berberine – take 500 mg, two capsules daily. Use with caution if you have ulcers, gastritis, or hypoglycemia.
- Allicin-C – follow supplement bottle recommendations.
- Neem – take two capsules two times daily with meals.
- Atrantil – follow supplement bottle recommendations.

Anti-BioFilm Protocol:

- PREFERRED: Symbiotics lactoferrin - follow supplement bottle recommendations (can increase up to two grams daily if needed).

OR CHOOSE ONE OF THE FOLLOWING FROM ANTI-BIOFILM AGENTS INSTEAD OF TAKING LACTOFERRIN

- **Calcium Disodium EDTA:** MRM Cardio Chelate – follow general supplement recommendations.
- **Fulvic Acid:** Food Grade fulvic acid – follow general supplement recommendations.
- **Guaifenesin:** Guai-aid – take one capsule every four to eight hours. Do not exceed four capsules daily. Guaifenesin is a systemic biofilm chelator; I do not recommend it as a first-line anti-biofilm agent in a protocol.
- **NAC:** Jarrow Formulas NAC Sustain – one tablet twice daily. NAC is a systemic biofilm chelator; I do not recommend it as a first-line anti-biofilm agent in a protocol. Do not supplement more than 1,200 mg daily, doses above this recommendation may make the NAC you take become a pro-oxidant.
- **Systemic Enzymes:** Interphase Plus, PRX Enzyme Formula, Neprinol AMD – follow general supplement recommendations.

Other protocol advice:

- Extra virgin coconut oil – consume two tablespoons daily.
- Reduce polyols and go on a gluten-free diet. For symptom relief consider a low-FODMAP diet.
- Galactomune – one scoop daily mixed well with filtered water at breakfast. Use with caution if you have yeast overgrowth or Th2 elevated issues.

Calcium disodium EDTA chelates iron out of the biofilm to break it up and pull it away from pathogenic bacteria.

The NAC or lactoferrin will do the same thing as the EDTA by chelating the iron out of the biofilm.

Coconut oil is used to reduce yeast overgrowth in the colon and inhibit archea overgrowth.

Moderate SIBO-C Protocol

For two to four weeks:

Choose two strong antimicrobial agents:

- Colloidal silver (Mesosilver, Sovereign Silver) – follow supplement bottle recommendations.
- Thorne Research Berberine – take 500 mg, two capsules daily. Use with caution if you have ulcers, gastritis, or hypoglycemia.
- Allicin-C – follow supplement bottle recommendations.
- Neem – take two capsules two times daily with meals.
- Atrantil – follow supplement bottle recommendations.
- Zane Hellas Oil of Oregano – follow supplement recommendations. Oil of oregano is a broad spectrum, systemic antimicrobial agent, do not use first in a protocol.

Anti-BioFilm Protocol:

- PREFERRED: Symbiotics lactoferrin - follow supplement bottle recommendations (can increase up to two grams daily if needed).

AND CHOOSE ONE OF THE FOLLOWING ADDITIONAL ANTI-BIOFILM AGENTS

- **Calcium Disodium EDTA:** MRM Cardio Chelate – follow general supplement recommendations.
- **Fulvic Acid:** Food Grade fulvic acid – follow general supplement recommendations.
- **Guaifenesin:** Guai-aid – take one capsule every four to eight hours. Do not exceed four capsules daily. Guaifenesin is a systemic biofilm chelator; I do not recommend it as a first-line anti-biofilm agent in a protocol.
- **NAC:** Jarrow Formulas NAC Sustain – one tablet twice daily. NAC is a systemic biofilm chelator; I do not recommend it as a first-line anti-biofilm agent in a protocol. Do not supplement more than 1,200 mg daily, doses above this recommendation may make the NAC you take become a pro-oxidant.
- **Systemic Enzymes:** Interphase Plus, PRX Enzyme Formula, Neprinol AMD – follow general supplement recommendations.

Other protocol advice:

- Extra virgin coconut oil – consume two tablespoons daily.
- Reduce polyols and go on a gluten-free diet. For symptom relief consider a low-FODMAP diet.
- Galactomune – One scoop daily mixed well with filtered water at breakfast. Use with caution if you have yeast overgrowth or Th2 elevated issues.

Calcium disodium EDTA chelates iron out of the biofilm to break it up and pull it away from pathogenic bacteria.

The NAC or lactoferrin will do the same thing as the EDTA by chelating the iron out of the biofilm.

Coconut oil is used to reduce or inhibit yeast overgrowth in the colon and reduce archea overgrowth.

Oil of oregano reduces archaea overgrowth.

Severe SIBO-C Protocol

For four weeks:

Choose three strong antimicrobial agents:

- Colloidal silver (Mesosilver, Sovereign Silver) – follow bottle supplement recommendations.
- Thorne Research Berberine – take 500 mg, two capsules daily. Use with caution if you have ulcers, gastritis, or hypoglycemia.
- Allicin-C – follow supplement bottle recommendations.
- Neem – take two capsules two times daily with meals.
- Atrantil – follow supplement bottle recommendations.
- Zane Hellas Oil of Oregano – follow supplement recommendations. Oil of oregano is a broad spectrum, systemic antimicrobial agent, do not use first in a protocol.

Anti-BioFilm Protocol:

- PREFERRED: Symbiotics lactoferrin - follow supplement bottle recommendations (can increase up to two grams daily if needed).

AND CHOOSE ONE OF THE FOLLOWING ADDITIONAL ANTI-BIOFILM AGENTS

- **Calcium Disodium EDTA:** MRM Cardio Chelate – follow general supplement recommendations.
- **Fulvic Acid:** Food Grade fulvic acid – follow general supplement recommendations.
- **Guaifenesin:** Guai-aid – take one capsule every four to eight hours. Do not exceed four capsules daily. Guaifenesin is a systemic biofilm chelator, I do not recommend it as a first-line anti-biofilm agent in a protocol.
- **NAC:** Jarrow Formulas NAC Sustain – one tablet twice daily. NAC is a systemic biofilm chelator; I do not recommend it as a first-line anti-biofilm agent in a protocol. Do not supplement more than 1,200 mg daily, doses above this recommendation may make the NAC you take become a pro-oxidant.
- **Systemic Enzymes:** Interphase Plus, PRX Enzyme Formula, Neprinol AMD – follow general supplement recommendations.

Other protocol advice:

- Extra virgin coconut oil – consume two tablespoons daily.
- Reduce polyols and go on a gluten-free diet. For symptom relief consider a low-FODMAP diet.
- Galactomune – one scoop daily mixed well with filtered water at breakfast. Use with caution if you have yeast overgrowth or Th2 elevated issues.
- 5-HTP supplement – start with 50 mg nightly and increase by 50 mg up to a max of 300 mg nightly depending on an improvement of motility. Do not use if you are on any medication that modulates serotonin levels (SSRI for example) or if you suffer from any mental health issues. Discontinue if you have any side effects and do not take longer than a few weeks.

Calcium disodium EDTA chelates iron out of the biofilm to break it up and pull it away from pathogenic bacteria.

The NAC or lactoferrin will do the same thing as the EDTA by chelating the iron out of the biofilm.

Coconut oil is used to reduce or inhibit yeast overgrowth in the colon and reduce archea overgrowth.

Oil of oregano reduces archaea overgrowth.

Mild SIBO-D Protocol

For two to four weeks:

Antibacterial

- PREFERRED: Nature's Way enteric coated peppermint oil - thirty to sixty minutes before meals, twice daily.

OR CHOOSE ONE OF THE FOLLOWING ANTIBACTERIAL AGENTS FROM THIS LIST

Choose one strong antimicrobial agent:

- Colloidal silver (Mesosilver, Sovereign Silver) – follow supplement bottle recommendations.
- Thorne Research Berberine – take 500 mg, two capsules daily. Use with caution if you have ulcers, gastritis, or hypoglycemia.
- Ceylon cinnamon oil – take one drop in one tsp. of extra virgin coconut oil or extra virgin olive oil, twice daily. Use with caution if you have hypoglycemia.

Anti-BioFilm Protocol:

- PREFERRED: Symbiotics lactoferrin - follow supplement bottle recommendations (can increase up to two grams daily if needed).

OR CHOOSE ONE OF THE FOLLOWING FROM ANTI-BIOFILM AGENTS INSTEAD OF TAKING LACTOFERRIN

- **Calcium Disodium EDTA:** MRM Cardio Chelate – follow general supplement recommendations.
- **Fulvic Acid:** Food Grade fulvic acid – follow general supplement recommendations.
- **Guaifenesin:** Guai-aid – take one capsule every four to eight hours. Do not exceed four capsules daily. Guaifenesin is a systemic biofilm chelator; I do not recommend it as a first-line anti-biofilm agent in a protocol.
- **NAC:** Jarrow Formulas NAC Sustain – one tablet twice daily. NAC is a systemic biofilm chelator; I do not recommend it as a first-line anti-biofilm agent in a protocol. Do not supplement more than 1,200 mg daily, doses above this recommendation may make the NAC you take become a pro-oxidant.

- **Systemic Enzymes:** Interphase Plus, PRX Enzyme Formula, Neprinol AMD – follow general supplement recommendations.

Other Protocol Advice:

- Extra virgin coconut oil – consume two tablespoons daily.
- Reduce polyols and go on a gluten-free diet. For symptom relief consider a low-FODMAP diet.
- Galactomune – one scoop daily mixed well with filtered water at breakfast. Use with caution if you have yeast overgrowth or Th2 elevated issues.

Calcium disodium EDTA chelates iron out of the biofilm to break it up and pull it away from pathogenic bacteria.

The NAC or lactoferrin will do the same thing as the EDTA by chelating the iron out of the biofilm.

Coconut oil is used to reduce or inhibit yeast overgrowth in the colon.

Moderate SIBO-D Protocol

For two to four weeks:

Antibacterial

- PREFERRED: Nature's Way enteric coated peppermint oil - thirty to sixty minutes before meals, twice daily.

OR CHOOSE TWO OF THE FOLLOWING ANTIBACTERIAL AGENTS FROM THIS LIST

Choose two strong antimicrobial agents:

- Colloidal silver (Mesosilver, Sovereign Silver) – follow supplement bottle recommendations.
- Zane Hellas Oil of Oregano – follow supplement recommendations. Oil of oregano is a broad spectrum, systemic antimicrobial agent, do not use first in a protocol.

- Thorne Research Berberine – take 500 mg, two capsules daily. Use with caution if you have ulcers, gastritis, or hypoglycemia.
- Ceylon cinnamon oil – take one drop in one tsp. of extra virgin coconut oil or extra virgin olive oil, twice daily. Use with caution if you have hypoglycemia.

Anti-BioFilm Protocol:

- PREFERRED: Symbiotics lactoferrin - follow supplement bottle recommendations (can increase up to two grams daily if needed).

AND CHOOSE ONE OF THE FOLLOWING FROM ANTI-BIOFILM AGENTS

- **Calcium Disodium EDTA:** MRM Cardio Chelate – follow general supplement recommendations.
- **Fulvic Acid:** Food Grade fulvic acid – follow general supplement recommendations.
- **Guaifenesin:** Guai-aid – take one capsule every four to eight hours. Do not exceed four capsules daily. Guaifenesin is a systemic biofilm chelator; I do not recommend it as a first-line anti-biofilm agent in a protocol.
- **NAC:** Jarrow Formulas NAC Sustain – one tablet twice daily. NAC is a systemic biofilm chelator; I do not recommend it as a first-line anti-biofilm agent in a protocol. Do not supplement more than 1,200 mg daily, doses above this recommendation may make the NAC you take become a pro-oxidant.
- **Systemic Enzymes:** Interphase Plus, PRX Enzyme Formula, Neprinol AMD – follow general supplement recommendations.

Other protocol advice:

- Extra virgin coconut oil – consume two tablespoons daily.
- Reduce polyols and go on a gluten-free diet. For symptom relief consider a low-FODMAP diet.
- Galactomune – one scoop daily mixed well with filtered water at breakfast. Use with caution if you have yeast overgrowth or Th2 elevated issues.

Calcium disodium EDTA chelates iron out of the biofilm to break it up and pull it away from pathogenic bacteria.

The NAC or lactoferrin will do the same thing as the EDTA by chelating the iron out of the biofilm.

Coconut oil is used to reduce or inhibit yeast overgrowth in the colon.

Severe SIBO-D Protocol

- Rifaximin – an antibiotic that only stays in the gut and is poorly absorbed.

OTHER ANTIBIOTICS THAT CAN BE USED OR ROTATED IF NEEDED:

- Tetracycline / Doxycycline – broad-spectrum antibiotic, follow moderate *Candida* protocol (Ch. 4) while on antibiotic to reduce the chance of developing *Candida* overgrowth.
- Cephalosporin – second generation or newer.
- Amoxicillin with Clavulanic Acid – use with caution in SIBO-C.

I recommend that if you use any other antibiotic than Rifaximin, you combine natural antimicrobial agents with the antibiotics to help increase efficiency. If you have SIBO-D, I recommend the use of ECPO, silver, and cinnamon.

Anti-BioFilm Protocol:

- PREFERRED: Symbiotics lactoferrin – follow supplement bottle recommendations (can increase up to two grams daily if needed).

AND CHOOSE TWO OF THE FOLLOWING ANTI-BIOFILM AGENTS

- **Calcium Disodium EDTA:** MRM Cardio Chelate – follow general supplement recommendations.
- **Fulvic Acid:** Food grade fulvic acid – follow general supplement recommendations.
- **Guaifenesin:** Guai-aid – take one capsule every four to eight hours. Do not exceed four capsules daily. Guaifenesin is a systemic biofilm chelator; I do not recommend it as a first-line anti-biofilm agent in a protocol.
- **NAC:** Jarrow Formulas NAC Sustain – one tablet twice daily. NAC is a systemic biofilm chelator; I do not recommend it as a first-line anti-biofilm agent in a protocol. Do not supplement more than 1,200 mg daily, doses above this recommendation may make the NAC you take become a pro-oxidant.
- **Systemic Enzymes:** Interphase Plus, PRX Enzyme Formula, Neprinol AMD – follow general supplement recommendations.

Other protocol advice:

- Extra virgin coconut oil – consume two tablespoons daily.
- Reduce polyols and go on a gluten-free diet. For symptom relief consider a low-FODMAP diet.
- Galactomune – one scoop daily mixed well with water at breakfast. Use with caution if you have yeast overgrowth or Th2 elevated issues.

Cycling of Antibacterial Agents and Anti-Biofilm Agents

If your SIBO symptoms do not get any better after one month of following any of the protocols above, or you fail your second breath test or your stool sample still shows overgrowth, you need to switch your antibacterial / anti-biofilm agents with ones that you have yet to use in the above protocols. Certain bacteria have different resistances and weaknesses to certain agents, so you might need to cycle agents to achieve better results.

You also might need to obtain prescriptions for antibiotics that are discussed in the Severe SIBO Protocol to complete your regimen. Always, let your doctor know what are you are taking to help overcome your SIBO.

For example, if you used ECPO and silver combined with lactoferrin and NAC to tackle your SIBO issues and saw no improvement, then you might want to switch to Allicin-C and berberine combined with systemic enzymes and guaifenesin.

If you show no overgrowth on a GI Effects stool test, and you pass a lactulose and glucose breath test after two months of the regimens and still have symptoms of SIBO, then you more than likely have other issues like possible yeast overgrowth or gallbladder issues.

Supplements to Reduce a Bacterial Herx Reaction

- Jarrow milk thistle – follow the general supplement bottle recommendations.
- Upgraded™ Activated Charcoal – follow the supplement bottle recommendations and do not take more than twelve capsules daily.
- L-glutamine - take 4,000 mg, daily with food (use with caution if you have a sensitivity to glutamic acid, deficiency in GABA, or severe leaky gut and brain).
- Take daily Epsom salt baths and maintain proper hydration to reduce toxins.

- Ingest a raw carrot salad to help reduce estrogen and endotoxin build up in the gut. Grate one raw organic carrot, and mix with one tablespoon of extra virgin olive oil, one tablespoon of extra virgin coconut oil, and one tsp of apple cider vinegar. Use with caution if you have histamine or fat malabsorption issues.

Supplements to Alleviate Brain Fog (Concentration and Memory Issues):

- Oxaloacetate – follow supplement bottle recommendations, use if you are suffering from brain fog.
- Pinella – follow the supplement bottle recommendations. Use Pinella if you are suffering from brain fog. There is alcohol in the tincture so use with caution if you are sensitive to it.

Supplements to Alleviate Th1 Inflammation and Pain (Gram-negative non histamine producing bacterial infections):

- Black cumin seed oil – one tablespoon with a meal. Use with caution if you have gastritis.
- Boswellia – follow supplement bottle recommendations.
- Thorne Curcumin – follow supplement bottle recommendations.
- Olive leaf extract - follow supplement bottle recommendations.

The milk thistle helps detoxify the liver.

Oxaloacetate has been shown to reduce brain fog symptoms and neural inflammation from endotoxin exposure.

Pinella has been shown to reduce brain fog symptoms and neural inflammation from endotoxin exposure.

Charcoal helps bind bacterial endotoxins.

The L-glutamine helps repair the intestinal healing.

Epsom salt baths help break down and eliminate toxins.

Black cumin seed oil, curcumin, boswellia, and olive leaf extract reduce Th1 inflammation.

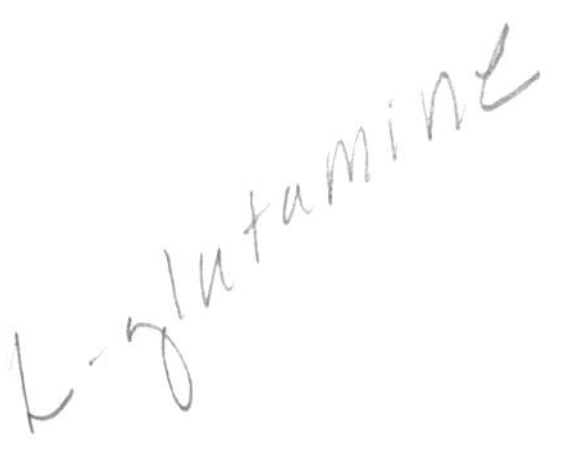

Rebuilding the Gut

Basic Protocol

This protocol should be used for most people unless otherwise indicated.

For a month:

- Jarrow L-glutamine – 8,000 mg, take in divided doses, three times daily on with food (use with caution if you have a sensitivity to glutamic acid, deficiency in GABA, or severe leaky gut and brain).
- Galactomune – one scoop daily mixed well with water at breakfast.
- Thorne Curcumin – follow the general supplement bottle recommendations.
- N-acetylglucosamine (do not use if allergic to shellfish or have yeast overgrowth) – follow the general supplement bottle recommendations.

For three months:

- Magnesium glycinate – 600 mg, taken before bed daily.

L-glutamine is the most abundant amino acid in the body and helps rebuild both the stomach lining and the gut.

The use of GOS will help regulate motility and improve probiotic bacteria colonization.

The curcumin is used to increase immune cells in the gut and heal inflammation.

The body makes n-acetylglucosamine to increase mucus production in the stomach and gut and to make a protective barrier.

Severe Protocol

For a month:

- Jarrow L-glutamine – 20,000 mg total. Take in three divided doses each day with food. Reduce by 5,000 mg each week until completion (use with caution if you have a sensitivity to glutamic acid, deficiency in GABA, or severe leaky gut and brain).
- Galactomune – one scoop daily mixed well with water at breakfast.
- Thorne Curcumin – follow the general supplement bottle recommendations.
- N-acetylglucosamine (do not use if allergic to shellfish or have yeast overgrowth) – follow the general supplement bottle recommendations.
- SeaCure white fish protein supplement (do not use if you are allergic to fish) – follow the general supplement bottle recommendations.

For three months:

- Magnesium glycinate – take 600 mg, taken before bed.

The increase in L-glutamine is to help the intestine heal faster.

The Seacure supplement is very high in amino acids that help heal the gut lining.

Stool Changes and Indications to Your Health

The color, shape, and smell of your stool can tell a lot about your digestive health and even the total health of your body. It is important for everyone to observe and make a note of these aspects of their stool health on a frequent basis. Everyone should do this every time you defecate if you have a chronic disease that can affect your digestion. Sometimes any of the following aspects of someone's stool being abnormal may indicate they have a severe health crisis occurring.

Stool Color

Mid to Dark Brown

A mid to dark brown is considered a normal healthy stool color. The reason for the brown color of the stool is the presence of bile in the stool. If the stool has a proper transit time in the intestines, then the stool should always be this color.

Black Tarry, Sticky Stools (Melena)

If you have black stools, then you may either have bleeding in the upper intestinal tract or stomach. Melena is usually a sign of a peptic or duodenal ulcer. The black color of the stools is caused by the oxidation of the iron in the hemoglobin of the blood in the stools. The oxidation of iron occurs during the stool passage through the ileum and colon until it is expelled out of the body. If the bleeding takes longer than fourteen hours to pass through the intestinal tract, it becomes dark.

If you are suffering from melena, then a diagnosis needs to be made by a qualified health professional to find the source of bleeding. Melena could also be caused by an overdose of anti-coagulant medications.

Less common causes of melena are the ingestion of bismuth subsalicylate, severe nose bleed, iron supplementation, consuming of dark foods (like black licorice), and blood ingested from the eating of certain foods (blood sausage).

Finally, melena caused by blood loss usually smells much worse than normal bowel movements. If the melena is not caused by blood loss, your feces should be a lot less sticky and should smell normal.

Red Stool Color (Hematochezia)

If you have a bright red stool, it is usually a sign of bleeding in the lower digestive tract or anus. The usual causes of hematochezia are hemorrhoids, straining while defecating, diverticulosis, IBD, and rarely colorectal cancer. Hematochezia can also be caused by ingestion of beets, which is a benign condition known as beeturia. Finally, red food dye can also turn stools bright red, so be aware of this if you have ingested anything containing it lately.

If hematochezia occurs a few times after you use the bathroom, constipation is the cause of the bleeding. If it frequently occurs, you might need to be medically evaluated.

Gray or Clay Colored Stool

Gray stools contain little or no bile. The pale color of the stool signifies biliary obstruction of the gallbladder or pancreas. It is usually a sign of obstruction of the bile duct from the gallbladder to the pancreas. This obstruction could be caused by something like a gallstone or even a tumor. In addition, antacids that contain aluminum hydroxide have been known to cause gray colored stool if frequently ingested.

The change from a normally colored stool to a gray colored stool is a slow process, and the stool will become pale over time. If you are passing a gray colored stool frequently, your gallbladder and pancreas need to be checked to see what is causing this reaction.

Yellow Stool

If your stool is yellow, it suggests that there is undigested fat in the stool. There are many possible causes of this including acute or chronic pancreatitis, obstruction of the pancreatic duct, GERD, diarrhea, lack of digestive enzymes, liver disease, and a gallbladder defect. If you have yellowing eyes or skin and stomach pain, yellow stools might indicate liver disease.

Yellow stool can also be a sign that fecal matter is passing through the digestive tract too quickly. Fecal matter moving too fast through the intestines can be caused by GERD, diarrhea, SIBO, or an infection of the intestines. Yellow stools usually appear greasy, smell horrible, and float in the toilet.

Green Stool

Green stool is usually either caused by diarrhea, pigment from ingesting food dye, or from ingesting green leafy vegetables. Iron supplements are also known to cause greenly colored stools.

Orange Stool

Most of the time an orange colored stool is caused by either ingestion of food that is high in beta-carotene or the medication, aluminum hydroxide. Orange stools rarely may be a symptom of the stool not absorbing bile salts. Diarrhea, gallbladder issues, gallstones, pancreatic issues, or liver issues can cause orange stools.

Stool Shape

The Bristol stool chart is accurate about the differences in stool shape and its relation to colon health. Stool type one and two are characteristic of someone suffering from constipation. On the other hand, stool type six and seven are characteristic of someone suffering from diarrhea. The best stool types to have are three-five with four being the best.

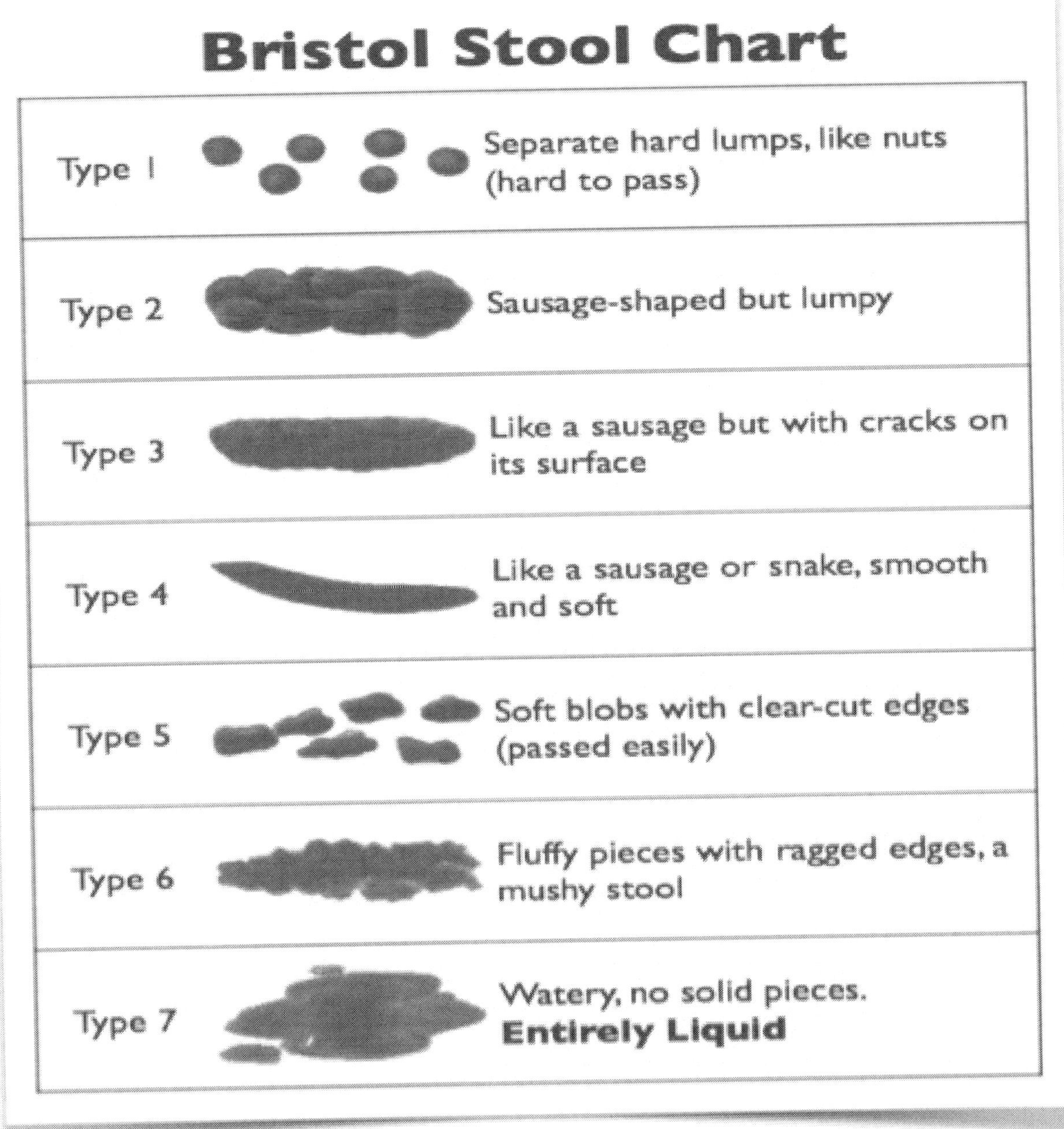

Stool Smell

Yes, it is perfectly normal for your stool to smell bad. However, if the smell of your stool is extremely rancid, then you might be suffering from a severe intestinal infection, *C. difficile*. If your stool smells like rotten eggs, you may be suffering from hydrogen sulfide overgrowth. In addition, if your stool smells like metal you might need to be evaluated for bleeding disorders.

Irritable Bowel Syndrome

The number of people diagnosed with IBS in the United States is greatly increasing every year. Recent statistics indicate that fifteen percent of the American population suffers from IBS, but much more go undiagnosed. Half of the Mexican population suffers from IBS, as well. IBS is also diagnosed three times more often in women than in men. There currently is not one known main conventional cause of IBS, and the number of cases is predicted to double in about twenty years.

There is evidence that IBS could be caused by bacterial, protozoan, or parasite infection. Get a Comprehensive Stool Analysis and parasite test from your doctor if you have IBS. I would also suggest getting an allergy test, SIBO test, and a HIDA scan (for gallbladder) to rule out these conditions with shared symptoms.

IBS symptoms include constipation, diarrhea, rosacea, bloating, gas, and abdominal pain. Proposed causes of IBS are either SIBO, yeast overgrowth, mass consumption of GMO's, stress, or hypothyroid / adrenal fatigue. Since IBS consists of a combination of leaky gut syndrome and SIBO, it can easily mimic different diseases. Celiac disease, fructose and lactose intolerance, inflammatory bowel diseases, and bile acid malabsorption (follow the bile acid malabsorption protocol (Ch. 4) if this is one of the symptoms) can all stem from IBS.

Following my protocols for SIBO and yeast (Ch. 9) should help most people reduce their IBS symptoms. Rosacea has been linked to both SIBO and IBS as a symptom in some scientific studies. IBS-D is strongly correlated with SIBO, where IBS-C may not occur from bacterial overgrowth.

Herbal IBS Protocol

- Iberogast – follow the general supplement bottle recommendations.
- Thorne Curcumin – follow the general supplement bottle recommendations.
- George's Always Active aloe vera – follow the general supplement bottle recommendations.

If You Are Constipated:

- Chia seeds – follow the recommended instructions.

- Uni-Fiber – follow the general supplement bottle recommendations
- Follow the cayenne pepper protocol (Ch. 18).
- Gaia natural laxative tea - follow the recommended boxed instructions for the consumption of the tea, rarely use.
- Stay hydrated.

If You Have Diarrhea:

- Upgraded™ Activated Charcoal – follow the general supplement bottle recommendations.
- Uni-Fiber – follow the recommended instructions.
- Rainforest Pharmacy sangre de drago – follow the general supplement bottle recommendations.

Iberogast can also be used to help with IBS. It contains peppermint oil, licorice and milk thistle, which help the most in the tincture. The peppermint oil eliminates opportunistic bacteria; the licorice is an anti-inflammatory, and the milk thistle cleanses the liver. Aloe vera soothes and protects the stomach and digestive tract.

Curcumin is used for proper bowel regularity and to reduce inflammation.

The laxative tea has senna, which is known as a stimulant laxative.

The Sangre De Drago has been clinically proven to help stop diarrhea.

The activated charcoal is used to bulk up the stools and to limit diarrhea.

Basic Stress / Adrenal Health Protocol

These protocols reduce stress and adrenal fatigue in the body. Stress causes the colon to spasm frequently. Try to get at least eight hours of sleep every night and try to be in bed before 10:00 p.m.

Male:

- Sodium ascorbate – take 2,000 mg, twice daily.
- Thorne Research B complex– take one capsule daily, do not use if you are an overmethylator.
- Magnesium glycinate – 400 mg, before bed.
- Drink a glass of warm distilled water with 1/8 tsp. sea salt upon waking.

Choose one of the three herbs:

- Life Extension ashwagandha extract (or any other ashwagandha containing the sensoril extract) - follow the supplement recommendations.
- Gaia Herbs holy basil – follow the supplement recommendations and take with a meal to prevent hypoglycemia.
- Rhodiola extract – follow the supplement recommendations.

The vitamin C and B5 are used to increase adrenal function and hormones.

The magnesium glycinate is to relax the body at night.

The herbs are to lower cortisol and to increase adrenal function.

The salt water is to regulate aldosterone levels upon waking to help the adrenal glands.

Female:

- Sodium ascorbate – take 2,000 mg, twice daily.
- Thorne Research B complex – once daily, do not use if you are an overmethylator.
- Magnesium glycinate – 400 mg, before bed.
- Drink a glass of warm water with 1/8 tsp. sea salt upon waking.
- Source Naturals Relora complex – follow the supplement recommendations.

In females, the magnolia bark in relora is recommended as the herb to use. This is because there are specific studies that show promotion and regulation of adrenal hormones in women. If a woman is allergic to relora, she may instead use any of the herbs recommended for men.

Constipation

Constipation causes multiple problems in the body and manifests itself in different ways. Constipation causes toxins to build up in the body from a lack of transit time in the body. The body tends to absorb toxins from slow moving waste in the colon. Slow moving waste also ferments longer and causes a greater growth of bacteria, gas, and heartburn by causing slow gastric emptying, excessive abdominal pressure, and bloating in the abdomen.

The main causes of constipation are a lack of magnesium, dehydration, lack of fiber, prescription drugs that cause constipation (opiates are a prime example), hypothyroidism, adrenal fatigue, and lack of exercise.

General Constipation Protocol

- Magnesium malate – 600 mg, daily.
- Stay hydrated - drink clean water with 1/4 tsp. of good quality sea salt or real salt in a glass of water once a day.
- Walk for at least thirty minutes a day.
- Drink a teaspoon of chia seeds soaked in water over the course of thirty minutes.
- Uni-Fiber – one tablespoon up to three times daily.
- Eat two green bananas daily.
- Follow stress and adrenal protocols (Ch. 9).
- Sodium ascorbate – take 2,000 mg, twice daily.
- Use a squatty potty when you defecate to retrain your body to squat when you use the toilet.
- Rarely: Gaia natural laxative tea - follow the recommended instructions.

Magnesium and vitamin C are osmotic laxatives. Make sure you drink water, so you do not become dehydrated.

Basic IBS Protocol for Constipation

- Magnesium malate – take 300 mg, twice daily with meals.
- Enzymedica Digestive Enzyme Gold – take one or two capsules with each meal
- Bulletproof® or Perfect Health® Diet.
- Jarrow L-glutamine – take 6,000 – 8,000 mg daily with food (use with caution if you have a sensitivity to glutamic acid, deficiency in GABA, or severe leaky gut and brain).
- Follow the average probiotic protocol (Ch. 13) for two to four weeks.
- Thorne Curcumin – follow the general supplement bottle recommendations.
- N-acetylglucosamine – follow the general supplement bottle recommendations (use with caution if you are suffering from yeast overgrowth).
- Drink a teaspoon of chia seeds soaked in water over the course of thirty minutes.

Other supplements used in protocol:

- Rarely: Gaia natural laxative tea - follow the recommended package instructions to consume the tea.

This protocol combines the SIBO protocol with the constipation protocol to relieve both constipation and the symptoms of IBS. This protocol should be taken for at least three months and then tentatively afterward if constipation symptoms return.

Diarrhea

Diarrhea is a medical condition in which someone has three or more loose bowel movements in a twenty-four hour period. The primary medical issues that develop when someone has diarrhea are electrolyte imbalance, dehydration, and malabsorption of nutrients. About thirty percent of people with IBS-D have bile acid malabsorption, so following the bile acid malabsorption protocol (Ch. 4) might be beneficial.

IBS-D is strongly correlated with SIBO. An overgrowth of bacteria produces excessive amounts of toxins, which irritate the TRPV-1 receptors in the bowels, which cause loose stools. Activation of TRPV-1 receptors also occurs during food poisoning or foodborne infections. Antidiarrheal supplements and medications should not be used if you have food poisoning unless needed because they can prolong your condition.

Basic IBS Protocol for Diarrhea

- Magnesium glycinate – take 400 mg, before bed.
- Enzymedica Digestive Enzyme Gold – one to two capsules with every meal
- Bulletproof® or Perfect Health® Diet.
- Jarrow L-glutamine - take 6,000 - 8,000 mg, daily with food (use with caution if you have a sensitivity to glutamic acid, deficiency in GABA, or severe leaky gut and brain).
- Follow the average probiotic protocol (Ch. 13) for two to four weeks.
- N-acetylglucosamine - follow the general supplement bottle recommendations (use with caution if you are suffering from yeast overgrowth).
- Upgraded™ Activated Charcoal – follow the general supplement bottle recommendations.

Taken for one month only:

- Nature's Way enteric coated peppermint oil - thirty to sixty minutes before meals, twice daily.

Anti-BioFilm Protocol:

- PREFERRED: Symbiotics lactoferrin - follow supplement bottle recommendations (can increase up to two grams daily if needed).

If diarrhea does not stop after a week:

- Rainforest Pharmacy sangre de drago – follow the general supplement bottle recommendations.
- In addition, consider following the bile acid malabsorption protocol (Ch. 4).
- Thorne Curcumin can also be used as long as it does not cause bowel upset and diarrhea.

The activated charcoal is used to bulk up the stools and to limit diarrhea.

The sangre de drago has been clinically proven to help stop diarrhea.

This protocol should be taken for at least three months and then tentatively afterward if the symptoms return.

Chronic Functional Abdominal Pain

Chronic functional abdominal pain is a condition where someone has the ongoing presence of abdominal pain, and there is no known medical explanation. CFAP shares some similarities to IBS, but there are no noticeable changes in bowel habits (diarrhea and constipation). Anyone with CFAP will have recurring bouts of severe abdominal pain. CFAP is a little-known disease that creates unnecessary frustration in affected people's lives because of the unknown cause of the disease.

It has been theorized that CFAP is not an abdominal problem but instead is a nervous system problem that might be caused by an infection. CFAP has been linked to different viral, bacterial, or protozoan infections. The condition may also develop from a traumatic event and has been linked to possible "brain-gut" dysfunction. If the pain starts after a traumatic event, then the person might need counseling to improve the CFAP. A neurotransmitter salvia panel may be beneficial in people with depression, anxiety, and have CFAP. Find a Naturopathic doctor that specializes in neurotransmitter imbalances and will be open to help "treat" people with CFAP using unconventional methods.

CFAP Protocol

- Follow the SIBO protocol (use peppermint oil) (Ch. 9).
- If there is no improvement after a month of the protocol, go to a doctor and ask about the use of Rifaximin.
- Relieve adrenal fatigue and hypothyroidism.
- Test for parasites and eliminate them with the parasite protocol (Ch. 4) if you are infected.
- Jarrow R-lipoic acid – take one capsule, twice daily with meals.
- Thorne Research B complex – take one capsule daily, do not use if you are an overmethylator.
- Thorne Curcumin - follow the general supplement bottle recommendations.
- Follow the cayenne protocol (Ch. 18).
- Magnesium glycinate – take 600 mg, taken at bedtime.

The SIBO and parasite protocols are to eliminate possible infection.

R-lipoic acid, magnesium, and the B complex are to help with nerve conduction.

Curcumin and cayenne are to help with inflammation and pain.

Ulcerative Colitis and Crohn's Disease

Ulcerative colitis and Crohn's disease are both inflammatory bowel diseases that bring both misery and torment to people diagnosed with them. These diseases drastically shorten both their quality and quantity of life. With proper diagnosis, knowledge, and protocol use, people with these diseases may overcome their disorders.

Ulcerative Colitis

Ulcerative colitis is a form of inflammatory bowel disease that is primarily located in the large intestine. In someone with ulcerative colitis, the colon ulcerates and can lead to open sores in the intestine. The constant ulceration in someone's large intestine causes the intestine to be in a state of excessive inflammation. The excess inflammation can cause constant diarrhea mixed with blood, intestinal cramps, severe intestinal pain, and rarely fever / infection. The excessive inflammation in the large intestine may cause symptoms similar to arthritis throughout the body, but systemic inflammation is less common in people afflicted with ulcerative colitis than those with Crohn's disease.

Tests used in the diagnosis of ulcerative colitis include blood tests for anemia or infection. Stool samples are also collected to check for excess white blood cells or pathogens in the stool. Sometimes a colonoscopy, flexible sigmoidoscopy (a lighted, flexible tube with a camera on the end), barium tests, and CT Scans are used for diagnostic purposes.

Crohn's Disease

Crohn's disease is ulcerative colitis' cousin and is an inflammatory disease of the entire digestive system. Unlike ulcerative colitis, which is only found in the colon, someone with Crohn's disease has many complex symptoms, which can make the diagnosis difficult, which is why Crohn's is discovered and treated in such late stages.

Digestive symptoms of Crohn's disease include abdominal pain, diarrhea (usually without blood), gallstones, frequent bowel movements (even more than twenty per day sometimes), bloating, and weight loss. Systemic symptoms include arthritis, inflammation of the eyes (uveitis, episcleritis), dermatitis, skin infections, depression, oral disorders, and nutritional deficiencies.

Tests used in the diagnosis of Crohn's disease are the same for someone with ulcerative colitis including blood tests for anemia or infection. Stool samples are also collected to check for excess white blood cells or pathogens in the stool. Sometimes a colonoscopy, flexible sigmoidoscopy (a lighted, flexible tube with a camera on the end), barium tests, and CT Scans are used for diagnostic purposes.

Ulcerative colitis and Crohn's disease are intermittent diseases with periods of exacerbated symptoms and periods where you might be symptom-free. Crohn's disease will usually have patchy areas of inflammation in/on the body where ulcerative colitis is usually localized to the large intestine.

Ulcerative colitis and Crohn's disease are not autoimmune conditions as mainstream medicine determines them to be. The diseases are caused by localized or systemic *Mycobacterium avium paratuberculosis* (*MAP*) infections.

Mycobacterium Avium Paratuberculosis and Ulcerative Colitis / Crohn's Disease

Mycobacterium is a genus of *Actinobacteria* that cause serious diseases in mammals (tuberculosis and leprosy are examples of *Mycobacterial* diseases). A *Mycobacteria* called *Mycobacterium avium paratuberculosis* is a pathogenic bacteria found in the gut of ruminant animals like cows and causes Johne's disease (*paratuberculosis*) in cattle.

Paratuberculosis causes diarrhea and wasting in the cattle. *MAP* also causes the cows to develop inflammatory bowel disease. Treatment of *paratuberculosis* in cattle is limited because of the cost of having to use human antibiotic treatments for the *Mycobacterial* infection. Usually, the most cost effective measure is to destroy the infected herd.

Common Infection Routes of MAP

MAP has recently been found as a zoological disease (a disease that can be transferred from animals to humans or vice versa). *MAP* can be transferred to humans when contact with infected cattle feces occurs, drinking improperly treated farm runoff water, ingesting beef, or ingesting milk and dairy products from infected cows. There are case studies identifying farmers infected with *MAP* after contact with aerosolized cow feces. *MAP* infections also originate from cattle farm runoff encountering municipal drinking water. *MAP* is a very resistant bacterium that can survive up to nine months in mud, a year in cow manure, and up to two years in water. Standard industrial water treatment such as filtration systems and chlorination may prove to be an ineffective treatment against eliminating *MAP*.

MAP also has been discovered in beef, but the levels are lower than other infection routes if the meat is prepared properly. Cow muscle tissue does not naturally contain many bacteria, but if the meat is not processed and prepared properly, feces can come in contact with the meat and infect it with *MAP*. *MAP* can also survive standard cooking temperatures, but it can be eliminated at prolonged temperatures around 165F. *MAP* also appears to be resistant to nitrates and smoke, as well.

Scientific literature indicates that humans are commonly exposed to *MAP* from the ingestion of milk and other dairy products. The proposed reason for the literature's conclusions is that the bacteria in milk are more invasive and populous than other routes of exposure. *MAP* is protected by the higher fat content of some dairy products. Fat globules protect *MAP* from stomach acid so that it can survive in greater numbers allowing it to reach the intestines. Raw dairy has a greater concentration of *MAP* bacteria than properly pasteurized dairy. The correlation between this data is unknown though because *MAP* can survive pasteurization. The research is mixed about if pasteurized milk and dairy products are safer and contain less *MAP* than if they are raw. I suggest anyone who is drinking dairy to consume pasture raised, vat pasteurized milk, for the healthiest way possible of trying to avoid *MAP*. Finally, *MAP* can also survive freezing (ice cream) for up to a year.

MAP is also found in other ruminant animals including goats, sheep, and deer, and I would avoid meat and dairy products from those animals as well if you have issues with *MAP*.

The Differences in the Development of Ulcerative Colitis or Crohn's Disease in MAP Infections

MAP is the primary cause of ulcerative colitis and Crohn's disease in humans. One of the deciding factors in whether anyone succumbs to ulcerative colitis or Crohn's disease seems to be the amount of their exposure to *MAP*. Lesser exposure to *MAP* over time leads to ulcerative colitis, where greater exposure to *MAP* causes Crohn's disease.

Scientific literature also shows the importance of someone's age at the time of infection. Adult humans tend to develop ulcerative colitis, and children tend to develop Crohn's Disease. Crohn's disease is usually undetectable in the body until early adulthood. Infant males and adult females, according to the literature, seem to contract Crohn's disease. The reason infant males might develop Crohn's disease instead of ulcerative colitis could be linked to their weaker immune systems, as opposed to infant females who have a higher functioning immune system. Adult males and infant females tend to contract ulcerative colitis instead of Crohn's.

The deciding factors of whether someone develops ulcerative colitis or Crohn's disease is the dose, the route of infection (drinking milk, contaminated water, handling, or breathing in aerosolized cow feces), the age in which one is infected, and the person's genetics and gender. Finally, in a major study *MAP* was found in the tissues of sixty percent of people with Crohn's disease and forty percent of people with ulcerative colitis. Sadly, the participants in this study re-diagnosed the people with ulcerative colitis and reclassified them with Crohn's disease. The researchers did this instead of concluding that *MAP* was the cause of both.

Rifabutin – An Antibiotic That Is Useful in the Treatment of MAP

Even though I believe natural antibacterial agents would eliminate *MAP* in the body, some people may also need to use conventional antibiotic therapy to help treat an active *MAP* infection. If any of the below protocols fail to help, reduce complications of a *MAP* infection, talk to your doctor about considering Rifabutin treatment.

Rifabutin

RANK: 4 POSSIBLY SAFE

Rifabutin was developed by the Italian drug company Achifar in 1975 and received FDA approval for use in the United States in the early 1990's. Rifabutin is used in the U.S. to treat tuberculosis infections. Rifabutin's mechanism of action is that it inhibits bacterial DNA-dependent RNA synthesis, which causes bacteria to fail to replicate. Finally, *Mycobacteria* appear to be very sensitive to Rifabutin's mechanism of action more than any other antibiotic.

Rifabutin has been found in a few studies including one phase three study, to relieve Crohn's disease symptoms, and complications even in people where a *MAP* infection was unknown.

Rifabutin also seems to lack rifampicin hepatotoxicity and major side effects. This means that Rifabutin "might" be a safer antibiotic for use. Rifabutin has similar side effects to other antibiotics like gastrointestinal upset and systemic allergic reactions.

Ulcerative Colitis (MAP Protocol)

Stage 1: One – Two Months

Antibacterial:

- PREFERRED: Nature's Way enteric coated peppermint oil - thirty to sixty minutes before meals, twice daily.

OR CHOOSE ONE OF THE FOLLOWING ANTIBACTERIAL AGENTS FROM THIS LIST

Choose one strong antimicrobial:

- Colloidal silver (Mesosilver, Sovereign Silver) – follow supplement bottle recommendations.
- Zane Hellas Oil of Oregano – do not use for first-time protocol. Oil of oregano is a broad spectrum, systemic antimicrobial agent, do not use first in a protocol.
- Thorne Research berberine – take 500 mg, two capsules daily. Use with caution if you have ulcers, gastritis, or hypoglycemia.
- Allicin-C – follow supplement bottle recommendations.
- Ceylon cinnamon oil – take one drop in one tsp. of extra virgin coconut oil or extra virgin olive oil, twice daily. Use with caution if you have hypoglycemia.

CHOOSE ONE OF THE FOLLOWING ANTIBIOFILM AGENTS

- **Calcium Disodium EDTA:** MRM Cardio Chelate – follow general supplement recommendations.
- **Fulvic Acid:** Food grade fulvic acid – follow general supplement recommendations.
- **Guaifenesin:** Guai-aid – take one capsule every four to eight hours. Do not exceed four capsules daily. Guaifenesin is a systemic biofilm chelator; I do not recommend it as a first-line anti-biofilm agent in a protocol.

- **NAC:** Jarrow Formulas NAC Sustain – one tablet twice daily. NAC is a systemic biofilm chelator; I do not recommend it as a first-line anti-biofilm agent in a protocol. Do not supplement more than 1,200 mg daily, doses above this recommendation may make the NAC you take become a pro-oxidant.
- **Systemic Enzymes:** Interphase Plus, PRX Enzyme Formula, Neprinol AMD – follow general supplement recommendations.

Other supplements in protocol:

- Consume food grade humic acid - follow the general supplement bottle recommendations.
- Pure Encapsulations zinc carnosine – one capsule with a meal, twice daily.
- Sodium ascorbate – take 4,000 mg, daily.
- Nordic Naturals fish oil - take 4,000 mg, daily.
- Thorne Curcumin- take once daily.
- Magnesium glycinate – take 400 mg, before bed.
- Optimize your vitamin D levels.
- Follow the Perfect Health® Diet, abstain from dairy and if needed ingestion of all ruminant animal (cow, goat, pig, sheep, and deer) products.

To control bleeding/diarrhea:

- Upgraded™ Activated Charcoal – follow the general supplement bottle recommendations.

If diarrhea persists after a week:

- Rainforest Pharmacy sangre de drago – follow the general supplement bottle recommendations.

If not any better in a month:

- Carnivora: follow the general supplement bottle recommendations.
- If a herx reaction occurs, follow the herx protocol (Ch. 9).
- Consider cycling antibacterial and antibiofilm agents, adding more of either as well. Consider the use of Rifabutin.

2: One - Six Months – Rebuilding the Gut / Body

- Remove carrageenan from your diet.
- L-glutamine - take 6,000 - 8,000 mg, daily with food (use with caution if you have a sensitivity to glutamic acid, deficiency in GABA, or severe leaky gut and brain).
- N-acetylglucosamine - follow the supplement bottle recommendations, use with caution if you have yeast overgrowth.
- Nordic Naturals fish oil - take 4,000 mg, daily.
- Thorne Curcumin - take once daily.
- Magnesium glycinate - take 400 mg, before bed.
- Thorne Research B complex – take once daily, do not take if you are an overmethylator.
- Jarrow Formulas methyl B12 – take one sublingual tablet, daily. Do not take if you are an overmethylator.
- Follow the Perfect Health® Diet, abstain from dairy and if needed ingestion of all ruminant animal (cow, goat, sheep, pig, and deer) products.
- Follow the advanced or severe probiotic protocol (Ch. 13).

Stage 3: One Year – General Advice

- Follow the Perfect Health® Diet, abstain from dairy and if needed ingestion of all ruminant animal (cow, goat, sheep, and deer) products.
- Magnesium glycinate – take 400 mg, before bed.
- Nordic Naturals fish oil - take 4,000 mg, daily.
- Thorne Naturals B complex – take once daily, do not use if you are an overmethylator.
- Follow the general probiotic regimen (Ch. 13).

Enteric-coated peppermint oil, colloidal silver, oil of oregano, zinc carnosine, and humic acid are strong antimicrobial agents and should reduce *MAP* colonization.

The lactoferrin is an even stronger antimicrobial and should only be used if symptoms have not resolved.

Carnivora can be used to help the body's natural immune system destroy the *MAP*.

Vitamin C helps strengthen the body's immune system.

The fish oil and curcumin help reduce inflammation in the body.

The magnesium helps the general integrity of the intestinal cells.

The activated charcoal helps absorb the toxins produced by *MAP* and helps bulk up the stools.

Sangre De Drago has been clinically shown to help relieve diarrhea.

L-glutamine is the most abundant amino acid in the body and helps rebuild both the stomach lining and the gut.

The curcumin is used to increase immune cells in the gut and heal inflammation.

The body makes N-acetylglucosamine to increase mucus production in the stomach and gut and to make a protective barrier.

The fish oil also helps reduce the inflammation.

The B complex and B12 help give the body the nutrients resulting from poor digestion.

Crohn's Disease (MAP Protocol)

Stage 1: One – Two Months - Reduction of *MAP* overgrowth / Reducing of Inflammation

Antibacterial

- PREFERRED: Nature's Way enteric coated peppermint oil - thirty to sixty minutes before meals, twice daily.

OR CHOOSE ONE OF THE FOLLOWING ANTIBACTERIAL AGENTS FROM THIS LIST

Choose one strong antimicrobial:

- Colloidal silver (Mesosilver, Sovereign Silver) – follow supplement bottle recommendations.
- Zane Hellas Oil of Oregano – do not use for first-time protocol. Oil of oregano is a broad spectrum, systemic antimicrobial agent, do not use for front line protocol.
- Thorne Research berberine - take 500 mg, two capsules daily. Use with caution if you have ulcers, gastritis, or hypoglycemia.
- Allicin-C – follow supplement bottle recommendations.
- Ceylon cinnamon oil – take one drop in one tsp. of extra virgin coconut oil or extra virgin olive oil, twice daily. Use with caution if you have hypoglycemia.

CHOOSE ONE OF THE FOLLOWING ANTIBIOFILM AGENTS

- **Calcium Disodium EDTA:** MRM Cardio Chelate – follow general supplement recommendations.
- **Fulvic Acid:** Food grade fulvic acid – follow general supplement recommendations.
- **Guaifenesin:** Guai-aid – take one capsule every four to eight hours. Do not exceed four capsules daily. Guaifenesin is a systemic biofilm chelator; I do not recommend it as a first-line anti-biofilm agent in a protocol.
- **NAC:** Jarrow Formulas NAC Sustain – one tablet twice daily. NAC is a systemic biofilm chelator; I do not recommend it as a first-line anti-biofilm agent in a protocol. Do not supplement more than 1,200 mg daily, doses above this recommendation may make the NAC you take become a pro-oxidant.
- **Systemic Enzymes:** Interphase Plus, PRX Enzyme Formula, Neprinol AMD – follow general supplement recommendations.

Other supplements in protocol:

- Consume food grade humic acid - follow the general supplement recommendations.
- Pure Encapsulations zinc carnosine – take one capsule with a meal, twice daily.
- Sodium ascorbate - take 4,000 mg, daily.
- Nordic Naturals fish oil – take 4,000 mg, daily.
- Thorne Curcumin - take once daily.
- Magnesium glycinate – take 400 mg, before bed.
- Carnivora: follow the general supplement bottle recommendations.
- Follow the Perfect Health® Diet or Bulletproof® diet.
- Optimize your vitamin D levels.

To control diarrhea:

- Upgraded™ Activated Charcoal – follow the general supplement bottle recommendations.

If diarrhea does not improve after two weeks into protocol:

- Rainforest Pharmacy sangre de drago – follow the general supplement bottle recommendations.

If there is no improvement after two weeks:

- Follow the Perfect Health® Diet, abstain from dairy and if needed ingestion of all ruminant animal (cow, pig, goat, sheep, and deer) products.
- If Herx reaction occurs follow herx protocol (Ch. 9).
- Consider cycling antibacterial and antibiofilm agents, adding more of either as well. Consider the use of Rifabutin.

Stage 2: One - Six Months – Rebuilding the Gut / Body

- Remove carrageenan from your diet.
- L-glutamine - take 6,000 - 8,000 mg daily with food (may increase dosage to 15,000 mg daily if needed) [use with caution if you have a sensitivity to glutamic acid, deficiency in GABA, or severe leaky gut and brain].
- N-acetylglucosamine - follow the general supplement bottle recommendations, use with caution if you have yeast overgrowth.
- Nordic Naturals fish oil - take 4,000 mg, daily.
- Magnesium glycinate – take 400 mg, before bed.
- Follow the advanced or severe protocol for probiotics for one month, then switch to the average protocol schedule for four months out of the year (at least have a one month break in-between) (Ch. 13).
- Follow the Perfect Health® Diet, abstain from dairy and if needed ingestion of all ruminant animal (cow, goat, pig, sheep, and deer) products.
- Thorne Research B complex – take once daily, do not use if you are an overmethylator.
- Jarrow Formulas Methyl B12 – Take one sublingual tablet, daily. Do not use if you are an overmethylator.
- BioCell collagen – take one capsule, daily.

If you have eye problems:

- Life Extension Super Zeaxanthin - follow the general supplement bottle recommendations.

Stage 3: One Year – General advice

- Follow the Perfect Health® Diet, abstain from dairy and if needed ingestion of all ruminant animal (cow, goat, pig, sheep, and deer) products.
- Magnesium glycinate – take 400 mg, before bed.

- Nordic Naturals fish oil – take 4,000 mg, daily.
- Thorne Research B complex – take once daily, do not take if you are an overmethylator.

Enteric-coated peppermint oil, colloidal silver, oil of oregano, zinc carnosine, and humic acid are strong antimicrobial agents and should reduce *MAP* overgrowth.

The lactoferrin is an even stronger antimicrobial and should only be used if symptoms have not resolved.

Carnivora can be used to help the body's natural immune system destroy the *MAP*. Carnivora supplementation is more important in people with Crohn's than those with ulcerative colitis because of the increased overall systemic inflammation damage. Vitamin C helps strengthen the body's immune system.

The fish oil and curcumin help reduce inflammation in the body.

The magnesium helps the general integrity of the intestinal cells.

The activated charcoal helps absorb the toxins produced by *MAP* and helps bulk up the stools.

Sangre De Drago has been clinically shown to stop diarrhea.

L-glutamine is the most abundant amino acid in the body and helps rebuild both the stomach lining and the gut.

The body produces N-acetylglucosamine to increase mucus production in the stomach and gut and to make a protective barrier.

The fish oil also helps reduce systemic inflammation.

The B complex and B12 help give the body the nutrients resulting from poor digestion.

The Biocell collagen will also help repair some of the systemic damage caused by Crohn's disease.

Super zeaxanthin helps the eyes function better.

Gluten Intolerance / Celiac Disease

What is Gluten and the Problem with Eating Wheat?

Gluten is a binding protein that is found in wheat and other related grain species such as barley and rye. Gluten is what gives elasticity to dough and helps wheat products rise, keep their shape, and gives wheat a chewy texture. Gluten contains gliadin and glutenin, which comprise eighty percent of the protein in wheat. Gluten is not destroyed by cooking or processing and is present in all wheat products.

Gluten is in almost every meal the average American consumes. Make sure you always check nutrition and ingredient labels for gluten before consuming.

If you dine out for your meals, check the restaurant's ingredient list before dining. Gluten is found in bread; most cereals, cookies, muffins, pancakes, waffles, most fried foods are coated in wheat flour, pies, cakes, gravy, pizza, pasta, wheat tortillas, and other foods that contain wheat flour. Remember, your food can be contaminated with gluten if it is fried in the same oil as food that contains gluten (for example, fries that are fried in the same oil that onion rings were fried in). Gluten can even be added to food secretly, like McDonald's French fries, where it is added as "natural flavoring." Finally, gluten proteins are not destroyed by cooking, heating, or cooling in any food product.

Gluten Intolerance and celiac disease are becoming more prevalent all over the world because wheat in the 1960's was selectively bred to contain more gluten. These new wheat plants were shorter and were quicker to harvest. The extra gluten and thicker gluten strands support higher grain yields. You can still purchase Einkorn Wheat (heirloom wheat) which has less gluten and gliadin than modern wheat. Einkorn Wheat tends to cause less of a reaction in your average person if they are sensitive to wheat (people with celiac disease still have to avoid it).

Upon digestion, gliadin is reduced to a collection of five polypeptides, which bind to the opiate receptors in the brain that makes eating wheat addictive. It also stimulates appetite and leads to further wheat cravings. Gliadin also has been shown to increase small intestinal permeability leading to leaky gut syndrome. Glutenin has been shown to bind with the leptin receptor in your stomach causing hunger. The binding of glutenin leads to less leptin being produced and circulating throughout the body. Leptin is the hormone of satiety, and it is what makes you feel full after eating a meal. Ingestion of glutenin makes you crave more food and often leads to overeating.

I know that you were taught to believe that whole wheat bread is better for you than standard white bread. The problem with whole wheat bread is that it also contains more gluten and more amylopectin A. Amylopectin A is a "complex" carbohydrate unique to wheat that is highly digestible by the enzyme amylase in your saliva and pancreatic secretions. Since amylopectin A is a carbohydrate that is easily digested, it quickly causes elevated blood glucose levels. After eating, two slices of whole wheat bread, your blood glucose increases more than eating two tablespoons of sugar.

All this information should cause even the average person who does not have a gluten intolerance to reduce or eliminate gluten from their diet. Even if you are not "allergic" to gluten, it can still eventually wreak havoc in your body nonetheless.

Gluten Intolerance

Gluten intolerance is different from celiac disease, in that gluten intolerance is more of an allergy where celiac disease is in the truest sense an autoimmune disease. With people who have celiac disease, gluten will make them ill and destroy their gastrointestinal tract. If you have gluten intolerance, ingestion of gluten can still cause digestive discomfort. When people are intolerant to gluten, they have symptoms ranging from migraines, abdominal bloating, abdominal discomfort or pain, diarrhea, nausea, vomiting, and weight loss after ingestion of gluten.

Unlike celiac disease, gluten intolerance might improve or be eliminated if you strengthen, repair the gut, and relieve any digestion related issues you may have. I still recommend that most people abstain from eating gluten because of the negatives associated with its consumption, though.

Testing for gluten sensitivity can be finicky; most people should avoid gluten if they have chronic health issues to see if they feel better eliminating it. I would eliminate gluten for at least two months to see if your chronic health problems improve.

Gluten Intolerance Protocol

- Adopt a gluten-free diet (Wheat Belly by: Dr. William Davis is a good gluten-free diet).
- Follow the gut rebuilding protocol (Ch. 9) for three months if you are diagnosed with gluten intolerance.
- Use Enzymedica GlutenEase digestive enzyme if you are eating a meal that might have some gluten cross-contamination. The DPP-IV enzyme in the formula might help break down gluten and help stop an over-response to the protein. The use of DPP-IV is not completely backed up by case studies yet, so it may not stop the reaction. If you still have a bad reaction to the gluten, follow the gut rebuilding protocol (Ch. 9) for an additional two weeks.
- Follow the average to advanced probiotic protocol (Ch. 13).
- Consider testing and treating SIBO, try a low-FODMAP diet.
- It might be possible to eliminate gluten intolerance by following the GAPS diet to completion (this can take three months to a year).

Celiac Disease

Celiac disease is different from gluten sensitivity. When someone with celiac disease encounters gluten, a person may have what I consider being a true autoimmune response. Most autoimmune conditions are caused by toxin exposure, unknown pathogens, lack of a nutritional element, or a poorly functioning immune system. There is disagreement though on whether the cause of this autoimmune reaction is a severe allergic reaction, if it is caused by genetics, or if severe leaky gut syndrome causes it because of constant contact with gliadin proteins.

If you have celiac, the disease itself is likely caused by severe leaky gut caused by gliadin overexposure, which leads to elevated inflammation. The inflammation and gliadin exposure is what triggers an autoimmune response. Does that mean that someone with celiac disease could be cured if you fix their leaky gut? More than likely their celiac disease would not resolve because gluten exposure in anyone that has celiac disease should always create leaky gut. In someone who has celiac disease, gluten and gliadin create an immune overreaction in their body. The overreaction response is more than likely due to their genetics, which causes the person afflicted to be unable to digest gluten or gliadin properly. The only "cure" for celiac disease is for the person to sustain lifelong abstinence from gluten.

When someone with celiac encounters gliadin, antibodies are produced from the exposure that interferes with the enzyme transglutaminase in the intestine. Transglutaminase modifies the gliadin protein to break it down properly. When this happens, the body's immune system continues to overreact from improperly digested gliadin proteins and creates a severe inflammatory response that further destroys the villi (villi are tiny hairs in the intestinal tract that move food along and help absorb nutrients) and the mucus barrier of the intestinal tract. The damage done to the intestinal tract can lead to nutritional difficulties, scarring, and infection. When the barrier of the intestinal tract is destroyed, gluten antibodies and proteins begin to spread to other parts of the body and wreak havoc systemically on someone's health through the bloodstream. The antibodies and proteins can even begin to attack the brain by weakening the integrity of the blood-brain barrier over time. The weakened blood-brain barrier and brain inflammation is the reason studies have found a correlation between undiagnosed celiac disease and schizophrenia in young adults!

Anyone with celiac disease has the same symptoms of someone who has gluten intolerance, or IBS. They will have chronic stomach and intestinal pain, bloating, and even mouth ulcers. They might also develop lactose intolerance, as well. The person might have trouble gaining weight, have intestinal polyps and infections, and develop vitamin deficiencies. The constant immune response created from the ingestion of gluten greatly damages internal organs over time. A poorly functioning thyroid gland is a good example of this. People with celiac disease are found to suffer from hypothyroidism because of poor thyroid health due to the excessive systemic gluten antibody damage to the thyroid.

People with celiac disease are not able to absorb nutrients, minerals, and fat-soluble vitamins like A, D, E, and K. Celiac disease has also been shown to be linked to SIBO because of the intestinal permeability and the breakdown of the protective mucus barrier allows bacteria to colonize the small intestine. Finally, they might have an IgA deficiency; an itchy rash on their skin, called dermatitis herpetiformis (appears as many blisters filled with fluid), and have abnormal liver function tests.

Diagnosis of this disease can be challenging, especially if someone with celiac disease started a gluten-free diet on his or her own. The intestines will eventually heal themselves, and antibody markers can return to normal after a couple of months. Blood tests can be used to measure IgG levels and anti-tTG antibodies (transglutaminase) to see if one is having an autoimmune reaction to gluten. An endoscopy or colonoscopy can be performed as well to look for lesions, and a biopsy can be done during those procedures.

Celiac Disease Protocol

- Adopt the Wheat Belly diet.
- Follow the SIBO protocol (Ch. 9) if SIBO is present.
- Remove carrageenan from your diet.
- Follow gut rebuilding protocol (Ch. 9) for three months if you are diagnosed with gluten intolerance.

- Use Enzymedica GlutenEase digestive enzyme if you are eating a meal that might have some gluten cross-contamination. The DPP-IV enzyme in the formula might help break down gluten and help stop a response to the protein. If you have a celiac reaction, follow the gut rebuilding protocol (Ch. 9) for an additional two weeks. DPP-IV is not completely backed up by case studies yet, so it may not stop the reaction.
- Thorne Research B complex – take the B complex three times a week, do not supplement if you are an overmethylator.
- Jarrow Formulas methyl B12 – Take 1,000 mcg, daily. Use another form like adenosylcobalamin if you are an overmethylator.
- Vitamin D optimization.
- Optimal Start – take three capsules daily in divided doses with food.
- Enzymedica Digestive Enzyme Gold – take one to two capsules with each meal (for at least three months).

Vitamin D production facilitates proper immune function. The vitamins are for nutritional deficiencies.

Appendicitis

What Is the Vermiform Appendix and Why Is It Important?

The vermiform appendix is a tiny narrow pouch that extends from the first part of the large bowel known as the cecum and is slightly after the ileocecal valve. A few other mammals have an appendix, rabbits being one such mammal. Lymphatic tissue (GALT) has been found in both the rabbit and human appendix. Finally, probiotic biofilm and colonization are found heavily concentrated in the appendix.

Our microbiome consists of probiotic microorganisms and opportunistic microorganisms that most of the time work together for the benefit of each other and the host. I know I have written a lot about the negatives of opportunistic bacteria biofilm formation, but probiotic bacteria also form biofilm to protect themselves from pathogens. Biofilm itself is not dangerous, but who is producing it is what matters. Our immune system determines if a bacteria is probiotic or opportunistic and helps maintain the probiotic biofilms. If the bacteria is determined to be a pathogen our immune system and our microbiome hopefully keeps it in check or eliminates it. Biofilm concentrations seem to be their highest inside of the appendix compared to the rest of the distal bowel. Biofilms are always shedding in our intestinal system, and our immune system reacts to it either positively or negatively depending on the strain. The shedding of probiotic biofilm may help to inoculate probiotic bacteria from our immune system further down the colon.

The location of the appendix, branching out from the end of the cecum, is essential to the protection of the probiotic bacteria that reside there. It avoids peristalsis pushed fecal matter to prevent colonization from pathogenic microorganisms that it may contain. The appendix appears to be critical in preventing post-infectious IBS or SIBO. When your intestines encounter a pathogen or toxins that pathogens produce, gut junctions quickly open up, and chloride ions and water are secreted to cause diarrhea in an attempt to flush the offending matter out of the intestinal tract. If you have your appendix, the fecal matter quick passes by leaving the beneficial probiotic colony protected and after the bowels have stabilized and the threat is mostly removed, the bacteria can help to recolonize the intestinal tract and aid prevention of overgrowth. However, if your appendix has been removed you have a greater chance to develop overgrowth or SIBO; it would be harder for your microbiome to bounce back and more opportunistic strains might take hold.

The appendix also contains lymphoid tissue that produces innate lymphoid cells. Innate lymphoid cells help to regulate homeostasis and inflammation within the body, and this concentration in the appendix and the cecum contribute to protecting us from allergies and autoimmune diseases caused by excessive inflammation from infections. The innate lymphoid cells produced in the appendix and cecum tend to be ILC3's. ILC3's are special in that they help to mediate the balance between probiotic and opportunistic pathogens by regulating inflammation, antimicrobial peptides, and the mucosal barrier.

Finally, the microbiome of the appendix seems to produce most of the melatonin that we find in the digestive tract. The highest concentration of melatonin in our gastrointestinal system is located in the appendix. The amount of melatonin produced by our gastrointestinal tract is four hundred times greater than what is produced by our pineal gland. Removal of the appendix may reduce the amount of melatonin produced by your digestive system. If you want to learn more about the importance of melatonin on increasing your digestive and overall health, read this blog.

Appendicitis

Appendicitis is a condition in which the appendix becomes inflamed. When appendicitis occurs, surgery is often required to remove the appendix from the body. There is no protocol to save your appendix once it reaches this stage because of the high risk of rupture. If your appendix ruptures, your chance of survival drops significantly. Included in this guide is advice to help keep appendicitis from occurring and what you should supplement for a healthy recovery if your appendix does happen to rupture.

The symptoms of appendicitis are severe abdominal pain, constipation, vomiting, and fever. The pain usually starts around the belly button, and over a period of time, moves to the right lower quadrant. If your appendix is inflamed, pain becomes very severe and can easily be found by pressing on the abdominal wall. If the appendix is inflamed, the person will experience sharp pain.

In some cases, no pain will present itself. If the cecum becomes distended, it will protect the appendix from abdominal pressure (this is known as silent appendicitis). A digital rectal exam can be given to determine if one has appendicitis if the appendix is pushed down into the pelvis. A positive case of appendicitis will cause a person to experience a sharp pain from tenderness in the rectovesical pouch.

Coughing can also be useful in diagnosing appendicitis. If the person coughs and it is extremely painful in the right lower quadrant, then they could be suffering from appendicitis (Dunphy's sign). Finally, if the sharp pain immediately goes away at any point in time, someone's appendix has ruptured and becomes a life-threatening medical emergency.

The use of blood tests, urine tests, X-rays, and ultrasounds are usually unreliable in the diagnosis of appendicitis. The most important clinical tests for appendicitis are symptom charting and physical examination. A CAT scan can also be used with great success in diagnosing appendicitis but should only be used as a last resort because of the dosage of ionizing radiation.

Finally, a scoring system known as the Alvarado score can be used to diagnose appendicitis. A score below five usually excludes the appendix in the cause of the pain. A score of five or six usually requires a CAT scan. A score of seven or higher is strong predictive of appendicitis.

Alvarado Score Chart

MIGRATORY RIGHT ILIAC FOSSA PAIN	1 POINT
ANOREXIA	1 POINT
NAUSEA AND VOMITING	1 POINT
RIGHT ILIAC FOSSA TENDERNESS	2 POINTS
REBOUND TENDERNESS	1 POINT
FEVER	1 POINT
LEUKOCYTOSIS	2 POINTS
SHIFT TO LEFT (SEGMENTED NEUTROPHILS)	1 POINT

The appendix has recently been discovered to have a purpose in overall human health. The appendix is a storage organ for probiotics in the large intestine. In theory, the main cause of appendicitis is constipation that backs up feces and opportunistic bacteria into the appendix. Eventually, the opportunistic bacteria take over the appendix, and the appendix becomes severely inflamed which leads to the condition known as appendicitis. Finally, the appendix might have been an extension of the cecum and aided in the digestion of cellulose.

How to Prevent Appendicitis and What to Do If You Have Yours Removed

Prevention of appendicitis is paramount, and constipation is its primary cause. Here are some tips to prevent appendicitis and what you can do to avoid an appendectomy hopefully:

- Relieve constipation. Use a squatty potty, eat a wide variety of seasonal fruits, vegetables, and starches (sans gluten) to increase microbiome diversity, make sure you are getting in enough magnesium, and ensure that you are staying well hydrated.
- Maintain microbiome diversity and MMC function using prebiotics occasionally like GOS or arabinogalactan.
- Squat when you defecate. The problems with sitting on the toilet instead of squatting are numerous. When you sit on the toilet, it makes a narrow anorectal angle. The tight anorectal angle obstructs the anus and causes you not to empty your bowels completely when you use the bathroom. When you do not completely empty your bowels, some stool is pushed back up into the colon when you stand up. Theoretically, feces back up eventually leads to appendicitis, from the irritation of the appendix from toxins and opportunistic bacteria that were supposed to be eliminated. Using a standard toilet in the industrial world might be the first correlation between the increase of appendicitis in the first world compared to third world countries where people mainly squat.
- If you do develop appendicitis, ask your doctor about relieving it with natural antimicrobial agents (oil of oregano for example) or antibiotics instead of having an appendectomy.

If you have had your appendix removed like me, there are things you can do to prevent the issues associated with its removal. If you develop food poisoning or a gastrointestinal infection, proper MMC regulation, reduction of intestinal inflammation, GOS supplementation, and probiotic supplementation may be needed to prevent post-infectious IBS or SIBO. Finally, good sleep hygiene is paramount because of the reduction of circulating melatonin due to appendix removal.

Diverticulosis & Diverticulitis

Diverticulosis is a condition in which there are pockets in the mucous lining of the colon trapping foodstuffs. There is a weakness in the muscle layers of the colon. Risk factors that can contribute to this disease include age, constipation, dietary fiber, and connective tissue disorders.

Symptoms of diverticulosis include abdominal cramping, abdominal tenderness, bloating, flatulence, irregular defecation, and bleeding. If the intestines become infected, the condition worsens from diverticulosis into diverticulitis.

Diverticulosis is diagnosed using an abdominal X-ray, CT scan, colonoscopy, barium enema X-ray, and MRI. There is currently no blood test that accurately diagnoses diverticulosis. Colonoscopies and barium enemas should not be used in the diagnosis of diverticulitis because of the risk that the bowel wall might perforate causing a massive systemic infection.

Diverticulosis Protocol

- Restrict nuts, seeds, and popcorn hulls.
- Use a squatty potty when defecating.
- Enteric coated peppermint oil – take one capsule on an empty stomach when intestinal spasms are felt.
- Uni-Fiber – take one tablespoon mixed with water up to three times daily to help cleanse the colon.
- L -glutamine – 7,500 mg, taken in divided doses mixed with water three times with food (use with caution if you have a sensitivity to glutamic acid, deficiency in GABA, or severe leaky gut and brain).
- Thorne Curcumin – follow the general supplement bottle recommendations.
- N-acetylglucosamine (do not use if allergic to shellfish) – follow the general supplement bottle recommendations, use with caution if you have yeast overgrowth.
- Grass-fed butter – consume a tablespoon each day with a meal.
- Magnesium glycinate – 600 mg, taken before bed.

Peppermint oil limits intestinal spasms.

Uni-Fiber cleans out the colon.

L-glutamine, curcumin, N-acetylglucosamine, and butter help maintain colon integrity.

Diverticulitis Protocol

- Follow the safe antibiotic guide (Ch. 19) if antibiotics are prescribed.
- If you choose not to take antibiotics, follow the severe SIBO protocol (Ch. 9).
- While intestines are infected, follow a low-residue diet.
- If surgery is needed, follow the surgery rebuilding protocol (Ch. 9) afterward.
- If a person is following a SIBO protocol, low-residue diet, or taking an antibiotic, follow the basic probiotic protocol (Ch. 13), as well.
- Remove carrageenan from your diet.
- After elimination of opportunistic bacteria, and completion of the SIBO protocol, follow advanced probiotic protocol (Ch. 13) for two weeks if antibiotics are prescribed again.

Proctitis

Proctitis is inflammation of the anus and lining surrounding the end of the rectum. Proctitis is usually caused by radiation from cancer treatments, infection, stress, or gluten intolerance. Symptoms of proctitis include straining to empty bowels, diarrhea, rectal bleeding, spasms, pain, and even mucus discharge in stool.

Diagnosis of proctitis is made using a proctoscope or a sigmoidoscope. A stool sample might also be needed to test for bacteria or infection. A colonoscopy and barium X-ray might be used after the proctitis is healed to determine the functioning of the colon.

Proctitis Protocol

- Use a squatty potty when defecating.
- If an infection is present, use the severe SIBO protocol (Ch. 9), or an antibiotic from the safe antibiotic guide (Ch. 19).
- Remove carrageenan from your diet.
- Enteric coated peppermint oil – take one capsule on an empty stomach when intestinal spasms are felt.
- Uni-Fiber – take one tablespoon mixed with water up to three times daily to help cleanse the colon.
- L -glutamine – take 7,500 mg mixed with water, in divided doses three times daily with food (use with caution if you have a sensitivity to glutamic acid, deficiency in GABA, or severe leaky gut and brain).
- Thorne Curcumin – follow the general supplement bottle recommendations.
- Follow the average probiotic protocol (Ch. 13) for two weeks.
- N-acetylglucosamine (do not use if allergic to shellfish) – follow the general supplement bottle recommendations, use with caution if you have yeast overgrowth.
- Grass-fed butter – consume a tablespoon each day with a meal.
- Magnesium glycinate – take 600 mg, taken before bed.

Peppermint oil limits intestinal spasms.

Uni-Fiber cleans out the colon.

L-glutamine, curcumin, N-acetylglucosamine, and butter help to maintain colon integrity.

Hemorrhoid

Hemorrhoids are vascular structures in the anal canal that sometimes swell and become inflamed. These structures help with stool control and act as a cushion composed of arteriovenous channels and connective tissue. Though the true causes of hemorrhoids are unknown, constipation is believed to be the main cause. Other causes and risk factors include prolonged straining or sitting, chronic coughing, and obesity.

Diagnoses of hemorrhoids are usually made by visual examination or a rectal exam using an anoscopy (tube device with a light on the end inserted into the rectum). There are two different types of hemorrhoids: internal and external.

Internal

Internal hemorrhoids usually present with painless, bright red rectal bleeding during or after defecation. The blood usually covers the stool (hematochezia) or is visible on toilet paper after wiping. The stool itself should be of normal color. Other symptoms include mucous discharge from the anus, itchiness, and fecal incontinence. Internal hemorrhoids only are painful if they have become thrombosed or necrotic which should be treated by a doctor. The degree of prolapse classifies internal hemorrhoids. Grade III and IV hemorrhoids usually warrant a visit to your doctor.

- Grade I: No prolapse. Just prominent blood vessels.
- Grade II: Prolapse upon bearing down but prolapse is reduced after ceasing defecation.
- Grade III: Prolapse upon bearing down and requires manual reduction by the person themself.
- Grade IV: Prolapsed and cannot be manually reduced.

External

If the hemorrhoid is not prolapsed, then it may go unnoticed. If the hemorrhoid becomes thrombosed, then it may become extremely painful. The pain will usually resolve within a few days. Itching and irritation may occur with an external hemorrhoid. Try to sit on a cushion if possible and try to reduce the pressure on the hemorrhoid.

Procedures and Surgery for Hemorrhoids

If my protocols do not reduce your hemorrhoid, then surgery might even be a need for relief. While most procedures for hemorrhoids are safe, sepsis and infections are possible. Surgery also poses more risks like uncontrolled bleeding, infection, anal strictures, fecal incontinence, and damage to nerves in the bladder causing urinary retention.

Rubber Band Ligation

Rubber band ligation is usually the primary treatment for those suffering from any hemorrhoidal diseases unless they have progressed to grade IV. In this procedure, an elastic band is tied around the hemorrhoid to cut off its blood supply. Within five to seven days, the hemorrhoid typically falls off. However, if the rubber band is too close to the dentate line, it will cause intense pain after it falls off. This method has a success rate of eighty-seven percent and a complication rate of about only three percent.

Sclerotherapy

When a sclerotherapy is performed, an agent is injected into the hemorrhoid to shrink the blood vessel. Usually, phenol is used for this procedure, which causes the hemorrhoid to shrivel up and disappear. The success rate for this procedure is seventy percent.

Cauterization

Cauterization is usually used only for hemorrhoids that are classified as either grade I or II. When a hemorrhoid is cauterized, a laser usually burns it so that it the blood flow is blocked, and it eventually falls off.

Excisional Hemorrhoidectomy

Excisional hemorrhoidectomy is a surgical excision of the hemorrhoid and is only performed in the most severe cases. It comes along with significant post-surgical pain that lasts for up to a month. However, if the hemorrhoid is thrombosed and has started to turn necrotic, this may be the most effective treatment. Application of glyceryl trinitrate ointment post procedure improves general healing and reduces pain.

Doppler-Guided Transanal Hemorrhoidal Dearterialization

Doppler-Guided Transanal Hemorrhoidal Dearterialization is a minimally invasive treatment that uses an ultrasound Doppler to locate arterial blood flow to the hemorrhoid. The arteries are then tied off, and the prolapsed hemorrhoid sutured to its original position. There is a slightly higher recurrence rate, but less complication and pain than having a hemorrhoidectomy.

Stapled Hemorrhoidectomy

Stapled hemorrhoidectomy involves the removal of the enlarged hemorrhoidal tissue following the remaining hemorrhoidal tissue and stapling it back into position. It is usually less painful and associated with faster healing than complete removal of hemorrhoid. This procedure has a greater recurrence rate than the above surgeries and is usually used only on grade II and III hemorrhoids.

Hemorrhoid Prevention Protocol

- Use a squatty potty when defecating.
- Maintain proper fiber ingestion.
- Remain hydrated.
- Magnesium malate – take 400 mg daily, with meals.
- Maintain a healthy body mass if possible.
- Have good posture when sitting; try to sit on the most comfortable furniture available if you have to sit for long periods.

Hemorrhoid Protocol

- Use a squatty potty when defecating.
- Make sure you are properly hydrated.
- Magnesium malate – take 600 mg daily, with meals.
- Aescin (horse chestnut) – follow general supplement bottle recommendations.

- Follow the average probiotic protocol (Ch. 13) for one week.
- Follow the cayenne pepper protocol (Ch. 18).
- Uni-Fiber – consume one tablespoon mixed in a glass of water, three times daily.
- Use witch hazel wipes after defecation.
- If the hemorrhoid is painful, take a warm sitz bath for twenty minutes.

The magnesium citrate and Uni-Fiber keep bowels loose and regulated.

The squatty potty prevents straining and constipation.

Cayenne pepper heals the hemorrhoid with anti-inflammatory factors and increases blood flow to the hemorrhoid.

Witch hazel shrinks the hemorrhoid.

Warm water in the bath increases blood flow to the hemorrhoid.

Hemorrhoid Surgery Protocol

- Use a squatty potty when defecating.
- Make sure you are properly hydrated.
- Magnesium malate – take 600 mg, daily with meals.
- Follow the critical probiotic protocol (Ch. 13) for two weeks. If herx symptoms appear, stop using the probiotic.
- Uni-Fiber – consume one tablespoon mixed in a glass of water, three times daily.
- Follow the basic rebuild gut protocol (Ch. 9).

Gastrointestinal Cancer

There is not a protocol one can follow for any specific form of cancer, but I can give you some possible ideas that you can further research for yourself. One day I will write a book more in-depth of alternative cancer therapies. Never follow any cancer protocol, without weighing your options and consulting a medical professional first.

- Antineoplaston therapy: http://www.burzynskiclinic.com/
- Carnivora: www.carnivora.com
- DCA: http://articles.mercola.com/sites/articles/archive/2012/08/04/dca-and-turmeric-on-cancer.aspx

- Royal Rife machine: http://rense.com/general31/rife.htm, http://rense.com/products/rifeb1.htm
- Hemp oil: http://phoenixtears.ca/
- Paw paw: http://www.pawpawresearch.com/
- Strict ketogenic diet: http://articles.mercola.com/sites/articles/archive/2013/03/10/ketogenic-diet.aspx, https://www.ncbi.nlm.nih.gov/pubmed/23755243
- IP6: http://ip6gold.com/
- IV vitamin C: http://orthomolecular.org/library/ivccancerpt.shtml, http://www.drhoffman.com/page.cfm/783

Books

- Cancer: Step Outside the Box
- World Without Cancer
- Cayenne: The Doctor Who Cures Cancer

Chapter 10

Magnesium

The Most Overlooked Mineral for Improving Digestive Health

Magnesium is essential to your digestive health because it is used in the production of the body's digestive enzymes. The colon also uses magnesium as an osmotic laxative and restores regularity to the bowels.

The majority of Americans are deficient in magnesium (deficiency could be as high as eighty percent), and this is contributing to the increasing cases of diabetes and heart disease. Many individuals have probably had magnesium serum blood tests, and the test results usually come back as normal. Unfortunately, they are never told that the results of the blood test reflect only about two percent of the total magnesium levels in the body, and the body magnesium levels normalize naturally through osmosis. If this level is not maintained, you could suffer from heart arrhythmia and even possibly have a heart attack! The body requires a lot of magnesium for healthy bones, organs, and cells.

Magnesium is essential for over three hundred enzymatic reactions in the body. It is used to regulate blood glucose, and to help prevent the development of diabetes. Magnesium relaxes arteries that carry blood throughout the body, which lowers blood pressure. Magnesium also chelates extra calcium in the body, which helps keep the arteries from hardening due to excessive calcium buildup. Finally, Magnesium supplementation lowers stress and anxiety levels.

The most bioavailable form is magnesium glycinate. The body absorbs the most elemental magnesium from the glycinated chelate and the extra glycine functions as both an amino acid and a neurotransmitter. Magnesium also relaxes nerves and relieves anxiety.

Possible Symptoms of Magnesium Deficiency

The following is a list of possible symptoms anyone might have if you suffer from a magnesium deficiency. It is also likely to be deficient in magnesium without any symptoms. Asymptomatic magnesium deficiency often occurs in young people and can depend on one's gender (men tend to have fewer symptoms than women do). Most people should at least supplement with 400 mg of elemental magnesium daily (as long as their kidney function is normal) because of the lack of magnesium in our diets, and the amount of antinutrients that make absorption difficult.

- Tingling in legs - magnesium deficiency is the main cause of restless leg syndrome
- Leg cramps (charley horses)
- Weakness
- Asthma
- Elevated blood pressure or pulse
- Heart disease
- Diabetes
- Dizziness
- Shaking
- Irregular heartbeat (palpitations)
- Constipation

Diagnostic Tests for Magnesium Deficiency

Here is a simple guide to determine what test you should have performed to determine if you are deficient in magnesium.

The Serum Magnesium Test

The serum magnesium test is the most common magnesium test performed and the most inaccurate. Two percent of the body's total magnesium concentration is in the blood plasma, and cellular osmosis keeps these levels consistent. If you score low on a plasma test, then you are in dire need of magnesium, and you are very deficient in your bones, organs, and muscles. Normal magnesium plasma levels are between 1.6 - 2.4 mEq/L.

Magnesium RBC Test

Magnesium RBC test is a more accurate test that quantifies the amount of magnesium stored in the red blood cells. This test measures intracellular magnesium levels and calculates the amount of magnesium that has been stored in your cells for the past four months. Results of 6 mg/dl or higher indicate strong magnesium reserves in the body.

Magnesium WBC Test

Magnesium WBC test is more accurate than the RBC test. Like the magnesium RBC test, the WBC test also measures intracellular magnesium levels. This test measures the amount of magnesium that is currently in your cells; it does not show an average of magnesium in the cells over a period like the RBC test. The availability of getting a magnesium WBC test is low, which makes this one of the hardest tests to recommend despite its excellent accuracy.

Magnesium EXA Test

Magnesium EXA test is the best test to determine magnesium deficiency and is performed by scraping your cheek buccal cells so that levels of magnesium stored in your cells, bones, and muscles can be determined. Like the WBC test, the EXA test is considered an intracellular magnesium test. The EXA test will account for ninety-nine percent of the body's total magnesium and is the most accurate diagnostic test for magnesium currently available.

Magnesium and Your Digestive Health

Magnesium is used in the body to activate digestive enzymatic reactions in your body as well as regulate the proper transit time of elimination. These enzymatic reactions in your body break down fats, proteins, and carbohydrates. Magnesium chloride increases your stomach acid to help you better assimilate food. If you have low stomach acid, magnesium chloride might be the type you want to use. Other forms of magnesium (unless chelated with an acid, either like citrate or malate) greatly reduce stomach acid, so they should be taken before bed as not to interfere with digestion.

Your intestines use magnesium as an osmotic laxative that means that your large intestine uses magnesium to regulate water in the bowl so that your stool becomes softer and easier to pass. Easier passing stools are why magnesium supplementation is great for someone who has constipation issues. Magnesium is very important for your digestive system as well as your overall health.

Different Forms of Magnesium

Recommended Forms of Magnesium

Magnesium Glycinate

Magnesium glycinate is the most bioavailable form of magnesium. The bounded glycine helps with sleep and provides a calm feeling. The glycinate form of magnesium is the least likely to cause loose stools. Take magnesium glycinate at bedtime.

Magnesium Malate

Magnesium malate is important for people who need more energy or suffer from chronic fatigue syndrome. Magnesium supplementation increases ATP, which is a molecule that provides energy to our cells. Malic acid has also been shown to increase ATP levels. Magnesium malate should be taken during the day with meals. The bound malic acid will slightly increase stomach acid and assimilation.

Magnesium Chloride

Magnesium chloride is one of the best forms of magnesium for people with GERD or stomach problems. It must be taken with food because of the chloride bond. When the salt is used in a biochemical reaction, the chloride is often used to make more hydrochloric acid in the stomach. Magnesium chloride may also be used topically as a spray for transdermal supplementation.

Magnesium Taurate

Magnesium taurate is a lifesaver for people with heart disease. The bound taurine increases heart function. Taurine can also cross the blood-brain barrier and support cognitive function. Take magnesium taurate at bedtime. Use with caution if you have an active CBS mutation expression.

Magnesium Sulfate

A magnesium sulfate supplement is effective for stopping pre-eclampsia when used in the bath as Epsom salt. Magnesium sulfate is reasonably absorbed, and the sulfur is good for the skin. Epsom salt baths are an effective usage of magnesium sulfate for muscle sprains due to skin permeability. Take magnesium sulfate by soaking in a bath or before bed.

Magnesium Arginate

Arginine is an amino acid that increases nitrogen levels in the blood. Magnesium arginate is very good for bodybuilders. Take magnesium arginate with meals throughout the day.

Magnesium Lysinate

Magnesium lysinate is a good source of magnesium and the amino acid lysine has been shown to be an excellent antiviral. Take magnesium lysinate before bed.

Magnesium Ascorbate

Magnesium ascorbate is a good source of magnesium and vitamin C. Magnesium ascorbate has the potential to cause some loose stools. Take magnesium ascorbate before bed.

Magnesium ZMK

Magnesium ZMK is a great form of magnesium that uses magnesium from several compounds in the Krebs cycle: citrate, fumarate, malate, succinate, and alpha-ketoglutarate. ZMK is great for athletes because it promotes recovery. A ZMK supplement should be taken before bed.

Magnesium Fumarate, Succinate, Alpha-ketoglutarate

See magnesium ZMK.

Magnesium Gluconate

Magnesium gluconate is a form of magnesium that is chelated with gluconic acid. Gluconic acid is produced from the fermentation of glucose. Magnesium gluconate has above average absorption in the body (better than magnesium citrate), but may cause loose stools. Take magnesium gluconate before bed.

Magnesium with Special Uses

Magnesium Citrate

Magnesium citrate is effective for bowel irrigation. It is also one of the most produced forms of magnesium in the supplementation industry. It causes some loose stools, and its absorption is average. Magnesium citrate should be taken with meals because the bound citric acid will slightly increase stomach pH. Citrate may interfere with ceruloplasmin.

Magnesium Orotate

Magnesium orotate is one least known forms of magnesium, but if you just had surgery or exercise constantly then this form will help with recovery. The bounded orotate will help muscle regeneration. Take magnesium orotate only for a short period because excessive orotate consumption will increase uric acid levels. Women should not use magnesium orotate if they are or are trying to become pregnant since it may be mutagenic (only found as a possibility in rats in vivo). Take magnesium orotate at bedtime.

Magnesium L-threonate

Magnesium L-threonate may greatly increase magnesium concentrations in the brain and spinal column for increased cognitive function. L-Threonate is an isomer of ascorbic acid, and new research has shown that it increases magnesium levels at about the same rate as magnesium sulfate. The main problem with using magnesium sulfate to increase magnesium levels in the brain is that sulfate should not be taken orally; sulfate mainly should be given though IV's or used topically, so it is harder to use to increase concentration. Take magnesium L-threonate at bedtime.

Magnesium 2-AEP

Magnesium 2-AEP is a form of magnesium that is chelated with phosphorylethanolamine, which is a vital component of the structure and integrity of cell membranes. Magnesium 2-AEP has been theorized to help people with MS because it helps cellular function, integrity, and helps protect the myelin in the brain. It has also been shown to suppress the immune system, so supplement with caution for long periods. Take magnesium 2-AEP with meals during the day.

Magnesium Peroxide

Magnesium Peroxide is only to be used as a colon cleanser. Take magnesium peroxide before bed.

Magnesium Phos 6X

Normally I do not recommend homeopathic supplements (if they work for some people I'm glad they do, but I would rather recommend nutraceuticals), but for homeopathic minerals, I feel they still can be beneficial because some of the trace mineral should still be left in the product. I would recommend using this remedy for anyone who is extremely sensitive to all forms of magnesium supplementation. If magnesium glycinate use still causes loose stools and magnesium chloride causes dermatological reactions, then this is the magnesium form for you to try. Magnesium phos contains some phosphorus so I would recommend if you have kidney problems to stay away from it. Taken before bed.

Magnesium Carbonate

Magnesium carbonate has one of lowest levels of assimilation of any of the magnesium chelations and is only used as a good osmotic laxative and antacid. Take magnesium carbonate at bedtime or if you have heartburn.

Magnesium Hydroxide

Magnesium hydroxide is poorly absorbed, and most of the magnesium in the supplement is released into the bowels. Most commercial preparations (milk of magnesia) have sodium hypochlorite (bleach) added so avoid those. Take magnesium hydroxide at bedtime for the laxative effects. Magnesium hydroxide also works as a great deodorant.

Magnesium Forms You Should Avoid

The following forms of magnesium either do damage in the body or are very poorly absorbed.

Magnesium Yeast Chelate

Magnesium yeast chelate is a "natural" form of magnesium that is claimed to be very easily assimilated by the body. What would possibly be wrong with recommending the chelation you may ask? Magnesium yeast is found in most of your "natural" vitamins including New Chapter, Garden of Life, and Megafood.

The main problem I have with this form of magnesium is that you have to ingest a lot of brewer's yeast (which some people are sensitive to) in the whole supplement to only get a tiny amount of magnesium. Most vitamins that use this form of magnesium have microscopic amounts of magnesium in their multivitamin (less than 100 mg elemental) or magnesium supplement. There are just a lot better options for magnesium supplementation out there.

Magnesium Aspartate

Excess aspartic acid is neurotoxic. ZMA supplements fall into this category, as well.

Magnesium Pidolate (Magnesium 5-oxo proline)

The excess glutamic acid in this supplement may be excitotoxic and neurotoxic if your glutamic acid pathways are hindered (upper gut overgrowth or GAD1 mutation).

Magnesium Oxide

Magnesium oxide is very poorly absorbed. Out of 400 mg, the body under ideal circumstances absorbs only eighty mg of elemental magnesium.

Magnesium Glycerophosphate

Magnesium glycerophosphate is chelated with phosphorus. The problem is that most people get too much phosphate in their diet. People with kidney problems should also stay away from this supplement because it is harder for them to eliminate excess phosphates.

Magnesium Lactate

Magnesium lactate should not be used by people who have kidney disease because the bound lactic acid causes more complications for the kidneys. There is no reason to take this form of magnesium at all; extra lactic acid is not good for anyone.

Magnesium Amounts in Food

Magnesium should always be supplemented because even if you eat a perfect diet, you will still have to eat a ton of nuts, brown rice, avocados, and spinach daily to keep from developing a deficiency. To take in around 400 mg a day, you would have to eat one cup of cooked spinach (157 mg), an ounce of pumpkin seeds (150 mg), an avocado (56 mg), and a cup of cooked brown rice (86 mg) a day on average (449 mg of magnesium total). These amounts also do not take into account the magnesium that is bonded to phytic acid in the pumpkin seeds, the brown rice, and that individual intestinal absorption of magnesium that is different for everyone.

Suppose you ate all of this food on a daily basis. You will only absorb 300 mg of magnesium from the food under ideal circumstances. Imagine if you had to take in 1,000 mg of magnesium daily. You would have to intake three cups of cooked spinach, three ounces of pumpkin seeds, three avocados, and three cups of brown rice throughout the day. Good luck!

Since ancient man did not take in much magnesium through food as much as modern man, why do we need to supplement it at all or in such large amounts? One theory is ancient water had a much higher mineral content and the water that ancient man consumed, therefore, had a higher concentration of magnesium. The plants, nuts, and animal meat and bones that ancient man consumed had a higher magnesium content because of unleached soil due to over farming. In addition, ancient man probably encountered fewer toxins and had less stress to deal with; this means they suffered from less magnesium wasting overall, as well.

The amount of magnesium absorbed by food, or supplements requires you to have a good functional digestive system. If you are suffering from poor digestion, the amount of magnesium you absorb from food will be limited. I would recommend eating food rich in magnesium such as spinach, avocado, and pumpkin seeds while you are supplementing with magnesium.

Food	Magnesium
Pumpkin Seeds - 1/4 cup	191 mg
Spinach - one cup cooked	157 mg
Swiss Chard - one cup cooked	151 mg
Sesame Seeds - 1/4 cup	126 mg
Halibut - four oz.	121 mg
Black Beans - one cup cooked	120 mg
Brown Rice - one cup Cooked	84 mg
Tuna - four oz.	73 mg
Scallops - four oz.	62 mg
Avocado - one cup	42 mg
Shrimp - four oz.	28 mg
Broccoli - one cup	19 mg
Cucumber - one cup	14 mg

Amount of Magnesium per Serving

Remember: Because of phytic acid levels, magnesium might not be as bioavailable in the body in food including beans, nuts, and seeds. For example, pumpkin seeds are high in magnesium, but the magnesium binds to the phytic acid, which blocks its absorption.

Elemental Magnesium

The supplementation dosage suggested in this chapter pertains to elemental magnesium. A supplement will usually have both the total amount of magnesium and the amount of its chelation on the front of the supplement. The elemental magnesium amount is found on the nutrition label. Elemental magnesium is the amount of actual magnesium you are getting when you take a supplement.

If the front of the supplement claims that four capsules are 2,000 mg of magnesium malate, and the back of the supplement states that you are getting 400 mg of magnesium, the 400 mg is the elemental amount of magnesium you will assimilate from the supplement. You also receive 1,600 mg of malic acid when you ingest the supplement as well. So out of that 2,000 mg of magnesium malate, 1,600 mg is made up of malic acid, and the other 400 mg of it is the elemental magnesium in the supplement.

Oral Magnesium Supplementation

Elemental magnesium's pH is neutral, but magnesium's pH changes depending on its chelation. If magnesium is chelated to an acid or a chelation that stimulates the production of HCL in the stomach, it needs to be taken with food. Magnesium that is bounded with an alkaline chelation should be either used as an antacid or taken before bed so not to hinder digestion. For this reason, I have broken up the different forms, and if they should be taken before bed or with a meal.

The general magnesium protocol for someone that weighs between one and two hundred pounds:

- Elemental magnesium – 800 mg for four to six months. Then, 600 mg daily thereafter.

If you weigh less than one hundred pounds:

- Elemental magnesium – 600 mg for two months, and then 400 mg thereafter.

The above recommendation is not the optimal amount of magnesium that anyone should take daily, but is a good standard protocol for you to follow.

The amount of magnesium you should supplement with is based on your weight. The average basis for good magnesium cellular saturation is between 10 – 14 mg per kilogram a day. The ideal magnesium intake for someone who is 200 pounds is about 1,000 mg - 1,400 mg of elemental magnesium daily for about four to six months until their magnesium levels are balanced. This number should be increased by 200 mg in times of elevated stress.

If you have loose stools at high levels of supplementation, then you should switch to supplementing with magnesium glycinate. If you continue to have loose stools with only glycinate supplementation, then you might need a mix of oral and transdermal to help increase your magnesium levels. Finally, if you are still having issues with magnesium sensitivity then a homeopathic magnesium supplement might be needed (follow the supplement instructions; the dosage of this supplement is not dependent on weight).

Proper kidney function is needed to excrete excess magnesium. If you have kidney disease, your renal function, and magnesium concentration levels should frequently be tested when on a magnesium protocol.

Transdermal Magnesium Supplementation

Transdermal magnesium can be very important if you want to raise the plasma levels of magnesium in your body quickly. Oral magnesium supplementation takes six to ten months to raise your magnesium levels to a normal range.

Transdermal supplementation, on the other hand, takes only three to four months. Taking Epsom salt baths twice a day can be one way to increase transdermal supplementation.

The best way to use transdermal magnesium is to use a magnesium gel-like MagneGel. MagneGel delivers approximately 150 mg of elemental magnesium per 1/4 teaspoon to the skin. I would suggest applying 900 - 1,200 mg transdermal daily for about four months. You can base the transdermal supplementation guidelines on the same oral weight recommendations that were listed above. If you weigh more than two hundred pounds, you will need to increase the amount you supplement.

Both Oral and Transdermal Supplementation

Another option is to use both oral and transdermal supplementation. I would take 600 mg of elemental oral magnesium daily, and use MagneGel once or twice a day if you weigh close to 200 pounds. This way, you would get around 1,000 - 1,400 mg of total magnesium intake a day. Follow this regimen for four months and then retest magnesium levels. Using both transdermal magnesium and oral magnesium may reduce oral absorption; this is why it is important to increase oral supplementation during the protocol.

Magnesium Dosage Based on Weight and Sex Recommendations

Remember, the amount of magnesium you should supplement depends on your weight. The basis for good magnesium cellular saturation is 14 mg per kilogram daily.

All of these magnesium dose recommendations are for someone that weighs roughly two hundred pounds (1,000 - 1,400 mg daily). If you only weigh a hundred pounds, I would divide the total magnesium intake daily to around 600 – 800 mg of magnesium daily to increase magnesium levels. If you weigh more than 350 pounds, you might want to increase daily magnesium intake to about 1,800 - 2,200 mg daily, as long as you have normal kidney function.

Women who are ovulating might want to increase their magnesium by about 150-200 mg daily when they are menstruating. Women who are pregnant might want to go more conservative on their dosages and take no more than 600 mg daily to be safe.

Building Magnesium Levels, When to Test, and Maintenance Dosage

Before supplementing with magnesium, it is prudent to have an EXA test or an RBC test performed. If your magnesium is low, then follow the recommendations from the guide above. Follow the chart below to determine how long you should supplement with magnesium.

Body's Stored Magnesium Levels	Magnesium Supplementation Type	Length of Average Supplementation
Very Low	Oral	10-12 Months
Very Low	Transdermal	6-8 Months
Very Low	Both	5-6 Months
Low	Oral	6-8 Months
Low	Transdermal	3-4 Months
Low	Both	2-3 Months
Average	Oral	4-6 Months
Average	Transdermal	2-3 Months
Average	Both	1-2 Months

Length of Average Magnesium Supplementation

If your magnesium levels are healthy, you should take daily supplementation of 400 - 600 mg elemental magnesium daily. Even if your magnesium levels are normal, and you have a specific, medical reason to increase your magnesium above these levels (chronic fatigue syndrome, nerve damage, and brain trauma, etc). You should be fine to increase supplementation as long as you have normal kidney function. You will need to get your magnesium levels frequently tested (every 2-3 months), to make sure hypermagnesemia does not occur.

Finally, if your magnesium levels are extremely low, IV magnesium supplementation might be needed on an emergency basis.

Hypermagnesemia

Hypermagnesemia is a rare condition in which a person has too much magnesium in their blood plasma. Hypermagnesemia usually does not occur in people that take supplemental magnesium, but it can occur if the person has impaired kidney function. IV magnesium bypasses the body's digestion entropy and has a greater chance of leading to overdose. In vivo, the body has many mechanisms in place to prevent an overdose from supplemental magnesium.

Diagnostic symptoms are usually a combination of low blood sugar and high calcium. Symptoms usually include weakness, vomiting, impaired breathing, hypotension, increased blood calcium levels, arrhythmia, lack of muscle reflexes, and bradycardia (slow heart rate). It is rare but possible that if one's plasma magnesium level is too high, the heart could stop, causing a "heart attack."

Treatment for hypermagnesemia includes giving IV calcium gluconate to inactivate free magnesium through a binding process. The calcium also reactivates the muscle cells because calcium is a muscle stimulator. Finally, dialysis might be needed in some cases to eliminate excess magnesium, and to help with kidney function.

Recommended Brands of Magnesium

- Best Glycinate: Pure Encapsulations magnesium glycinate
- Best Malate: Jigsaw magnesium malate / Other Recommendations: Now magnesium malate, Jarrow Formulas Magnesium Optimizer malate, Source Naturals magnesium malate
- Best Citrate: Natural Calm / Other Recommendations: Pure Encapsulations magnesium citrate, Now magnesium citrate, Source Naturals magnesium citrate
- Best Chloride: Trace Minerals Research ionic magnesium
- Best Peroxide: New Earth Oxy-C magnesium peroxide
- Best Ascorbate: Now magnesium ascorbate powder
- Best Orotate: Advanced Research magnesium orotate
- Best Taurate: Cardiovascular Research magnesium taurate
- Best Dermal Magnesium: Designs for Health MagneGel
- Best Magnesium Sulfate: Epsoak epsom salt, Kirkman magnesium sulfate cream
- Best 2AEP: Advanced Research 2AEP magnesium
- Best Arginate: Advanced Research Magnesium Arginate with Aspartate (It is the only one I can find, but it does have aspartate in it, use sparingly)
- Best Lysinate: Doctor's Best high absorption magnesium

- Best Magnesium L-Threonate: Life Extension magnesium L-threonate / Other Recommendation: Jarrow Formulas MagMind
- Best Magnesium "Blend": Solaray vegan magnesium / Other Recommendation: Source Naturals Ultra Mag
- Best Magnesium for Athletes: ZMK supplement

Chapter 11

All About Zinc!

Quite a few people ask me if they could only afford one supplement for stomach discomfort (ulcers, *H. pylori* infection, or gastritis suffers) which supplement would I recommend to them for their troubles? If I had to choose one digestive supplement that could handle those multiple stomach issues and more, it would be zinc carnosine. Zinc carnosine is a supplement that is the chelation of the mineral zinc with the amino acid carnosine.

Zinc is an essential trace mineral that can decrease wound healing time and is also important for maintaining the integrity of the immune system. The immune system uses zinc to help develop and maintain the function of neutrophils, macrophages, killer cells, and B/T cells. Zinc is also a crucial component in the production of the antioxidant enzyme CuZnSOD. Copper and zinc combine with the superoxide dismutase enzyme to produce CuZnSOD. CuZnSOD is a chelated enzyme that has both strong antioxidant and anti-inflammatory properties. Zinc, in studies, has also been known to shorten the duration of childhood diarrhea. It is theorized that zinc increases immune function and toxin elimination.

Finally, zinc is used in the body in the production of testosterone (limits the DHEA aromatization into estrogen), growth hormones, and insulin-like growth factor-1. Zinc is a very important supplement in their daily lives, so I recommend taking 30 mg Now L-Opti zinc daily, to ensure proper hormone regulation.

Forms of Zinc

Recommended Forms of Zinc

Zinc L-monomethionine

Zinc L-monomethionine is the form of zinc that I recommend the most (yes, even more than zinc glycinate). Zinc L-monomethionine is a highly absorbed form of zinc with multiple benefits. Zinc L-monomethionine is highly absorbed because it is bounded with the l isomer of methionine. Methionine is an essential amino acid, which means your body cannot produce this amino acid, and it must be supplemented through the diet. Methionine has two isomers (isomers are molecules with the same molecular formula, but different chemical structures) D and L. The D isomer is synthetic and is created during supplement production. The L isomer is natural and is what the body recognizes as methionine. Therefore, the L isomer has a higher absorption. The extra methionine provided by the zinc supplement is used in the body to make cysteine, carnitine, taurine, lecithin, SAM-e, and phosphatidylcholine.

Methionine, when converted into SAM-e eventually degrades into a byproduct known as homocysteine (excess homocysteine has been linked to being a possible factor in developing heart disease). Homocysteine then is immediately inactivated and turned into either the amino acid cysteine or methionine in the body before any damage can be done as long as adequate B12 and glycine are provided. Methionine is beneficial to the body in supplemental form as long as you take a good B vitamin complex or take a supplement that contains the amino acid glycine. I recommend the Optizinc brand of L-methionine supplements.

Zinc Glycinate

Zinc Glycinate is a zinc supplement that is chelated with the amino acid glycine. Glycine reduces anxiety in the body and promotes a feeling of well-being. Check your supplement to see if the glycinate chelate in your supplement is made from the TRAACS Albion process of manufacturing chelates (the supplement should have the TRAACS or Albion logo). Choose a glycinate product that uses TRAACS so you can get the best quality glycinate available.

Zinc Monomethionine

Zinc monomethionine is the brother of Zinc L-monomethionine and also has great absorption. Zinc monomethionine is not absorbed as well in the human body compared to L-Methionine because it contains both of the D and L isomers. When using this supplement a B vitamin complex supplement or glycine supplement may be needed as well to help with absorption and monomethionine regulation. I recommend the Optizinc brand of monomethionine supplements.

Zinc Picolinate

Zinc picolinate is a zinc supplement that is chelated with picolinic acid. Picolinic acid is a compound that is an isomer of niacin and is a carbolite of the amino acid tryptophan. Zinc picolinate has superior absorption, and picolinate absorption is superior to even gluconate chelates.

ZMK

ZMK is a great form of zinc that uses compounds from the Krebs cycle also bonded to magnesium including citrate, fumarate, malate, succinate and alpha-ketoglutarate. ZMK is great for athletes because it speeds up recovery. A ZMK supplement should be taken before bed.

Zinc Gluconate

Zinc gluconate is a form of zinc that is chelated with gluconic acid which occurs from the natural fermentation of glucose. Zinc gluconate has above average absorption in the body. Zinc gluconate is the type of zinc that is found in products like throat lozenges and nasal spray that are used to shorten the duration of the common cold. The zinc gluconate nasal sprays have been linked to permanent loss of the sense of smell in some people and should be avoided.

Zinc Orotate

Like magnesium orotate, zinc orotate is one of the least known forms of supplemental zinc. The extra orotate will help with muscle regeneration and repair. Women should avoid it if they are or are trying to become pregnant since it may be mutagenic (only found as a possibility in rats in vivo, and rats are biologically different than humans. Therefore, zinc orotate might be safe after all).

Avoid These Forms of Zinc

Zinc Oxide

Zinc oxide has a poor absorption rate in the human body. Zinc oxide's poor absorption properties are why it is used as a sunscreen and a skin protectant. I only recommend the use of zinc oxide skin care products, but limit the products made with nano zinc oxide which can be absorbed and nano zinc oxide safety has not been fully studied yet.

Zinc Aspartate

Aspartic acid is neurotoxic. This recommendation includes ZMA supplements.

Zinc Citrate

Zinc citrate is zinc chelated with citric acid. Zinc citrate has average absorption and increases stomach acid levels. An animal study showed that the citric acid in the zinc citrate supplement could offset some of the absorption problems if the zinc supplement is taken with a meal high in phytic acid. Excess citric acid may hinder ceruloplasmin production by the body.

Zinc Pyrithione

Zinc pyrithione is often used in anti-dandruff shampoos. Its mechanism of action for eliminating yeast is the disruption of the membrane transport by blocking the proton pump that energizes the transport chain. Zinc pyrithione can cause irritation and allergies, and its use should be limited to topical use only.

Carnosine

Carnosine is both an amino acid and an antioxidant. Most carnosine in the diet comes from the ingestion of red meat. Carnosine is believed to protect the organs from oxidative stress and advanced glycation end products (AGEs). AGEs are produced during the breakdown of glucose, fructose, and galactose by the body for assimilation. Excess AGEs that are produced in the body have been linked to a wide range of diseases from diabetes, cardiovascular disease, and Alzheimer's disease. Sadly, the amount of carnosine in most zinc carnosine supplements is tiny and is broken down easily by the enzyme carnosinase, so the effects of the supplemental carnosine would be minimal.

Zinc Carnosine

Zinc binds quickly to stomach tissue if taken on an empty stomach. If zinc is taken on an empty stomach, it can cause severe stomach pain and gastritis. It has been theorized that zinc ions are highly soluble in stomach acid and have corrosive, antimicrobial, and immune stimulating properties that irritate the stomach tissue because of the direct absorption of the zinc ions. If you chelate zinc with carnosine, the chelation slows down the absorption and elimination of zinc from the stomach. Zinc is then able to repair the stomach and intestinal tissue without irritating it so zinc carnosine may be taken on an empty stomach as needed. Zinc carnosine also protects the stomach lining from an opportunistic *H. pylori* infection, and NSAID damage that causes ulcers that can come from the long-term use of the medication.

Supplemental Restrictions and Toxicity

High doses of zinc carnosine cause zinc toxicity and lower immune system functioning over time. Symptoms of zinc toxicity include nausea, vomiting, abdominal pain, frequent colds, increased cholesterol levels, and chills. If I had to take a maximum dose of zinc carnosine, I would take no more than 450 mg of zinc carnosine (one hundred mg of elemental zinc) a day total for two weeks. Most supplement instructions recommend taking zinc carnosine twice a day for a total of seventy-five mg of zinc carnosine daily (fifteen mg of elemental zinc).

If you supplement with zinc, I would recommend no more than sixty mg of elemental zinc daily. If you supplement with sixty mg of zinc, I will suggest that as long as you did not suffer from adrenal fatigue that you should supplement with two mg of Pure Encapsulations copper glycinate daily. Zinc and copper influence one another in the body and a good supplementation ratio are for every fifteen mg of zinc, one mg of copper is needed (15:1 ratio).

Excessive copper buildup and toxicity make adrenal fatigue symptoms worse, so limit copper intake during zinc supplementation until adrenals have healed. Zinc carnosine is one of my top three favorite digestive health supplements; everyone should keep a bottle in their medicine cabinet so they can take it when needed.

Zinc Supplement Recommendations

- Recommended Zinc Carnosine Supplement (It is also what I take daily): Peptic Z/C, Other Recommendations: Doctor's Best Pepzin GI, Enzymedica Acid Soothe
- Recommended Form of Zinc L-methionine: Now L-Opti zinc
- Recommended Form of Zinc Glycinate: Numedica zinc glycinate / Other Recommendation: Now Foods zinc glycinate
- Recommended Form of Zinc Monomethionine: Life Extension Opti zinc / Other Recommendation: Zinc Balance
- Recommended Form of Zinc Picolinate: Zinc picolinate
- Recommended Form of Zinc Citrate: Pure Encapsulations zinc citrate / Other Recommendations: Thorne Research zinc citrate
- Recommended Form of Zinc Gluconate: Pure Formulas Liquid Zinc Gluconate
- Recommended Form of Zinc Orotate: Advanced Research Labs zinc orotate

Chapter 12

Lower the pH of Your Stomach

Lowered stomach acid production, or increased stomach pH, facilitates overgrowth of pathogens and protein fermentation and malabsorption, which increases gastric pressure and causes stomach distension. I know that is counter to everything you have heard from mainstream medicine. Most people are told that they have too much stomach acid, which causes GERD. You see advertisements all the time on television for acid reducing medication like PPI's. You know the commercials with Larry The Cable Guy telling you if you take a PPI you can eat a million hot dogs, ride four wheelers, and not suffer any GERD. Betaine HCL supplementation improves GERD symptoms for most people compared to PPI use, yet PPI's are advertised everywhere.

The primary cause of GERD is not increased stomach acid but instead is from elevated gastric pressure. For GERD to occur, the LES (lower esophageal sphincter) has to be weakened, increase gastric pressure has to force stomach acid and pepsin into the esophagus, and uncontrolled excessive inflammation has to happen. Generally, throughout the day we reflux occasionally, from esophageal pressure changes, swallowing, and consuming of food. That being said, for most people our esophagus can easily handle the reflux episodes and inflammation. For others, they cannot, and they develop reflux conditions like GERD.

So How Does Low Stomach Acid Production / Elevated Stomach pH Cause GERD?

Lowered stomach acid production facilitates overgrowth of pathogens, protein fermentation, and malabsorption, which increase gastric pressure and stomach distension. The increase in gastric pressure and stomach pressure weakens the LES and causes GERD.

Stomach acid is produced by our stomach to help limit pathogen overgrowth, digest protein, activate digestive enzymes, signal an increase in mucin production in the stomach, and increase absorption of B12 later in the gastrointestinal tract (intrinsic factor). So without proper stomach acid production, what happens to our digestion?

Microorganism overgrowth eventually occurs and leads to further digestive issues. Protein that is maldigested influences the microbiome, leading to overgrowth producing excessive amounts of hydrogen gas, causing distension, esophageal pressure changes, and LES weakness. Protein is broken down ineffectively from lack of stomach acid, causing excessive protein fermentation from overgrowth leading to increased hydrogen gas production and distension. Upper gut bacteria are also able to use glucose from our food as a source of fuel and increase hydrogen production leading to stomach distension. A hiatal hernia may eventually develop from worsening stomach distension increasing further pressure on the LES and esophagus. The increased pressure would further weaken the LES and worsen GERD.

Overgrowth in the stomach and esophagus may lead to reduced probiotic *Akkermansia muciniphila* colonization in the upper gut, which combined with reduced stomach acid production result in a reduction of mucosal barrier health in the stomach and esophagus. Increased endotoxin production from Gram-negative overgrowth can increase inflammation in the stomach, causing gastritis, and increase inflammation in the esophagus, causing the symptoms of GERD. The esophagus is also able to produce limited quantities of bicarbonate (using carbonic anhydrase) to protect itself from reflux; its capacity is reduced if repeated reflux events are occurring. The worsening combination of increased inflammation (endogenous cytokines and chemical injury) from constant refluxing (due to increased gastric pressure) into the esophagus, reduction of mucosal integrity, and endotoxin inflammation causes the symptoms of GERD from excessive esophageal inflammation.

All of these issues occur from decreased stomach acid production. Most people are then prescribed PPI's which reduce stomach acid further (the less stomach acid for a time, the less chemical injury to the esophagus). For a while, inflammation in the esophagus and stomach is reduced from a lack of chemical reflux. Overgrowth worsens over time and eventually, from increased inflammation, GERD symptoms occur again, for some stronger than ever and the cycle repeats itself. The PPI dosage is increased, symptoms abate, then later return worse than ever until the PPI's dose is maxed out. A truly vicious cycle.

Betaine HCL, Does it Improve Digestion?

Betaine HCL might improve digestion, but there is not much diagnostic information available that shows taking betaine HCL reduces stomach pH and increases stomach acid production, but we do have promise. We do have an excellent study that measures gastric re-acidification using betaine HCL to try to improve the absorption of certain medications that require proper stomach acid for the breakdown. Prior studies have shown that absorption of certain drugs depend on stomach acid which explains why some medications like ketoconazole or antibiotics are recommended not to be taken with antacids. In a prior study, people taking the PPI omeprazole were given Coca-cola (pH of 2.5) and ketoconazole to see if it would increase absorption of the medication, which it did.

In the study, volunteers were given the PPI rabeprazole for five days, and their gastric pH was monitored throughout the study using Heidelberg pH capsules. The pH of the stomach was more alkaline in most of the volunteers who took the PPI for five days. When the volunteers in the study took 1,500 mg of betaine HCL, their stomach pH decreased to around one for more than an hour with no noted side effects. In people with healthy digestion, this level of stomach pH frequently occurs when we ingest our meals. Also, it did appear that at least short term use of betaine HCL does not create a negative feedback loop of decreased gastrin production leading to reduced production of stomach acid, marked by standard blood gastrin tests results during the study.

In people with low stomach acid levels, the use of betaine HCL in the short term can help decrease stomach pH, reduce overgrowth, and improve protein digestion. It is still best (until we get more data on long term gastric acid negative feedback loop and betaine HCL use) to improve endogenous stomach acid production by supplementing with bitter herbs like gentian and ingesting enough pure salt (chloride is used to make HCL). If you have ulcers or severe gastritis supplementation with betaine HCL should be done with caution to prevent worsening of symptoms. Finally, in people with *H. pylori* overgrowth increasing stomach acid production may cause severe inflammation from increased endotoxin and ammonia production from *H. pylori* and increased burrowing of the bacteria into the mucosal barrier. Use with caution in systemic stomach overgrowth, or if you have ulcers / gastritis. Supplementation with zinc carnosine, l-carnitine, and activated charcoal may reduce these issues.

Betaine HCL Protocol

The protocol for taking betaine HCL is simple and can improve your digestion. Start out with two capsules taken during a meal. If you feel like you have severe gastritis or feel pain, stop immediately! If your heartburn is worse, continue to increase the dose by one capsule every day for a week to see if it improves; if not, discontinue the betaine HCL. Increase the dosage of betaine HCL with every meal by one capsule until you feel a slight warm feeling in your stomach. The next meal, take one capsule less and continue taking the same dosage until you get that warm feeling again, then continue to decrease the dosage. Never take more than fourteen capsules in one meal. If you get severe gastritis or pain, consume 1/2 teaspoon of baking soda mixed well first in a glass of filtered water to buffer the pH for relief, and then consult with your gastroenterologist.

Premier Labs betaine HCL without pepsin is the brand I recommend. If you cannot order it, consider using Doctor's Best betaine HCL with pepsin and gentian.

Pepsin is the main enzyme used by the stomach to digest protein. Pepsinogen activates and converts into the enzyme pepsin in the presence of stomach acid. Pepsin helps break down protein into amino acids the body can absorb and then becomes inactivated, by turning back into pepsinogen when it is mixed with bicarbonate released from the pancreas in the small intestine. This transformation protects the rest of the intestinal system from the pepsin and stomach acid. If you have silent reflux, pepsin is your main issue, and you want to avoid supplements with the enzyme. Some people also have adverse reactions to porcine based pepsin but can tolerate betaine HCL without it.

Lower stomach pH will ensure that the stomach microbiome is kept in balance, and protein digestion improves!

Apple Cider Vinegar

To help reduce the pH of the stomach if you have a less acidic stomach (pH of 4) take a teaspoon of organic apple cider vinegar with the mother in a glass of warm non-chlorinated water ten minutes before a meal. Drink with a straw so tooth enamel is not damaged. Do not use if you are suffering from severe esophageal inflammation or gastritis. The low pH of the ACV may aggreviate the tissue and cause pain and or burning.

Chapter 13

Probiotic, Prebiotic, and HSO Guide

Probiotics are live organisms that may have a health benefit to the host organism. Bacteria and yeast both compose the human gut flora and exist in many other parts of the body too. You have more bacteria living on and in your body now then you do other cells!

Probiotic Bacteria vs. Opportunistic Bacteria Theory

Bacteria in the gut maintain proper gastrointestinal function, break down lactase, and manufacture and absorb vitamin K, vitamin B12, thiamine, riboflavin, and biotin. Probiotic bacteria also keep in check or even destroy opportunistic bacteria, and help ferment carbohydrates for digestion in the large intestine. Digestion probiotics are mainly found in the large intestine and can become opportunistic bacteria if they are transplanted into the small intestine, which causes a condition called SIBO. This can usually happen if the mucus lining of the intestines is disrupted or if antibiotics leaving the surviving bacteria to become opportunistic eliminate most of the probiotics in the intestines. This occurs because the intestine's natural balance of probiotic bacteria has shifted.

All probiotics, given the chance, become opportunistic bacteria and cause intestinal infections. This can occur if the conditions are just right in the intestines and their numbers are numerous. If probiotic bacteria do not maintain a proper balance in the intestines, health problems usually arise. Opportunistic bacteria can be either probiotic bacteria that become infectious because of different circumstances or foreign bacteria that are exposed to its host and become infectious. An infection of opportunistic bacteria in the gut only happens if someone is in a critical health crisis, has been given a drug to disrupt intestinal health or immune system function, or has an immune system lowering condition. Caution needs to be observed when supplementing probiotics (the proper amount and type needed) so that the chance of opportunistic infections are kept to a minimum. Nonetheless, for the average person, probiotics are still very important to help relieve digestive ailments / disorders.

Probiotics are found in the natural gut flora of humans. For most HSO's it is unknown if they are part of the natural gut flora in humans. HSO's are bacteria that are found in soil. If you add, HSO's to your gut, they will both attempt to assimilate or become opportunistic and wreak havoc in your intestines. Some HSO's are more harmless than others are and may work together with probiotic bacteria. I still cannot recommend any HSO because very few of them currently are 100% proven to be part of natural human gut flora. If they were, it would make the HSO's probiotics instead.

Different Strains of HSO's

Bacillus coagulans

Bacillus coagulans is a Gram-positive, rod-shaped, endospore forming, L-lactate producing bacteria. *B. coagulans* can survive stomach and bile acids and pass through into the colon. It is truly unknown like most HSO's if it would germinate and become flora in the intestinal tract without constant ingestion. The reported benefits of taking *B. coagulans* and most spore-forming probiotics themselves might come from the ingestion of spores and the immune regulating reaction to them, instead of them germinating and colonizing the gut. Finally, *B. coagulans* possibly even when it germinates may only reside in the gastrointestinal tract for a few days before it is eliminated from the body (similar to the transient probiotic properties of *S. boulardii*).

Bacillus coagulans was originally misidentified as *Lactobacillus sporogenes* when it was discovered in the early 1930's. There is still a debate about the correct genus of the bacteria between probiotic supplement manufacturers and microbiologists. One study about the debate states:

"In any case, the use of the term Lactobacillus sporogenes seems to aim to deliberately confound consumers, trying to benefit from association with the extensive literature on the safety and health benefits of the genus Lactobacillus"

The author of the study also brings up similar concerns I have about fully recommending *B. coagulans*:

"For this reason the use of the wrong nomenclature of L. sporogenes becomes once more questionable, since it seems to try to get advantage from the old tradition of safety of lactobacilli to remedy to the lack of safety reports on B. coagulans."

The conclusion of the report is that probiotic companies that mislabel *B. coagulans* as *L. sporogenes* are doing it for their advantage since the reclassification of the bacteria occurred a long time ago, and anyone who is selling a probiotic product should know about correct nomenclature for safety.

However, here are some possible positives about *B. coagulans* if it colonizes the gut:

- Lower inflammatory responses.
- Produces bacteriocins (hopefully, it reduces opportunistic, not probiotic growth).
- Reduces opportunistic biofilm.
- Produces the SCFA butyric acid from carbohydrate fermentation.
- Lowers intestinal pH by producing L-lactate (instead of the problem causing D-lactate).
- May reduce *Klebsiella* overgrowth and rheumatoid arthritis symptoms.
- Survives stomach and bile acids.
- Relieves diarrhea and gastroenteritis.

- Increases probiotic colonies of *Faecalibacterium prausnitzii*.

So my main issue with Bacillus coagulans much like any probiotic is the question, "Is there enough science to back up the claims to improve your digestive health?" Maybe, but more studies will be needed.

Is it known to cause infection? Currently, compared to other *Bacillus* HSO's, no.

Does it have the risk of it developing opportunistic capability (horizontal gene transfer for example)? Yes, but unlikely.

Is it properly labeled and uncontaminated? Depends on the individual strain and the supplement, this is a risk with all probiotic supplements. However, the risk is greater with HSO's.

Is it normal flora? No.

I need more information before I can fully recommend *B. coagulans*. One study however on its safety mentions:

"In conclusion, the studies described in this paper were conducted as a comprehensive safety assessment of GanedenBC30™, a commercially available probiotic strain of B. coagulans. As part of a pre-clinical safety evaluation program, several tests have been performed. GanedenBC30™ demonstrated no evidence to suggest mutagenicity or genotoxicity in a number of commonly utilized genetic toxicity assays. No treatment-related mortality, morbidity or clinical symptoms resulted from an acute oral toxicity study using a single dose of 5000 mg/kg. In a subchronic oral toxicity study, GanedenBC30™ in daily doses of 100, 300 and 1000 mg/kg bw/day for 90 days was well tolerated and did not cause either lethality or toxic clinical symptoms in either male or female rats. The NOAEL derived from the results of the 90-day study is 1000 mg/kg. Since the concentration of the B. coagulans used was 1.36×10^{11} CFUs/g, this corresponds to 1.36×10^{11} CFUs/kg. For an average 70 kg human being, this corresponds to 95.2×10^{11} CFUs. Because the suggested human dose is in the range of 100×10^{6} to 3×10^{9} CFUs, this gives a safety factor ranging from 3173 to 95,200 times. Based upon scientific procedures and supported by history of use, GanedenBC30™ is considered safe for chronic human consumption."

Granted some of the studies were disclosed as being sponsored in some fashion by the largest producer of *Bacillus coagulans*, Ganeden Biotech, so there may be some conflict of interest even though it was disclosed and none were listed. Either the HSO for research was supplied by them, or some of the people listed as working on the study were employed by the company. More studies in the future need to be made without their involvement.

In conclusion, I can not fully recommend *B. coagulans* yet as a probiotic. I will list some recommendations for supplements that you can use that contain it, but I will not use affiliate links because I do not recommend it completely.

- Seeking Health – Bacillus coagulans probiotic
- Thorne – Bacillus coagulans probiotic
- Vital Proteins – collagen with probiotic

Bacillus licheniformis

Bacillus licheniformis is one of the worst offending soil based "probiotics" and is known to cause food poisoning, septicemia, peritonitis, and ophthalmitis. *Bacillus licheniformis* is not native human flora but appears to be native flora in birds. *Bacillus licheniformis* is a ubiquitous organism and likely enters the human digestive system many times a day. While data regarding its ability to survive in the human gastrointestinal tract is sparse, it is likely that the spores pass without activating.

Bacillus licheniformis is known to cause spontaneous abortions in cattle and sheep as well as contaminate dairy (a cause of food poisoning) with toxins produced from the animals from ingestion of spoilage. *B. licheniformis* is a spore former and likely to survive all industrial processing of milk, such as the manufacture of milk powder and whey concentrate. Toxins produced by *B. licheniformis* interfere with mitochondrial function and over-activate the TRPV1 receptors in the intestines causing diarrhea.

Not all strains of *Bacillus licheniformis* appear to contain toxin-expressing genes, but with most probiotic supplements not labeling the strains of bacteria used, it is hard to know what you are taking in. Some "probiotic" supplements have removed it from their formulations in recent years; Garden of Life's Primal Defense is a prime example of the change of heart.

People may criticize me for being overly cautious when it comes to other "HSO" probiotics and their chances of causing infections. There have been some cases involving *Bacillus licheniformis* causing infections in people who are hospitalized or after surgery and it has even been associated with food poisoning. *Lactobacillus acidophilus* might have a few cases of septicemia infections in recorded literature, but it is a more widely used probiotic and the worst it would cause is an easier to identify and treat infection compared to most "HSO's."

Endospores are dormant, tough encapsulations that protect the bacteria from your immune system, antibiotics, antibacterials, and even probiotics. Bacteria can also lie dormant in endospores until their environment becomes favorable for faster reproduction and survival. Bacterial endospores may also become opportunistic in a host; share in a commune with the gut flora for a time. Bacterial endospores can survive without nutrients for a long time and are resistant to UV radiation, desiccation, high temperatures, extreme freezing, and most chemical disinfectants.

Since bacteria in the *Bacillus* genus are spore forming, it becomes hard to eliminate them if they become opportunistic. Most proponents say that the endospore aspect of *licheniformis* is a good quality in a "probiotic." Their reasoning behind this recommendation is that since *Bacillus licheniformis* is encapsulated in an endospore, the bacteria can survive stomach acid when ingested and propagate easily in the intestines.

Bacillus licheniformis has been shown to be immunostimulatory in some cases and produces bactericides to help eliminate other bacteria. Some non-HSO bacteria also produce bactericides to help reduce the total bacterial load in the intestines, but most of those bacteria are easy to eliminate if they cause an infection. If *Bacillus licheniformis* becomes opportunistic, its bactericides may target normal probiotic flora and reduce their populations increasing its virulence.

Bacillus subtilis

I will not recommend any probiotic that contains any strains from the *Bacillus* genus, including *Bacillus subtilis*, to my clients. I will not even recommend the world-renowned probiotic Primal Defense. Primal Defense comes highly recommended for digestive ailments by most of the experts in the natural health blogosphere. I believe that the risk of supplementing with this particular "probiotic" is too great, compared to any benefit towards your health that you may obtain from it. *Lactobacillus plantarum* would give you most of the same benefits. These benefits include being acid stable (*plantarum* survives stomach acid), being immunostimulatory, being an anti-inflammatory substance producing probiotic, and being a bactericide (a substance that eliminates opportunistic bacteria) producing probiotic as well. *Lactobacillus plantarum* would also be a much easier bacteria to eliminate if it did become opportunistic, compared to any HSO.

The most common bacteria claimed to be a probiotic in the *Bacillus* genus is *Bacillus subtilis*. *Bacillus subtilis* is extremely common and is found mainly in soil, in either decomposing plant matter or dirt. You might even recognize *subtilis'* cousin from the genus *Bacillus*. The bacteria goes by the name *Bacillus anthracis* (a.k.a. anthrax). Now granted, there is a big difference in the opportunistic and destructive capabilities of *anthracis* versus its gentler cousin *subtilis*. But, both bacteria share a common characteristic: endospores.

Endospores are dormant, tough encapsulations that protect the bacteria from your immune system, antibiotics, antibacterials, and even probiotics. Bacteria can also lay dormant in endospores until their environment becomes favorable for faster reproduction and survival. Bacterial endospores may also become opportunistic in a host, share in a "probiotic" communal with other true probiotics for a time, or slowly replicate more bacteria. Bacterial endospores can survive without nutrients for a long time and are resistant to UV radiation, desiccation, high temperatures, extreme freezing, and most chemical disinfectants. Since bacteria in the *Bacillus* genus are spore-forming, it becomes hard to eliminate them if they become opportunistic. Most proponents say that the endospore aspect of *subtilis* is a good quality in a "probiotic." Their reasoning behind this recommendation is that since *Bacillus subtilis* is encapsulated in an endospore, the bacteria can survive stomach acid when ingested and propagate easily in the intestines. *Bacillus subtilis* is also known to be immunostimulatory and produces bactericides to help eliminate other bacteria.

In the rare case that *subtilis* became opportunistic, it would be almost impossible to eliminate using standard antimicrobials. Antimicrobials that are used in eliminating *Bacillus* infections include both conventional antibiotics and natural antibacterial agents; have issues in eliminating a *Bacillus* opportunistic infection successfully on their own. Biofilm chelators need to be used to help break down the bacterial endospores so that antimicrobial agents can eliminate the opportunistic *Bacillus* infections. Strong biofilms and endospores are the main reason I am reluctant to recommend this probiotic, because if *Bacillus subtilis* becomes opportunistic, it can be very hard to eliminate from the body.

A few known clinical case studies mention opportunistic *Bacillus* infections occurring in people with compromised immune systems. One of the case reports theorizes that the main reason for such few known clinical reports of infection associated with *Bacillus subtilis* is because most doctors recognize it as a probiotic bacterium. Therefore, the bacteria are not tested as the cause of disease or death in most potentially infected people. One study also mentions that *Bacillus subtilis* may cause liver toxicity in some people. Most proponents will say that it is fine to supplement with *Bacillus subtilis*, because unless your immune system is compromised, or it becomes opportunistic, it is considered a beneficial intestinal probiotic. The problem with this idea is that no one can predict when his or her immune system may become compromised.

A possible scenario when one's immune system could become compromised is as follows. You could get into a massive car accident, and because of an injury to your intestinal area, your immune system would become compromised. You are then given antibiotics to stop the sepsis. From taking the antibiotics, you destroy your natural probiotic gut flora. *Bacillus subtilis* survives. Because it is in a protective spore, and later becomes opportunistic. Antibiotics are then rendered ineffective due to the bacterial endospores, and you die from the opportunistic *Bacillus subtilis* infection. Do you not believe that it is possible that this scenario can happen? Just replace *Bacillus subtilis* with another endospore bacterium, *Clostridium*. *Clostridium* also sometimes becomes opportunistic during massive antibiotic use, and it then becomes the superinfection *Clostridium difficile*, which may also be very deadly to eliminate.

Theoretical Endospore Bacteria Elimination Protocol

I would strongly recommend you use a combination of the safest possible antibiotics and biofilm chelators to eliminate this serious infection. The following protocol, however, is a great natural protocol to follow for some relief, hopefully.

Antibacterials

- Nature's Way enteric-coated peppermint oil – three times daily, taken thirty minutes before each meal.
- MesoSilver - follow supplement bottle recommendations.
- Zane Hellas Oil of Oregano - follow supplement bottle recommendations.

Biofilm Chelators

- Symbiotics lactoferrin - take two - six capsules daily in divided doses with meals daily.
- Jarrow Formulas NAC Sustain – one tablet twice daily. NAC is a systemic biofilm chelator; I do not recommend it as a first-line anti-biofilm agent in a protocol. Do not supplement more than 1,200 mg daily; doses above this recommendation may make the NAC you take become a pro-oxidant.

What About Bacillus subtilis That Are Ingested in Some Food Products?

There is some evidence that *Bacillus subtilis* might be a very small part of the normal gut flora of humans. *Bacillus subtilis* being normal gut flora has been theorized because soil is only known to be a reservoir for the bacteria, and it needs a host to live in to be able to propagate fully. Some human intestinal biopsy samples have shown that *subtilis* does populate the gut in some humans, but not all of the biopsies in the study showed *subtilis* as normal human intestinal flora. In addition, the Japanese do use *Bacillus subtilis* to produce a fermented soybean product known as natto. However, the amount of *Bacillus subtilis* in a large serving of natto is only about 10 million, which is a drop in a bucket compared to the trillions of bacteria that live in your digestive system. Therefore, the amount of *Bacillus subtilis* that the Japanese inoculate themselves with by consuming natto is very small. Most probiotic supplements that use HSO's would have billions of *Bacillus subtilis* and other members of the *Bacillus* genus all in one supplement. On average, the Japanese do not consume natto on a daily basis, but most people supplement with probiotics regularly and the amount of *subtilis* they ingest during a period of supplementation may cause opportunistic problems in the future.

I hope I have convinced you to leave HSO probiotics alone and try to supplement other safer non-spore forming probiotics. Remember, any probiotic can become opportunistic. Therefore, if you decide to take a probiotic supplement, make sure the species can be easily eliminated.

Other Soil Based Organisms and the Risks Associated With Their Supplementation

There are other soil-based organisms used in soil based probiotic supplements, they include:

HSO's That Are Not Considered Normal Human Flora or Have Non-Existent Human Interaction Research

- *Azospirillum brasiliense*
- *Azospirillum lipoferum*
- *Bacillus brevis*
- *Bacillus macerans*

- *Bacillus pumilus*
- *Bacillus polymyxa*
- *Bacteroides lipolyticum*
- *Bacteroides succinogenes*
- *Kurthia zopfii*
- *Myrothecium verrucaria*
- *Pseudomonas calcis*
- *Pseudomonas denitrificans*
- *Pseudomonas glathei*
- *Streptomyces fradiae*
- *Streptomyces cellulosae*
- *Streptomyces griseoflavus*

Acinetobacter Genus

Acinetobacter is a genus of Gram-negative bacteria that are commonly found in soil. Some *Acinetobacter* is also part of normal human flora. Many *Acinetobacter* bacteria are opportunistic bacteria and have been known to cause many different opportunistic infections. Their biofilms play an active role in periodontal infections, sepsis, and urinary tract infections. *Acinetobacter* bacteria are also highly resistant to most antibiotic treatments.

I do not recommend using any probiotic that has any members of the *Acinetobacter* genus if possible. The most common form of *Acinetobacter* used in probiotic formulations is *Acinetobacter calcoaceticus*. Even though *Acinetobacter calcoaceticus* is found in normal intestinal flora, it is extremely opportunistic if given the chance and is very resistant to antimicrobial agents. Supplementing with *Acinetobacter calcoaceticus* would be equivalent to supplementing with *Clostridium*, both are probiotic flora under normal circumstances, and both can easily become opportunistic and cause serious infections if given the opportunity (lowered immune system, multiple strong antibiotic use).

Arthrobacter Genus

Arthrobacter is a genus of Gram-positive bacteria that are commonly found in soil. Unlike the soil organism *Bacillus subtilis*, this bacteria does not form endospores; they do however form biofilm. I would consider most bacteria from the *Arthrobacter* genus to be safer than some of the other soil-based organisms. *Arthrobacter* bacteria are known to be part of the human flora on the skin and mucosal lining.

Like any probiotic bacteria, bacteria from the *Arthrobacter* genus have been known to cause infections. Those include *Arthrobacter woluwensis*, which has been implicated as a cause of endocarditis in people with heart valves, and *Arthrobacter cumminsii*, which may be a cause of urinary tract infections.

Supplementation of any probiotic from the *Arthrobacter* genus should be done with caution for the time being because of the lack of safety studies and the unknown knowledge if these bacteria are normal probiotic flora in the intestines.

Azotobacter Genus

Azotobacter is a genus of Gram-negative, motile, oval, soil-based bacteria that forms thick walled cysts. Cysts are related to endospores; they both protect the bacteria from heat, drying, UV, antimicrobials, etc. Bacterial cell wall thickening forms bacterial cysts. Cysts are formed so that the bacteria can be protected as it lies dormant waiting to be able to replicate safely. Cysts are not as strong as endospores, but still can be difficult to eradicate.

I cannot recommend any probiotic with *Azotobacter* bacteria because of the resistant nature of the cysts, as well as no studies have been done to show if any bacteria from the *Azotobacter* are part of natural human flora, or if any of the bacteria are safe for supplementation.

Brevibacteria Genus

Brevibacteria is a genus of Gram-positive soil-based bacteria that is found naturally as part of the human skin flora. *Brevibacteria linens* are the bacteria known as the common cause of excessive foot odor.

I do not recommend this soil-based organism because it is currently unknown if it is normal flora of the human intestinal tract. This bacteria genus though does appear safer compared to other soil based organisms. There are no known infections associated with this genus, and they do not develop cysts or endospores for protection.

Enterococcus faecalis

Enterococcus faecalis is a Gram-positive, soil based bacteria that inhabits the gastrointestinal and urinary tract of humans. *Enterococcus faecalis* is the main probiotic found in Dr. Ohhira's probiotic. Doctor Ohhira's probiotic strain of *Enterococcus faecalis* is a specific strain known as TH10. *Enterococcus faecalis* TH10 may be a safer strain of *Enterococcus faecalis*, but there are not enough studies or evidence to show that this strain will not cause severe opportunistic infections like other strains of the same bacteria. In defense of Dr. Ohhira's probiotic, many people have taken the probiotic, and it has helped their digestive woes. There are, however, anecdotal reviews of people who have taken the probiotic and have had UTI's and other infections that might have been caused by the probiotic as well. For this very reason, I do not recommend Dr. Ohhira's probiotic anymore in any of my protocols (the probiotic also contains carrageenan, which is inflammatory to the gut). I believe that there are safer probiotics available that people can supplement to help their digestive system.

Though *Enterococcus faecalis* is normal probiotic bacteria in the intestinal tract, this bacteria can easily become opportunistic and cause health issues. *Enterococcus faecalis* can become opportunistic and has been known to cause life-threatening sepsis in humans. *Enterococcus faecalis* infections have been known to cause endocarditis, UTI's, sepsis, root canal infections, and meningitis. *Enterococcus faecalis* are also known to be highly antibiotic resistant, suppress immune function by suppressing lymphocytes, and they form biofilms as well. Since *Enterococcus faecalis* has been shown in multiple clinical studies as being opportunistic bacteria and has multiple resistances to eradication, I cannot recommend this probiotic for supplementation currently, even the TH10 strain without more data.

Phanerochaete chrysosporium

Phanerochaete chrysosporium is a soil-based fungus that is responsible for white rot fungus in plants. *Phanerochaete chrysosporium* degrades lignin in dead plants so that they further decay and become soil.

Phanerochaete chrysosporium has been implicated lately as an opportunistic fungus that can cause invasive fungal infections. Emerging medical literature implicates *Phanerochaete chrysosporium* in fungal lung infections that are very difficult to resolve.

Phanerochaete chrysosporium also degrades different toxic substances including benzene, pesticides, and toluene. In theory, this sounds like a good idea within the human body; degrade the poisons so the body can easily eliminate them. The main issue with this process is that since the degradation is not occurring in the liver for proper elimination. The degradation would theoretically occur in the intestines which if you are suffering from leaky gut, the toxins would be absorbed into the bloodstream. *Phanerochaete chrysosporium* degrades benzene into cation radicals that are one of the main causes of benzene toxicity in the body by wreaking havoc on a cellular level causing severe free radical damage. Stay away from this fungus if all possible.

Pseudomonas fluorescens

Pseudomonas fluorescens is a Gram-negative soil based organism that is recognized as either a friendly HSO or an extremely opportunistic bacterium depending on the research. *Pseudomonas fluorescens* is present in low populations in few people's intestinal flora. *Pseudomonas fluorescens* infections were once considered to be rare, and mainly occur in people with compromised immune systems. *Pseudomonas fluorescens* was considered to be for the longest time the "harmless" *E. coli Nissle* of the opportunistic *Pseudomonas* genus, compared to its highly infectious cousin *Pseudomonas aeruginosa*. Recent information though changed the opinion of many microbiologists that no long consider *Pseudomonas fluorescens* as innocent.

Different Strains of Non HSO Probiotics

Bifidobacteria Genus

The *Bifidobacteria* genus of probiotics is a genus of Gram-positive, non-motile, anaerobic bacteria. They inhabit the gastrointestinal tract, vagina, and oral cavity of mammals. They are major native flora of the digestive tract and compose about 6% of the bacteria in adult stools. *Bifidobacteria* along with lactobacillus help maintain gastrointestinal integrity, help break down lactose and FOS, produce some of the B complex vitamins, and also absorb nutrients.

Bifidobacteria animalis – A type of *Bifidobacteria* found in mammals. This probiotic strain is patented in the yogurt Activa. It has been shown to survive digestion and colonize the digestive tract. It has also been shown to reduce colonic transit time keeping you regular. It has also been shown in studies to help with diarrhea and protects the intestines from zinc deficiency, which has been implicated as one of the causes of leaky gut syndrome. In a recent case study in 2006, it was shown to help prevent opportunistic infection from some strains of *Salmonella*.

Bifidobacteria bifidum - A type of *Bifidobacteria* that is usually found in the colon and vagina of humans. The probiotic has been shown to help maintain healthy flora balance, bolster the immune system, and help digest carbohydrates. Recent studies have shown that *bifidum* may help with allergies in some people and may help suppress allergic reactions through proper immune function.

Bifidobacteria breve – A type of *Bifidobacteria* found in the colon and vagina of humans. Cases of people with IBS have been shown to have a shortage of this important probiotic. Lack of this bacterium in women has also been linked to vaginal yeast infections (*Candida* overgrowth) as well. In breastfed infants, *breve* has been shown to make up a majority of their gut bacteria. *Breve* ferments sugar in the digestive tract and also helps produce lactic acid.

Bifidobacteria infantis – A type of *Bifidobacteria* that is found in both infant and adult human colons. This bacterium helps make acids that impede colonization of opportunistic bacteria by lowering intestinal pH. Studies have shown it to be beneficial in eliminating symptoms associated with IBS.

Bifidobacteria longum - A type of *Bifidobacteria* that is found as natural flora in the intestinal tract of humans. *Bifidobacteria longum* is also known to be one of the first colonizing probiotics in newborns.

Bifidobacteria longum is important to the metabolism, fermentation, and digestion of some carbohydrates in the intestinal tract including oligosaccharides. *Bifidobacteria longum* can break down and ferment amino acids and break down bile salts into amino acids and bile acids to that they can be reabsorbed back into the body.

Bifidobacteria longum has been shown in studies to help improve lactose intolerance, prevent diarrhea, alleviate some food allergies, and help fight colonization of opportunistic bacteria in the colon. Finally, *Bifidobacteria longum* have been shown in studies to be able to help scavenge free radicals in the intestines and help prevent colorectal cancer.

E. coli Nissle

E. coli have a bad rap when you think of bacteria because most people know *E. coli* as one of the opportunistic strains that cause food poisoning. Most *E. coli* are harmless and are probiotic bacteria in humans. They help produce vitamin K2 in your intestines. One specific strain, *E. coli Nissle* has been shown to be extremely beneficial to human gut flora.

The mutaflor strain was isolated by a German professor, Alfred Nissle in 1917 during the First World War when he found the strain in soldier excrement. Hitler was even known to use it to help with his gastrointestinal disturbances. It has been recently shown to help ulcerative colitis go into remission. My speculation is that it reduces *Mycobacterium avium paratuberculosis* colonization.

E. coli Nissle has also been shown in helping relieve chronic constipation, pouchitis, IBS, and *C. difficile* pseudomembranous colitis.

I find it hard to recommend mutaflor for most people because it has limited availability in the USA due to problems with FDA registration. I hope that it becomes available soon so more people to help their digestive disorders can use it.

Lactobacilli Genus

Like *Bifidobacteria, Lactobacilli* inhabits the gastrointestinal tract, vagina, and oral cavity of mammals. *Lactobacillus* is an opportunistic bacterium in one's oral cavity and has been shown to cause dental caries. They are excellent at converting lactose and other sugars into lactic acid in the digestive tract and can help inhibit some opportunistic bacteria growth by lowering pH levels. Some forms of *Lactobacilli* that are supplemented can die off after supplementation is stopped, so you must continue your supplementation to maintain benefits.

Lactobacillus acidophilus – The most widely recognized probiotic and a type of *Lactobacillus* that is found in the mouth, intestines, and vagina of humans. *Acidophilus* is good for people who have lactose intolerance because the bacteria can produce extra lactase in the human gut. *Acidophilus* can also have positive effects on the Immune System including, increased cytokine activity, phagocytic activity, and antibody production. It has also been shown to help with allergies.

Lactobacillus brevis – A type of *Lactobacilli* that is used in the fermentation of sauerkraut and sourdough bread and is also found naturally in the human gut flora. Clinical studies of *brevis* have shown that it provides anti-inflammatory benefits to the human digestive system. In addition, some studies show that it might help with abdominal cancer prevention as well. Make sure it says on the package before purchasing that they are live cultured and not heat-treated.

Lactobacillus bulgaricus – A type of *Lactobacilli* that is used in the productions of Swiss cheese and yogurt and is found in normal human gut flora. *Bulgaricus*, like most *Lactobacilli* bacteria, help produce lactic acid to decrease intestinal pH ranges and helps make up the mucus barrier of the intestines. *Bulgaricus* can draw away toxins in the intestinal tract as well keep opportunistic bacteria in check. *Bulgaricus* can also withstand stomach acid and bile salts as well and does not have to be enteric coated. It has some anti-cancer properties as well.

Lactobacillus casei – A type *of Lactobacilli* that is found in the intestinal flora and oral cavity of humans. Just like other forms of *Lactobacilli*, it decreases pH by making lactic acid and helps keep opportunistic bacteria in check. It is found commonly in yogurt and cultured cheese.

Lactobacillus gasseri - A type *of Lactobacilli* that is found in vaginal flora. It seems to help with weight maintenance, maintaining a healthy microbiome, and helps to compete with *H. pylori* to reduce its colonization.

Lactobacillus helveticus – A type *of Lactobacilli* that is used in the production of cheese including mozzarella, cheddar, parmesan, and Swiss. It is found in the human intestinal tract and is also a lactic acid producing bacteria. *Helveticus* has shown to increase calcium absorption. In addition, *Helveticus* fermented milk peptides have been shown in studies to reduce arterial stiffness and lower blood pressure.

Lactobacillus plantarum – A type of *Lactobacilli* that is found in the human large intestine. It is used in the production of sauerkraut, kimchi, pickles, and sourdough bread. *Plantarum* is an excellent probiotic which has shown useful in the elimination of the symptoms associated with IBS. It can reform the gastrointestinal mucus barrier, and inhibits opportunistic bacteria by making bactericidal peptides. *Lactobacillus plantarum* also prevents allergies, especially to soybeans. Finally, *Lactobacillus plantarum* stimulates the immune system by producing the amino acid L-lysine in the intestine.

Lactobacillus reuteri – A type of *Lactobacilli* that is found in the human large intestine, oral cavity, and human breast milk. This bacterium is important in infant immunogenesis. Breastfeeding is one way for an infant to receive this important probiotic. *Reuteri* is also found in the adult human flora, but is very sensitive to antibiotics, and it might be totally wiped out in some adult human's flora. *Reuteri* has been shown to help prevent infections of the colon, and it stimulates the immune system, relieves babies that have colic, and may even help eradicate *H. pylori* infections in the stomach.

Lactobacillus rhamnosus – A type of *Lactobacilli* that is found in the human large intestine, and urinary tract, and vagina. It is similar to the other forms of *Lactobacilli*. It decreases pH by synthesizing lactic acid and keeps opportunistic bacteria in check. *Rhamnosus* helps women with UTIs by excreting biosurfactants that keep opportunistic bacteria from attaching to the urinary tract wall. The opportunistic bacteria are then eliminated from the body.

Lactobacillus salivarius – A type of *Lactobacilli* that is typically found in the oral cavity of humans. It can also be found in the human intestinal system. *Salivarius* keeps opportunistic bacteria in the oral cavity in check so that dental caries will not occur.

Saccharomyces boulardii

Saccharomyces boulardii is a strain of beneficial yeast that is a soil based organism and is only found as normal gut flora in humans that eat lychee fruit on a regular basis.

S. boulardii was discovered in the 1920's by a French biologist, Henri Boulard, while he was in Southeast Asia looking for a strain of heat-resistant yeast to help production of wine. A cholera outbreak occurred during his exploration. Boulard noted that natives would either chew on the skins of lychee / mangosteen fruit or make tea with the skins to relieve diarrhea. He later isolated *S. boulardii* from lychee fruit.

S. boulardii has been shown to help greatly with diarrhea that is food-borne, or bacterial related and has been shown to help immensely with people with *C. difficile* infection.

I do not consider *Saccharomyces boulardii* to be a soil based organism anymore. Even though it is not technically part of the natural intestinal flora of humans like most other non-HSO probiotics, I consider *Saccharomyces boulardii* to be a rare, important exception.

S. boulardii should be used with caution in people who have severely compromised immune systems because of the chance of systemic fungal infection (fungemia). If fungemia occurs, follow the advanced *Candida* protocol (Ch. 4) advocated earlier in the book as well as the yeast herx protocol (Ch. 4). *S. boulardii* also causes allergic symptoms in some people with yeast allergies.

S. boulardii also has been shown to help people suffering from acute diarrhea, IBD, and travelers' diarrhea.

Streptococcus Genus

The *Streptococcus* genus of bacteria is a spherical, Gram-positive bacterium that also produces lactic acid. It is found all over the body, but it can be a beneficial probiotic in the oral cavity and gut of humans. Several strains of *Streptococcus* bacteria are known as opportunistic bacteria. These bacteria can cause strep throat, bacterial pneumonia, and other infections. The two main probiotics from the genus are not usually opportunistic and are important to human health.

Streptococcus salivarius – A type of *Streptococcus* that is found in the oral cavity and the upper respiratory system of humans. *Streptococcus salivarius* is one of the first bacteria to colonize a human infant and common exposure to the bacteria is harmless. Studies have shown that it can help prevent oral infections as well as help keep the opportunistic bacteria *Streptococcus pyogenes* (cause of strep throat) at bay and reduce the number of infections.

Streptococcus thermophilus – A type of *Streptococcus* that is used in conjunction with *Lactobacillus bulgaricus* to make yogurt. In addition, it is a lactic acid producing bacteria that inhabits normal gut flora. It also can endure high temperatures and pasteurization. *Thermophilus* can also help humans assimilate the milk protein casein during digestion. It can also help reduce intestinal inflammation and help prevent the transformation of nitrates into nitrites in the intestines.

Brands Recommended for Specific Probiotics

- *Bifidobacteria animalis*: HMF Intensive probiotic
- *Bifidobacteria bifidum*: HMF Intensive probiotic, Renew Life Probiotics, Pure Encapsulations Pure Probiotic, GutPro, Jarrow Formulas Jarrow Dophilus, Natren Healthy Trinity
- *Bifidobacteria infantis*: Klaire Labs Therbiotic infant formula, Renew Life probiotics, GutPro
- *Bifidobacteria breve*: Renew Life probiotics, Pure Encapsulations Pure Probiotic, Jarrow Dophilus EPS, GutPro
- *Lactobacillus acidophilus*: Enzymedica Pearls, Natren Healthy Trinity, HMF Intensive, Jarrow Formulas Jarrow Dophilus
- *Lactobacillus bulgaricus*: Natren Healthy Trinity
- *Lactobacillus brevis*: Garden of Life RAW probiotics (If you are female: Klaire Labs – Ther-Biotic women's formula)
- *Lactobacillus casei*: Health Aid ImmunProBio

- *Lactobacillus gasseri* : GutPro
- *Lactobacillus helveticus*: Xymogen Probio Defense, Garden of Life RAW probiotics
- *Lactobacillus plantarum*: Ideal Bowel Support Jarrow Formulas, GutPro
- *Lactobacillus reuteri*: BioGaia reuteri (If you are female: Jarrow Formulas FemDophilus)
- *Lactobacillus rhamnosus*: Allergy Research Group rhamnosus, Culturelle, (If you are female: Jarrow Formulas FemDophilus)
- *Lactobacillus salivarius*: Allergy Research Group *salivarius*, Pure Encapsulations Probiotic G.I., GutPro
- *E-coli Nissle*: Mutaflor
- *Streptococcus salivarius*: Jarrow-Dophilus oral probiotic gum
- *Streptococcus thermophilus*: Pure Encapsulations Probiotic G.I.
- *Saccharomyces boulardii*: Florastor, Jarrow Formulas Saccharomyces boulardii

Probiotic Protocols

Basic Protocol – Should only be used if you have great digestive health and no issues.

- Choose one probiotic.
- Take before bed with a glass of non-chlorinated water.
- Jarrow Dophilus EPS – take two capsules daily (do not use with histamine or D-lactate sensitivity).
- GutPro Capsules – take two capsules daily.

If you are a woman, you might want to try either: Fem-Dophilus - take one capsule daily, Jarrow Dophilus – take one capsule daily.

Average Protocol – The average person should use this protocol or people with mild digestive problems.

- Choose one probiotic.
- Take before bed with a glass of non-chlorinated water.
- Natren Healthy Trinity – take one capsule daily (do not use with histamine or D-lactate sensitivity).

- Jarrow Dophilus EPS – take four capsules daily (do not use with histamine or D-lactate sensitivity).
- GutPro Capsules – take three capsules daily.
- D-lactate free Custom Probiotic – use one baby scoop and mix it with filtered water.

If you are a woman you might try: Fem-Dophilus - take two capsules daily, Jarrow Dophilus – take two capsules daily / Raw Probiotics Women – take one capsule daily (do not use with histamine or D-lactate sensitivity).

Advanced Protocol – A person with medium to severe digestive problems should use this protocol.

- Choose one probiotic.
- Take before bed with a glass of non-chlorinated water.
- Natren Healthy Trinity – take two four capsules daily (do not use with histamine or D-lactate sensitivity).
- VSL # 3 – take one capsule daily (do not use with histamine or D-lactate sensitivity).
- D-lactate free Custom Probiotic – use one adult scoop and mix it with filtered water.

*Severe Protocol - **A person only under direct doctor's supervision for SEVERE abdominal symptoms should use this protocol.***

- Requires a Prescription: VSL#3DS – follow supplement box instructions (do not use with histamine or D-lactate sensitivity).

Prebiotics

Prebiotics are nondigestible food ingredients or supplements that stimulate the growth of probiotic bacteria and may help improve your immune system. Feeding probiotics in the hope that they naturally populate your large intestine should be done with the utmost caution. You do not want their numbers to increase so greatly that they become opportunistic, and SIBO occurs.

The use of prebiotics is not always beneficial to people with digestive issues. If prebiotics are incorrectly supplemented as probiotics sometimes are, they may cause you to either develop SIBO or worsen your digestive ailments. In people with SIBO, most prebiotics will ferment and create more gas that will cause your symptoms to worsen.

I still believe in some cases prebiotics may be more useful for you to supplement instead of using probiotics to promote the natural replenishment of your probiotic flora. Many different prebiotics can be used to help replenish your gut flora. I recommend the use of galacto-oligosaccharides mainly.

Different Types of Prebiotics

Prebiotics That I Rarely Recommend

Fructo-oligosaccharide / Inulin

Inulin is a group of natural polysaccharides. Inulin is found in many different plants and belongs to a dietary class known as fructans. Foods that naturally contain inulin are chicory, onion, bananas, garlic, asparagus, wheat, tomatoes, and Jerusalem artichoke. Inulin is fermentable in the intestines and helps provide "food" for bacteria to reproduce.

Remember the link that I mentioned between prebiotics and SIBO? If you research fructans and many of the different foods that were listed earlier, you will eventually find information that points you to FODMAPs. FODMAPs are fermentable foodstuff that is known to contribute to SIBO symptoms and increase abdominal gas in certain people.

Most people with SIBO go on an anti-FODMAP diet to help eliminate the excess bacteria they have in their small intestine. Fructans (inulin, FOS) are considered the greatest contributor to SIBO in most people and, therefore, should be avoided in people with SIBO.

Fructo-oligosaccharides are oligosaccharide fructans that are either sourced from different foods containing inulin or are made from the yeast *Aspergillus niger* reacting to fructose.

FOS's are also fermentable in the gut like inulin and provide nutrients for bacteria to reproduce.

FOS's and inulin both feed probiotic bacteria and opportunistic bacteria in the gut. They have been found to feed the probiotic bacterial genus *Bifidobacteria.* Though increasing *Bifidobacteria* in the colon may be healthy, overpopulation of the bacteria may lead to SIBO. In addition, both prebiotics have been found to feed different potential opportunistic bacteria including *Klebsiella*, *E. coli*, and *Clostridium*. Increased populations of *Klebsiella* in the intestines have been linked to intestinal permeability (leaky gut). FOS and inulin can also feed yeast like *Candida*, so people with active yeast infections should also limit their intake.

If you choose to use either FOS's or inulin as your prebiotic, I recommend to use it only for a very short period, and if you develop SIBO, follow the SIBO protocol (Ch. 9).

Lactulose

Lactulose is a synthetic, non-digestible sugar that is used in the treatment of constipation and people with liver disease. Lactulose is a disaccharide formed from one molecule of fructose and galactose. Lactulose is an osmotic laxative.

Lactulose is considered a prebiotic because the intestines do not absorb it and bacteria in your intestines break lactulose down and ferment it for food. In studies, lactulose helps support proper amounts of *Lactobacillus* and *Bifidobacterium* flora in the intestines. Unlike inulin and FOS, lactulose seems to hinder the growth of some opportunistic bacteria including *E. coli*, and *Staphylococcus*. Finally, lactulose appears to be indigestible by most yeasts including *Candida*.

Lactulose may contribute to developing SIBO if taken in large doses. Lactulose as a cause of SIBO seems to be less likely than FOS or inulin. Even though, lactulose tends to be more specific in the bacteria that it helps populate I cannot recommend it because of its strong laxative nature. It is also more likely to cause flatulence and requires a prescription for its use.

Xylo-oligosaccharide

Xylo-oligosaccharides are polymers of D-xylans that are derived from enzymatic hydrolysis of xylans that occur in plant or starch matter. Xylans are a kind of hemicellulose that is found in the cell walls of plants. Unlike the other prebiotics listed above, it is unknown if XOS's are indigestible by the human body.

The main reason I cannot recommend XOS's is that there is not much literature or studies for me to recommend its use. One in vivo study of only five humans showed that XOS's increased *Bifidobacteria* populations greatly, but this is hardly an appropriate sample size for broad conclusions. In addition, another study concludes the supplementation of XOS's might be beneficial in people with type 2 diabetes in improving overall blood glucose levels.

Xylooligosaccharides may contribute to SIBO, and it is unknown about its selectivity of bacteria. I cannot recommend the supplementation of XOS's currently at this time.

Honorable Mention Prebiotics

Arabinogalactans

What Are Arabinogalactans?

Arabinogalactans are polysaccharides that are found in plants and even mycobacterial cell walls. Arabinogalactan consists of chains or arabinose and galactose monosaccharides. You can either ingest arabinogalactans through diet or prebiotic supplements. Good sources of arabinogalactans found in diet are:

- Carrots
- Radishes
- Pears
- Corn
- Tomatoes
- Coconut meat and milk

Arabinogalactans are also found in some common herbs that people use to improve their health. They include:

- Echinacea purpurea
- Curcuma longa
- Viscum album (Mistletoe)

The Supposed Benefits of Ingesting Arabinogalactans

There are reported various benefits of ingesting arabinogalactans for improving your immune system and your digestive health.

Ingesting arabinogalactans improve your digestive system in multiple ways as a reduced fermentation potential prebiotic fiber. The prebiotic fiber has shown in studies to favor butyrate production (an important SCFA for intestinal mucosal integrity), increase production of the SCFA propionate, and slightly increase production of the SCFA acetate, lower colonic pH, and decrease the generation / absorption of ammonia in the digestive system. It has also been shown to favor selective probiotic bacteria including *Bifidobacteria* and *Lactobacillus* and seems to discourage the growth of opportunistic *Clostridia* and *E. coli*. It is unknown if *Klebsiella* ferments the prebiotic, but in studies, it appears that it does up-regulate the immune system to keep opportunistic Gram-negative bacteria like *Klebsiella* in check. Arabinogalactan ingestion might also reduce bacterial adherence and biofilm formation. The benefits on the microbiome of ingesting arabinogalactans seem to be comparable to my recommended prebiotic, GOS.

Arabinogalactans have been shown to increase immune system function in in-vitro studies. It appears that the immune modulating properties of Echinacea purpurea might be from the arabinogalactans that the herb contains. Arabinogalactans have been shown to:

- Enhance function of natural killer cells. NK cells help our bodies by preventing cancer metastasis (regulate cytotoxicity) and fight viruses.
- Mistletoe has reported anti-cancer effects which may stem from its concentration of arabinogalactans.
- Increase macrophage activation against pathogens.
- Increased production of TNF-alpha, interleukin-1, and interferon-beta to help our immune system fight pathogens.
- Have anti-metastasis properties (in-vitro, and in-vivo animal studies).
- Reduce pediatric occurrences of otitis media.

Potential Negatives of Ingesting Arabinogalactans

Ingestion of arabinogalactans in food sources, in supplemental form, or in herbs may have specific benefits to improve your health. There are sadly some proposed drawbacks to its use.

Arabinogalactans are also a component of mycobacteria cell walls. The mechanism of action for the antitubercular drug ethambutol might occur from inhibition of mycobacteria arabinogalactan synthesis. Ethambutol reduces mycobacteria concentrations by counteracting the enzyme arabinosyl transferase, reducing arabinogalactan synthesis, and increasing cell wall permeability. It is unknown if ingesting arabinogalactans while suffering from a mycobacterial infection, especially if you are suffering from for example an *MAP* overgrowth of the gut (ulcerative colitis), would cause any issues or increase in mycobacterial strength or concentration. That being said there are probably different arabinogalactan receptors between what the mycobacteria produce and what we ingest. That being said I would caution anyone with mycobacterial infections to reduce their consumption and do not supplement with this prebiotic fiber until more studies can be done.

There are not many studies on which opportunistic organisms may use arabinogalactans as a source of fuel. We know through studies that opportunistic overgrowth of *Clostridia*, *E. coli*, and possibly *Klebsiella* do not prefer the prebiotic and that it may reduce their concentration in the gut. Some yeast can ferment arabinose, so if you have yeast overgrowth and react negatively to arabinogalactans, I would reduce or eliminate the amount of the prebiotic you ingest.

Finally, there was one in-vivo study done with arabinogalactan ingestion that does cast doubt on some of its ability to help improve digestive health. In the study only *Lactobacillus* was shown to increase through supplementation, SCFA amounts did not improve, and *Clostridia* increased slightly as well. I do have issues with this study: they sampled fecal flora instead of colonic flora biopsies; it can be difficult to obtain SCFA information from fecal samples because most are reabsorbed by the gut; they used significant amounts of arabinogalactan (fifteen and thirty grams), and it was generously sweetened with aspartame (could have an adverse effect on the microbiome). That being said the study's authors marked one important conclusion, the more arabinogalactan one consumes (thirty grams in the study), the greater chance of fermentation side effects like bloating and flatulence, and it seems that an increased dosage does not correlate to its effectiveness, just length of time.

Arabinogalactan Supplementation Recommendations

If you want to try arabinogalactans as a prebiotic, I suggest you take in five to ten grams daily for at least a month to see if you have any improvement in your overall health. Not everyone can tolerate prebiotics, so if it causes excessive side effects like flatulence and bloating after a few days of consuming it, it might be best to try lower doses or discontinue its use.

Most arabinogalactan supplements are sourced from the bark of the larch tree.

- Recommended Powder – Foodscience of Vermont Arabinogalactan Powder
- Recommended Capsules – Pure Encapsulations Arabinogalactan

Isomalto-oligosaccharide

Isomalto-oligosaccharides are a mixture of short-chain carbohydrates (glucose oligomers linked with isomaltose) that have been shown to have prebiotic and digestion-resistant properties. ISO's are sourced from different starches using enzyme-catalyzed hydrolysis. ISO's also seem to cause low amounts of flatulence; they have anti-dental caries properties and have a low glycemic index. The final fermented by-products of ISO's are SCFA's (short chain fatty acids) that help nourish the gut and facilitate growth and repair. Finally, ISO's have been shown to increase *Bifidobacteria* populations in the gut naturally.

I cannot fully recommend ISO's yet because it is currently unknown if the prebiotic is selective, meaning that it might also increase some opportunistic bacteria / yeast greatly. I also cannot recommend ISO's yet because one of the source materials used to produce the prebiotic is wheat. Now granted, there should not be any gluten left in the final product. ISO's still might aggravate some people's medical issues if they are allergic to wheat, not just gluten, so it should always be avoided unless their source is known.

Mannan-oligosaccharide

Mannan-oligosaccharides are a glucomannoprotein complex that is sourced from certain fungi including *Saccharomyces cerevisiae* using enzymatic hydrolysis. MOS has been shown in vivo animal studies to inhibit bacteria with type one fimbriae (opportunistic *E. coli* and *Salmonella* are examples*)* from adhering to the intestines so that they can propagate. MOS's have also been shown to limit *Clostridium* populations in the gut as well. MOS's are known to block the opportunistic bacterium *Clostridium perfringens* from adhering to the intestines, which is a known cause of foodborne illness. Finally, MOS supplementation has been found in vivo animal studies to increase villi and intestinal mucosal health.

Theoretically, MOS should be able to be fermented by *Bifidobacteria* and *Lactobacilli* and, therefore; should help increase their populations.

In humans, mannan-oligosaccharides have primarily been studied in the relief of bacterial urinary tract infections. The use of MOS in the relief of bacteria UTI's has been recommended in studies. The relief occurs by blocking bacteria from adhering to the urinary tract thus eliminating them from the body.

I hope that MOS will be studied more in humans for improving digestion so that we know if the in vivo animal studies carry over. Also in some in vitro studies, MOS's have been shown to feed and encourage the propagation of opportunistic *Candida albicans*. If you have a yeast allergy, you might also be allergic to MOS since it is derived from *Saccharomyces cerevisiae,* so avoid supplementation.

Honestly, I would still consider the use of the Jarrow probiotic Jarrow Formulas Saccharomyces boulardii & MOS if I were suffering from an opportunistic *Clostridium* infection including *Clostridium difficile*, because of the amount of research concluding that both would be effective against the bacterium.

My Recommended Prebiotic – GOS

Galacto-oligosaccharide

Galacto-oligosaccharides are a chain of galactose (monosaccharide sugar) units that are produced by the enzymatic hydrolysis of lactose. Like other prebiotics, GOS's are unabsorbed by the intestines and are fermentable in the gut by bacteria. Galacto-oligosaccharides seem to be the gold standard of prebiotics, and I recommend them for use in most cases of poor intestinal health.

Galacto-oligosaccharides have been shown in studies to increase naturally gut flora populations of *Bifidobacteria* and *Lactobacilli*. *Bifidobacteria* seem to benefit greatly from GOS supplementation and increase more in number with it than any other prebiotic. Also, try to use a GOS supplement that was produced from *Bifidobacteria* enzymes for a greater synergistic effect.

GOS's have also been shown to be very selective and limit the growth of opportunistic *E. coli*, *Salmonella*, *Typhimurium*, and *Clostridia* in the gut. The process of fermenting GOS's in the colon produces antimicrobial agents that help eliminate opportunity bacteria and limit their ability to adhere to the intestinal tract. GOS's can also restore proper bowel function and relieve chronic constipation with its use. Finally, GOS's improve intestinal mucosa and villi function and can help relieve leaky gut.

Galacto-oligosaccharides have been shown in studies to cause the least amount of flatulence compared to other prebiotics. Only in levels way above the recommended supplementation range (greater than fifteen grams), were flatulence and diarrhea reported. Even in large doses of twelve grams daily, no digestion discomfort was reported. GOS are selectively fermented and as such have a low chance of causing flatulence or SIBO. GOS's are not even considered to be a FODMAP like most of the other prebiotics are.

There are even more reasons to supplement galacto-oligosaccharides than just improving overall gut health. GOS's have been shown to reduce allergy severity, reduce the chance of infectious diseases, improve calcium / magnesium absorption, increase bone density, and even reduce the severity of the common cold and the flu when supplemented.

The only GOS supplement I currently recommend is Galactomune by Klaire Labs. It does contain beta glucans so use with caution if you are allergic to yeast. I recommend taking two scoops daily in place of the probiotics listed in above protocols if you choose to supplement with GOS.

Why Use Probiotic Supplements? Why Not Use Natural Probiotics in Food?

Natural probiotics should be supplemented in people with certain digestive conditions, and in people who are sensitive to probiotic supplements. Natural probiotics consumed in food have a symbiotic relationship with probiotics taken as supplements. If you do decide to get your own probiotics from food, the probiotic food should only be prepared by yourself and not commercially obtained. Ferment your own vegetables, make coconut milk kefir or make probiotic yogurt.

The reason that someone needs this symbiotic relationship is that for most people, supplements and natural probiotics alone cannot fix their issues. Some natural compounds and probiotics will be missing from supplemental probiotics. Natural probiotics might not contain the right probiotic strains, be acid stable enough, or enteric coated. Both forms of probiotics might be needed to alleviate your digestive concerns.

What is Kefir?

Kefir is a fermented milk product that originated from the Caucasus mountain region. It is a slightly tangy beverage full of probiotic yeast and bacteria. It is made by adding kefir grains (a "grain" is a combination of bacteria, yeast, proteins, lipids, and carbohydrates) to a liquid medium (either ruminant dairy, coconut milk / water, or water). "Controlled" fermentation occurs to produce the actual kefir product.

Since kefir is a fermented beverage, it is rich in many different vitamins, minerals, SCFA's, and amino acids. Kefir contains:

- B vitamins (thiamin, folate, B-12, biotin)
- Vitamin K2
- Calcium
- Magnesium
- Phosphorus
- Propionic acid
- Acetate
- Vitamin A
- Vitamin E
- Amino acids (methionine, cysteine, tryptophan, phenylalanine, tyrosine, isoleucine, threonine, lysine, valine)
- Lactoferrin
- Probiotic bacteria and yeast

Why I Am Hesitant in Recommending Kefir

Kefir has helped many people recover from their digestive woes and improve their overall health. That being said, using it on a daily basis may be hiding digestive issues if it brings constant relief. There are issues with its use including:

- **Histamine intolerance** – Some kefir contains strains that produce histamine. If you are suffering from histamine intolerance, then you want to stay away from kefir that contains: *Lactobacillus bulgaricus, Lactobacillus casei, Lactobacillus helveticus, and Lactobacillus reuteri* (might be ok for some people with histamine intolerance, converts histidine to histamine).
- **SIBO** – I do not recommend the ingestion of probiotics when motility is compromised.
- **Yeast and aldehyde sensitivity** – The yeast in the probiotic drink can produce aldehyde. Aldehydes are broken down in the body by the enzyme aldehyde dehydrogenase in the liver. The body's production of aldehyde dehydrogenase depends on bioavailability of molybdenum, liver function, and genetics (ALDH genes). People with yeast sensitivities do not have enough aldehyde dehydrogenase and because of this react negatively to products containing yeast and mold.
- **D-lactate sensitivity** – Many of the lactic acid producing bacteria in kefir produce D-lactate. L-lactate is the primary lactic acid produced within the body and is readily metabolized. D-

lactate is also produced by our bacteria and our metabolism, but in lesser amounts. When D-lactate is over produced and leaks out into the bloodstream from our gut, medical problems including delirium, ataxia, slurred speech, trouble concentrating, and brain fog can occur. Though true D-lactate acidosis is rare (short bowel syndrome), issues from too much D-lactate being in the blood can occur. *Lactobacillus acidophilus, L. bulgaricus, L. fermentum, L. delbrueckii subsp lactis* are examples of D-lactate producing probiotics.

- **Contamination** – Production of fermented foods always comes at a likelihood of contamination. Granted, the risk of contamination of a foreign strain is manageable in a controlled environment. Microorganisms, however, are mostly everywhere and are hard to keep out of a medium that is tailored to their growth.
- **Immunocompromisation** – Immunocompromised individuals should ingest probiotic foods or probiotic supplements with caution because of potential opportunistic effects.
- **Casein sensitivity** – Casein is a protein found in some dairy products (milk, cheese, kefir). Casein can be a hard to digest protein and can cause inflammation and digestive issues for some people. Casein also contains the opioid peptide casomorphin, which can slow motility and possibly cross the blood brain barrier causing proposed issues (cravings, histamine intolerance, further slowing of motility). There are claims of differing beta-casein proteins, known as A1 and A2. A1 proteins are mostly found in U.S. and Canadian dairy and may be more reactive in the gut because of the release of beta-casomorphin-7 upon its digestion. Also, A1 beta-casein contains histidine at position 67 of its makeup instead of proline that may affect its digestion and possible triggering in people who are histamine intolerance. However, studies are differing in the reactions of A1 or A2 casein in the human body. To be the most health conscious, if possible, I would consume milk or dairy products produced from A2 dairy.
- **Lactose intolerance** – Lactose is a disaccharide sugar found in some forms of dairy. Not all dairy kefir contains lactose. Some people are lactose intolerant, and ingestion of the sugar causes digestive symptoms including diarrhea, abdominal cramps, gas, and bloating.
- ***MAP*** (*Mycobacterium avium paratuberculosis*) – If you suffer from ulcerative colitis or Crohn's disease you should avoid all dairy products including kefir produced from dairy. If you are suffering from either condition, you should have little issue with dairy free kefir.

Final Thoughts on Kefir

Kefir is fine to ingest occasionally for most people as long as you do not have any of the above issues.

Homemade kefir might be a better option because you can control the strains used and the type of starter material (dairy, coconut, or water). It is possible to produce a kefir overlooking most of these issues from home. You could produce for example either water or coconut kefir from D-lactate free / low histamine producing probiotics and yeast. In doing so, you would avoid issues with D-lactate sensitivity, histamine intolerance, and casein / lactose intolerance. If I were to produce kefir at home, this is what I would make so that I could ingest the best possible kefir.

What about producing kefir without using yeast? Well, kefir technically is supposed to have yeast in it; producing kefir without yeast is more akin to producing yogurt, I am sorry to say.

That being said, if you were suffering from SIBO, yeast sensitivity, or severe immunocompromisation there might be no version of the drink that you would be able to tolerate. I cannot recommend kefir ingestion if you fall into these categories.

Microbial Ingestion and Our MMC

We ingest microbes on a constant basis through swallowing, eating food, drinking water, and clearing our sinuses. What is our first line of defense? What keeps us from getting sick when we are swallowing all these microbes all the time? The answer is our mitigating motor complex, or MMC for short.

The Stomach

Gastric acid eliminates many of the microbes that we ingest because they cannot survive the low pH of the fluid. Our stomach also produces pepsinogen that is activated in the presence of gastric acid (pepsinogen becomes pepsin) to help us digest proteins. Pepsin also inhibits bacterial growth by proteolysis, which is breaking down bacterial proteins necessary for their survival.

Small Intestine

Some parts of the small intestine are relatively sterile environments like our stomach compared to the rest of our body. There are some bacteria in the small intestine, but they exist in small numbers because of proper MMC function. Our large intestine is a perfect place for bacterial growth; it is an anaerobic competitive environment with many carbohydrates that can be fermented for energy. Bacteria in the large intestine do not have to deal with strong peristalsis waves that occur in the small intestine, immune system components to reduce their populations, or deal with the harsh components of chemical digestion (stomach acid, bicarbonate, bile, and pepsin that are still found in the duodenum).

The few microbes that survive stomach acid and pepsin in the stomach are further reduced by bile in the duodenum. The jejunum of the small intestine contains more microbes than the duodenum and the stomach because it is a very alkaline environment. Large amounts of mucus are secreted by goblet cells in the jejunum to help trap opportunistic microbes during digestion. If the MMC is functioning properly, goblet cells are also able to produce acidic mucus, which can be used to trap further and eliminate pathogens. Like the jejunum, the ileum also contains more microbes than the duodenum and stomach, but it contains GALT lymphoid tissue known as Peyer's patches. Peyer's patches produce leukocytes that help combat opportunistic microbes in the lower intestinal tract.

Large Intestine

Even though half of the small intestine contains more microbes than the stomach, there are defense mechanisms in each section to help eliminate opportunistic microbes and push the microbes that survive where they belong into the colon. Strong MMC contractions push what organisms survive into the large intestine through the ileocecal valve where they either become healthy flora or are eliminated by the body through our feces.

Failure of the MMC

In most people with SIBO, stomach acid levels are below normal (which is why PPI are indicated as a cause of bacterial / yeast overgrowth). Lower stomach acid and pepsin levels mean that more bacteria survive after consumption and enter the small intestine unchallenged.

Less bile is also produced in people that are suffering from overgrowth that further hinders microbial reduction. Microbial toxins that are ingested or caused by overgrowth damage the interstitial cells of Cajal that control the MMC. When these cells are damaged, gastric and small intestine emptying slows and the ileocecal valve has issues opening and closing properly.

Bacterial overgrowth also leads the goblet cells to produce too much mucus, and by doing so further pull microbes into the small intestine that lead to their survival in an overwhelmed system. The immune system is so overwhelmed that they cannot eliminate the microbes that are trapped in mucus. The goblet cells eventually exhaust themselves, leading to bacteria producing biofilms, which replace beneficial mucus, causing small intestine ulceration.

Bacteria move freely from the large intestine into the small intestine further causing issues because of a faulty functioning ileocecal valve. The ileocecal valve connects the small intestine and the large intestine and prevents waste and bacteria from back flowing into the small intestine during proper digestion. When we suffer bacterial overgrowth, the ileocecal valve malfunctions further hindering digestion and MMC function.

Probiotics and Poor MMC function

So where do probiotics fit into this equation and why should we avoid them if we are suffering from overgrowth or poor MMC?

If you have issues with your MMC, the probiotic bacteria you ingest will end up in your small intestine instead of your large intestine where they belong. The bacteria could then become opportunistic, produce hydrogen gas, and worsen SIBO symptoms, or die off causing herx reactions. Either way, they will contribute more to your digestive woes instead of improving them.

Histamine Intolerance and Probiotics

Probiotics are important in maintaining our gut flora, but they can still cause issues just like any supplement and most issues with supplementation go unreported on the natural health blogosphere. Everyone writes about the pros of taking probiotics, but what are the cons?

Histamine is an organic compound produced by the body. Histamine is produced during immune responses and as a neurotransmitter down regulator. Histamine produced by the stomach and the intestines help to regulate their function. There are four types of histamine receptors in the body, and activating each receptor performs a different task.

- **H1** – blood vessel dilation, smooth muscle contraction of the bronchi and GI tract, stimulation of vagus nerve, increases histamine and arachidonic acid release, decreased AV node conduction of the heart, helps form nitric oxide, improves eosinophil function.
- **H2** – stimulates nasal and intestinal mucosa, relaxes the LES, increases vascular permeability, stimulation of suppressor T cells, increases stomach acid production, reduces neutrophil and basophil function, increases lymphocytes, and increases the activity of NK cells.
- **H3** – increases histamine in the brain as a neurotransmitter, suppresses norepinephrine release at parasympathetic nerve endings, stimulates nasal mucus, reduces bronchoconstriction and gastric acid.
- **H4** – enhances the function of eosinophils, mast cells, and neutrophils.

As you can see, different histamine receptors have different effects on our digestive health, which is why it is important for its production and activation and deactivation of certain receptors to be in balance.

Most people make histamine out to be a monster. Too much histamine is the cause of my seasonal allergies. Histamine overproduction is the only cause of my anaphylactic reaction when I eat shrimp, which I am allergic to. Excess histamine is the reason I have heartburn, so I take a histamine receptor two antagonist like Pepcid to relieve my digestive woes. The main problem is not directly the histamine in all of these individual issues; the real problem is why too much histamine was released or is circulating throughout the body during these health issues.

The body needs the correct balance of histamine so that your digestive system, immune system, neurotransmitter system, cardiovascular system, and nervous system work properly.

Proper ingestion of omega 3 fatty acids (fresh fish only), vitamin D3, vitamin B6, magnesium, and vitamin C can help the body maintain proper histamine balance. Some people also require taking mast cell stabilizers like quercetin (use with caution if you have a COMT mutation), or cromoglicic acid to help improve histamine intolerance symptoms. If you are suffering from having a histamine imbalance, you should try a histamine reduced diet to see if your issues improve. Finally, some people supplement directly with the DAO enzyme which breaks down histamine in the body with differing success.

If you are supplementing probiotics and have histamine issues, you should only supplement histamine-degrading probiotics instead of histamine-producing probiotics until the imbalance corrects itself. The intestines and stomach require histamine for proper function. It is totally unknown if these probiotics increase histamine levels in vivo in humans, I would still limit them if needed. Histamine-producing probiotics should not be used until the body can maintain proper levels of histamine.

Histamine Producing / Degrading Microorganisms

Histamine Modulators / Producers:

- *Candida*
- *Citrobacter*
- *Clostridium perfringens*
- *E. coli*
- *H. pylori*
- *Klebsiella pneumonia*
- *Klebsiella oxytoca*
- *Lactobacillus bulgaricus*
- *Lactobacillus casei*
- *Lactobacillus reuteri*
- *Morganella morganii*
- *Proteus mirabilis*
- *Staphylococcus*
- *S. thermophilus*

Histamine Degraders:

- *Bifidobacterium infantis*
- *Bifidobacterium longum*
- *Lactobacillus gasseri*
- *Lactobacillus rhamnosus*
- *Lactobacillus salivarius*
- *Lactobacillus plantarum*

Probiotic Supplements Without Histamine Producing Bacteria:

- BM
- Gutpro

What is the Difference Between L-lactate and D-lactate?

Lactic acid bacteria in our gut produce both L-lactate and D-lactate by carbohydrate fermentation.

L-lactate is produced in our body from lactic acid bacteria in our microbiome and is a natural byproduct produced during the Kreb's cycle for metabolism. L-lactate is also up-regulated during exercise because of the increased need for mitochondrial energy and oxygen to support our muscles. L-lactate is oxidized back into glucose by our liver and is further used for energy production by our body. Finally, our brain can metabolize lactate for energy.

D-lactate is not produced by our body and is only produced by the lactic acid bacteria in our microbiome. There is no issue with the D-lactate that is produced by the lactic acid bacteria within our gut. Little D-lactate is produced by these bacteria unless there is a significant overgrowth of these bacteria or severe carbohydrate malabsorption. Also, most microbiome produced D-lactate is eliminated through our stool or broken down by the enzyme D-lactate dehydrogenase.

The Issue with D-lactate Overproduction and Leaky Gut

D-lactate acidosis does exist in medical literature but is a very rare occurrence. It is documented to occur in short bowel syndrome, a medical condition where carbohydrate malabsorption occurs from the absence of the small intestine causing overgrowth of lactic acid bacteria. Increased D-lactate over time produced by these bacteria and having leaky gut issues creates D-lactate acidosis. Symptoms of D-lactate acidosis include:

- Delirium
- Ataxia
- Violent behavior
- Slurred Speech
- Brain Fog
- Headaches
- Fatigue
- Reduction of mitochondrial function
- Leaky gut

D-lactate acidosis has also rarely been diagnosed in people with severe leaky gut including people suffering from IBD.

Is it possible for people who ingest D-lactate probiotics or probiotic food to develop a buildup of D-lactate in the blood and cause issues similar to D-lactate acidosis? Possibly, if they have a severe enough leaky gut and brain that allow the D-lactate to cross the intestinal barrier and the BBB.

Most of the studies, however, with D-lactate acidosis and SBS show that it takes awhile for the body to build up enough D-lactate from excessive carbohydrate fermentation to cause severe notable health issues. In most cases, the body can metabolize D-lactate quickly and reduce concentrations of it in the bloodstream before it causes issues. Finally, severe leaky gut and brain would also need to occur for side effects of excessive D-lactate in the bloodstream to be noticed.

Reduction of SCFA production has been theorized in people with D-lactate overgrowth which may contribute to the development of leaky gut. The reduction of SCFA is also hypothesized to cause a reduction of neurotransmitters and ATP being produced by the gut microbiome causing neurological and lack of energy symptoms.

Finally, many people have adverse side effects from ingesting probiotics that produce D-lactate, which include the strains, *Lactobacillus acidophilus*, *L. bulgaricus*, *L. fermentum*, and *L. delbrueckii subsp lactis*. Their sensitivities from ingesting these probiotics, however, might stem from other issues besides D-lactate sensitivity. That being said, if you suffer from headaches, brain fog, or fatigue when ingesting D-lactate producing probiotic strains, I would avoid them and search out a D-lactate free probiotic.

Probiotic Supplements and Mislabeling

When culturing probiotic supplements, issues can arise: contamination, horizontal gene transfer (one bacteria transfers genes to another; antibiotic resistance is an example of this), and mislabeling of strains to name a few. This section is going to tackle the issue of the mislabeling of strains and how that can be harmful to your health.

Mislabeling of different strains in probiotic supplements has occurred since they were brought to market. Sometimes mislabeling is not directly the manufacturer's fault since nomenclature of strains changes occasionally. *Bacillus coagulans* was originally misidentified as *Lactobacillus sporogenes* when it was discovered in the early 1930's. There is still a debate about the correct genus of the bacteria between probiotic supplement manufacturers and microbiologists. One study about the debate states:

"In any case, the use of the term Lactobacillus sporogenes seems to aim to deliberately confound consumers, trying to benefit from association with the extensive literature on the safety and health benefits of the genus Lactobacillus."

And to stir up the people who believe I am too harsh on HSO's, from the same study:

"For this reason the use of the wrong nomenclature of L. sporogenes becomes once more questionable, since it seems to try to get advantage from the old tradition of safety of lactobacilli to remedy to the lack of safety reports on B. coagulans."

The conclusion of the report is that probiotic companies that mislabel *B. coagulans* as *L. sporogenes* are doing it for their advantage since the reclassification of the bacteria occurred a long time ago, and anyone who is selling a probiotic product should know about correct nomenclature for safety.

Colony forming unit amounts in probiotics have also been mislabeled. Most of the stated colony forming units on probiotic supplement levels are far below what can be cultured or considered to be "live" probiotics. There was a recent study done to determine whether or not the amount of probiotics that were alive coincided with the amount listed on the label. In the study, only one probiotic out of the five was able to culture the amount that was claimed to be alive in the supplements, and that probiotic was able to culture a lot more than was stated in the supplement.

So if most of these probiotics are dead when we are ingesting them, why do some people still see a benefit when taking them? It would appear that even dead probiotics show possible benefits for some people because our immune system reacts to them, up-regulates itself, and begins to fight overgrowth. That being said, would it not be better to take immune stimulants or a good prebiotic like GOS to stimulate the growth of our probiotic flora to tackle the overgrowth instead?

Probiotics, Th1 / Th2 Reactions, and our Immune System

More research is needed to determine exactly how probiotics modulate our immune system. We barely have an understanding of how pathogens affect our immune system and most of what conventional medicine believes is incorrect. Cytokines are proteins that our cells secrete to signal immune reactions. Cytokine release regulates inflammation, histamine production, gene expression, and identification / elimination of pathogens by our immune system. One of the major releases of cytokines by our immune system occurs from our helper T cells.

We are briefly going to talk about the Th1 and Th2 divisions of helper T Cells and how they relate to your state of health.

Th1

Th1 cells are what is known as cell-mediated immunity and help us fight off Gram-negative bacteria, mycobacteria, and viruses. When our body comes in contact with these organisms or has a chronic infection or overgrowth of them, the Th1 cells of our immune system become active. Inflammation occurs, and certain cytokines are released to try to help deal with the infection, TNF-a, IFNy, and IL-2. In chronic infections or overgrowth, our Th1 cells remain overactive and cause dominance in our immune system. Certain symptoms occur including, inflammation and brain fog after ingesting food (usually after a few hours), brain fog, fatigue (sometimes after meals and from exposure to sunlight), SIBO, IBS, joint pain, inflammation, hypothyroidism (low T3), rosacea, reduction in frequency of colds and infections, and ulcers. There are "autoimmune diseases" that are linked to Th1 dominance; I will go into more on that in a later book update, but here is some more information.

Th2

Th2 cells are what is known as antibody-mediated immunity and help us fight off Gram-positive bacteria, *H. pylori*, yeast, mycotoxins, mycobacteria, and parasites. When our body comes in contact with these organisms or has a chronic infection or overgrowth of them, the Th2 cells of our immune system become active. Histamine reactions and inflammation occurs. Certain cytokines are released to try to help deal with the infection, IL-4, IL-5, IL-6, IL-10, IL-13. In chronic infections or overgrowth, our Th1 cells remain overactive and cause dominance in our immune system. Certain symptoms occur including, inflammation, histamine intolerance, asthma, allergies, anaphylaxis, hives, post nasal drip, GERD, multiple chemical sensitivity, low pregnenolone, and ulcers. There are "autoimmune diseases" that are linked to Th1 dominance; I will go into more on that in a later book update, but here is some more information.

There is a test that can be done to determine if you are Th1 / Th2 dominant by measuring certain cytokines.

Which Probiotics Stimulate Which Th Response

Certain probiotics increase or decrease Th1 or Th2 responses by our immune system. If you are Th1 dominant for example, you would not want to take probiotics that increase Th1 responses; it can increase inflammation and symptoms. You instead would want to take probiotics that lower Th1 and maybe even probiotics that lower Th1 and increase Th2 to balance your immune system.

Probiotic Strains That are Believed to Manipulate Th1

TNF-a

Increases

- *L. bulgaricus*
- *L. casei Shirota*
- *L. plantarum*
- *L. reuteri*
- *L. rhamnosus*
- *L. salivarius*

Decreases

- *Bifidobacterium breve*

IFN-y / IL-12

Increases

- *B. bifidum*
- *E. coli (TG1)*
- *L. acidophilus*
- *L. casei Shirota*
- *L. johnsonii*
- *L. paracasei*
- *L. plantarum*
- *L. reuteri*
- *L. rhamnosus GG*
- *L. salivarius*

Probiotic strains that may help people with Th1 issues: *Bifidobacterium breve, L. delbrueckii subsp. bulgaricus, L. helveticus R389, S. thermophilus.*

Probiotic Strains That are Believed to Manipulate Th2

IL-4 / IL-5

Decreases

- *Bifidobacteria*
- *L. casei*
- *L. lactis*
- *L. gasseri*
- *L. paracasei*
- *L. plantarum*
- *L. reuteri*
- *L. rhamnosus GG*
- *L. salivarius*

IL-6

Increases

- *B. lactis*
- *L. bulgaricus*
- *L. casei Shirota*
- *L. helveticus R389*
- *L. rhamnosus*

IL-10

Some of these probiotic strains would lower TNF-a by increasing IL-10. If you notice, some are noted to increase TNF-a, which might cause a net equalizing effect. If you have an elevated TNF-a gut condition like ulcerative colitis or Crohn's disease, it might be worth trying these probiotic bacteria to see if it improves your condition even if it is known to increase TNF-a.

Increases

- *Bifidobacteria*
- *L. acidophilus*
- *L. casei*
- *L. delbrueckii subsp. Bulgaricus*
- *L. helveticus R389*
- *L. rhamnosus*
- *S. thermophiles*

Probiotic strains that may help people with Th2 issues, *Bifidobacterium* (may increase IL-10 in some people which may cause Th-2 issues, avoid *B. lactis*), *L. lactis, L. gasseri, L. paracasei, L. plantarum, L. reuteri, L. rhamnosus, L. salivarius*.

Should Probiotics Be Used Every Day?

The answer is no.

Probiotics and prebiotics should be used as a supplementary tool to improve your digestive health, not be your holy grail. I know this statement is totally against mainstream alternative medicine. Here is why it is true:

1. Your body can replenish its natural flora most of the time on its own if you are in overall good health and eliminated opportunistic infections.
2. Overuse of probiotics and prebiotics cause SIBO.
3. You may introduce the wrong probiotic bacteria, and that may cause more digestive issues. Supplementing probiotics with success is a coin flip. The information in this guide might help you make better choices, but even what seems like the best choice at the time may go wrong.
4. Any probiotic can become opportunistic, anytime.

In some cases, including repeated SIBO infections, probiotics and prebiotics should not be supplemented and natural flora replenishment may need to be facilitated. This decision should always be made on an individual basis.

With all this being said, I still believe that probiotics and prebiotics can be used to help improve your digestive health. Both tools have to be used carefully, and if any negative symptoms occur, you can try to switch probiotics or prebiotics to see if it alleviates the problem. If it does not, discontinue them both and see if that helps. If you are still having issues like flatulence and heartburn, consider following the SIBO protocol (Ch. 9) recommendations.

Probiotics and prebiotics should be supplemented in most people for no longer than a month. The lowest dose of probiotics possible should be used to improve intestinal integrity or alleviate digestive concerns, as well. Remember if long-term probiotic use is needed, more than likely digestive concerns are not being addressed properly, and more diagnostic work may be needed. Rarely, would I recommend long-term probiotic use in most cases.

Chapter 14

Opportunistic / Infectious Gastrointestinal Bacteria

Probiotic bacteria are very important for keeping opportunistic or infectious bacteria at bay so that the immune system can eradicate the pathogens. Nonetheless, if infection numbers of opportunistic bacteria are greater than the immune system can handle, illness will occur.

Foodborne Infection vs. Food Poisoning

In bacterial foodborne gastrointestinal illnesses, there is a difference between classical food poisoning and foodborne infections. Food poisoning occurs after the consumption of food containing bacterial toxins (examples include *E. coli*, *B. cereus*, and *Clostridium botulinum*). Most bacteria that cause food poisoning become inactivated upon ingestion by stomach acid and do not usually infect their hosts. The toxins they produce cause the actual illness. The main symptom of toxin-related food poisoning is diarrhea because of the activation of TRPV1 receptors in the gut by the toxins. The activation of the TRPV1 receptors causes loose stools because of a defense mechanism of the body trying to rid itself of the offending toxins. Vomiting, tachycardia, and headaches may also occur with food poisoning. Low-grade fever can also occur, but it is rare. *Clostridium botulinum* toxin poisoning is a serious medical emergency and causes symptoms like paralysis and breathing trouble. Symptoms of food poisoning can occur in foodborne infections, but the overall range of symptoms most of the time are self-limiting (except for *Clostridium botulinum*).

Foodborne bacterial infections occur when the contaminated food or water acts as a delivery system and reservoir for the bacteria (*Campylobacter*, *H. pylori*, *Salmonella*, *Shigella*, and *Listeria monocytogenes*) so that the bacteria can propagate and cause an infection. Once the bacteria colonize, they rapidly produce toxins in the bowel. Similar symptoms of food poisoning occur including diarrhea, vomiting, tachycardia, and headaches. Elevated fever and chills are one of the main symptoms that separate foodborne illnesses and food poisoning. Foodborne bacterial infections regimen choices depend on the severity of the infection, and some may require hospitalization and antibiotic use.

Antibiotic therapy is contraindicated in true food poisoning because the toxins ingested, not a bacterial infection, is what makes you ill. Most of the time there is no infection associated with true food poisoning. Antitoxins and hospitalization may be needed in a severe case of food poisoning. Foodborne infection, on the other hand, may need antibiotic therapy and hospitalization depending on the severity of the bacterial infection. Anti-diarrheal medicine should also be avoided unless necessary. Use of Antidiarrheal medication has been linked to poor outcomes and longer hospitalization because diarrhea is a defense mechanism by the body to eliminate toxins and bacteria through the bowels.

One of the most important things you can do while ill is to remain hydrated especially if you are vomiting and have diarrhea. I recommend every hour at least drinking a mixture of 1/2 - one teaspoon of Real Salt, 300 mg of potassium gluconate, and 200 mg of magnesium glycinate in a ten – twelve ounce glass of filtered water.

Foodborne Infection Protocol

- S. boulardii Jarrow Formulas with Lactobacillus reuteri or you can use Jarrow Lactobacillus plantarum – take while infected, on a daily basis at night with a glass of filtered water.
- Upgraded™ Activated Charcoal – two capsules every thirty minutes until vomiting and diarrhea stop. No more than twelve capsules per day.
- Sodium ascorbate - 4,000 mg, daily.
- Follow SIBO antibacterial and biofilm elimination protocols (Ch. 9).

If the diarrhea does not stop in a few days, or if diarrhea is very serious:

- Rainforest Pharmacy sangre de drago – follow the general supplement bottle recommendations.

The activated charcoal is to absorb the toxins produced by the bacteria.

Sangre de drago has been shown clinically to stop diarrhea.

The vitamin C is to help detoxify the body.

Probiotics, natural antibacterial agents, and anti-biofilm agents may help eliminate opportunistic bacteria causing the food poisoning.

Food Poisoning Protocol

- Upgraded™ Activated Charcoal – two capsules every thirty minutes until vomiting and diarrhea stop (no more than twelve capsules per day).
- Sodium ascorbate - 4,000 mg – 8,000 mg, daily.

- Jarrow Formulas NAC Sustain – one tablet twice daily. NAC is a systemic biofilm chelator; I do not recommend it as a first-line anti-biofilm agent in a protocol. Do not supplement more than 1,200 mg daily; doses above this recommendation may make the NAC you take become a pro-oxidant.
- Jarrow Formulas milk thistle – follow supplement bottle recommendations.

If diarrhea does not stop in a few days, or if the diarrhea is very serious:

- Rainforest Pharmacy sangre de drago – follow the general supplement bottle recommendations.

The activated charcoal is to absorb the toxins produced by the bacteria.

Sangre de drago has been shown clinically to stop diarrhea.

The vitamin C, NAC, and milk thistle is to help detoxify the body.

Opportunistic / Infectious Gastrointestinal Bacteria

Bacillus cereus

Bacillus cereus (like its "cousin" *Bacillus subtilis*) is a soil-based, Gram-positive bacterium. Many different strains of *Bacillus cereus* are implicated in opportunistic human infections, including foodborne illness. The bacteria are best known for causing food poisoning in improperly cooked or stored rice (also known as "fried rice syndrome"). *Bacillus cereus* is also found in the guts of chickens and pigs, and undercooked meat from those animals may cause an infection.

Symptoms of *Bacillus cereus* toxin ingestion usually appear a few hours after ingestion of contaminated food products. Symptoms may take longer to develop if an infection develops from *Bacillus cereus* endospores. *Bacillus cereus* infection / poisoning are very common foodborne illnesses because in order for the endospores to be inactivated, the food has to be cooked at a temperature greater than 212F for a while. The cooked food also has to be properly refrigerated and stored, so inactive endospores do not activate, produce toxins, and germinate causing illness.

Infection of *Bacillus cereus* usually results in severe nausea, vomiting, and diarrhea. The emetic form of *Bacillus cereus* food contamination usually presents itself very quickly after food ingestion (one to five hours after eating). Most of the time, the emetic form of *Bacillus cereus* food contamination comes from the toxins that the bacteria produce from improper cooking and storing rather than an actual infection. On the other hand, the diarrheal form of a *Bacillus cereus* infection usually comes from an active infection (from endospore germination) and manifests itself in eight to sixteen hours after consumption of contaminated food.

A foodborne infection of *Bacillus cereus* is usually self-limiting, and most cases resolve within a day or two. If you have the self-limiting form of the infection, I suggest that you follow my food poisoning protocol (Ch. 14). Rarely, a *Bacillus cereus* infection may require hospitalization, because of both an active infection and the toxins the bacteria produce. If this is the case, I recommend combining my food poisoning protocol (Ch. 14) with my anti-biofilm protocol (Ch. 9) in combination with conventional antibiotic therapy to help eliminate illness caused by the bacteria.

Campylobacter jejuni

The *Campylobacter* genus is a Gram-negative, opportunistic spiral bacterium. *Campylobacter jejuni* is the species that is mainly associated with foodborne illnesses out of this genus. *Campylobacter jejuni* is commonly found in animal feces, and naturally colonizes the digestive tract of many bird species. *Campylobacter jejuni* is also found in the digestive tracts of cattle as natural flora in lesser amounts.

Symptoms of an opportunistic *Campylobacter jejuni* infection usually appear within a few hours of the ingestion of compromised food products. *Campylobacter jejuni* also produces a toxin (cytolethal distending toxin) that hinders lymphocytes for a short time and limits immune system functioning so that the bacteria can easily further propagate unchecked. Infection of *Campylobacter jejuni* usually results in self-limiting enteritis, abdominal pain, diarrhea, fever, and malaise. Symptoms usually persist for twenty-four hours and for at most a week. Rarely, *Campylobacter jejuni* infection can lead to Guillain-Barre syndrome, so make sure you eliminate it or support your body's immune system as soon as possible.

Severe infections may cause bloody diarrhea and high fevers and may be needed to be treated with hospitalization and antibiotic therapy. *Campylobacter jejuni* also forms biofilms, so anti-biofilm protocols (Ch. 9) combined with antibiotic therapy may help speed up recovery rates from infection.

As long as you are not suffering from a severe infection, follow the food poisoning protocol (Ch. 14) or SIBO protocol (Ch. 9) depending on the severity of symptoms.

Clostridium Genus

The *Clostridium* genus is a Gram-positive, endospore-forming probiotic / opportunistic bacteria that are known for causing devastating infections in the human body.

Clostridium botulinum

Clostridium botulinum is an opportunistic bacteria that's toxin is known as the cause of botulism. *Clostridium botulinum* produces strong neurotoxins that create multiple serious medical issues within the body upon digestion. These toxins are what cause the health issues; *Clostridium botulinum* in most cases is easily inactivated by stomach acid and eliminated from the body upon digestion. Botulism is a serious medical condition that needs to be evaluated and treated by medical professionals in a well-equipped hospital.

Most *Clostridium botulinum* toxin poisonings come from homemade canned foods, because of improper technique and knowledge of canning methods. Improperly canned food is a perfect place for *Clostridium botulinum* to thrive because of the long shelf life of most canned food that contributes to its growth and toxin production. Most cans are also stored at room temperature, and there is very little to no oxygen in a vacuumed sealed can or jar, which helps facilitate growth.

Growth and toxin production of *Clostridium botulinum* is quite rare because its growth requires a low acidic, low salt, low sugar environment, which is lacking in most modern canned foods. Most canned foods receive a boiling water bath for a few minutes before and after canning so that *Clostridium botulinum* is eliminated.

Throw out any cans or jars that are passed the use by date, leaking or bulging, damaged or cracked, have a rancid smell, or are moldy to prevent *Clostridium botulinum* illness.

Most honey also contains *Clostridium botulinum* spores that can cause a lesser infectious disease in infants known as infant botulism. Honey should never be fed to any child under the age of one because of the risk of the disease. Proper stomach acid levels inactivate *Clostridium botulinum* spores in honey easily for anyone over the age of one. Most infants recover from infant botulism without any long-term issues.

Signs of a *Clostridium botulinum* toxin poisoning include muscle weakness (especially of the facial, cranial, and breathing muscles), double vision, difficulty chewing and swallowing, breathing issues, nausea, vomiting, and autonomic nervous system problems. Treatment usually consists of supportive care in a hospital ICU, and the use of antitoxins and mechanical ventilation may become necessary. Most *Clostridium botulinum* hospitalizations take one to two months before you are released and lasting muscle weakness and neurological issues may persist for months to years afterward.

Clostridium difficile

Clostridium difficile is a probiotic / opportunistic Gram-positive bacteria that are found in the natural gut flora of humans. Usually, it is kept in check by other probiotic bacteria so that it does not have the opportunity to become opportunistic; but, when gut flora is severely disrupted, *Clostridium difficile* becomes opportunistic leading to a *Clostridium difficile* infection.

Clostridium difficile is mostly antibiotic resistant, creates biofilms in the colon, and causes a reconstruction of the colon itself, a medical condition called pseudomembranous colitis. This form of colitis is an extreme inflammation of the colon. Exogenous mucous membranes are produced by the bacteria causing even more bowel problems and may lead to a life-threatening condition called toxic megacolon.

Clostridium difficile infections are extremely serious and should be treated in the hospital. There are supplements that may help prevent the infection from occurring, and supplements that can be taken to help recover during or from an infection, but there are no supplements that can eliminate an infection on its own for safety reasons. If you are hospitalized or are on strong antibiotics for a period, supplementation of small amounts of probiotics (five – ten billion) should be considered to help prevent opportunistic *Clostridium difficile* infection. You can also supplement with vitamin D, zinc, and vitamin C to help boost your immune system to help prevent and opportunistic infection.

Symptoms of a *Clostridium difficile* infection include diarrhea, abdominal pain, fever, and a distinctive stool odor. If you have any of these symptoms and have had recent antibiotic treatment, then it is likely you have a *Clostridium difficile* infection. *Clostridium difficile* is typically diagnosed with a stool sample or culture, and a Toxin ELISA test.

Clostridium difficile Elimination Protocol

- Antibiotic Rifaximin – take as directed (push for the use of Rifaximin if possible, it has been shown through multiple studies that it can help eliminate *Clostridium difficile* with fewer side effects then Flagyl or Vancomycin).
- ***If you cannot use Rifaximin, try to use Flagyl first instead of Vancomycin if at all possible. My recommendation is that Vancomycin should be used as a last resort, but always check with a doctor first.***

Anti-BioFilm Protocol

- Symbiotics lactoferrin - follow supplement bottle recommendations (can increase up to two grams daily if needed).
- EDTA – follow supplement bottle recommendations.
- Jarrow Formulas NAC Sustain – one tablet twice daily. NAC is a systemic biofilm chelator; I do not recommend it as a first-line anti-biofilm agent in a protocol. Do not supplement more

than 1,200 mg daily; doses above this recommendation may make the NAC you take become a pro-oxidant.

Other supplements in protocol:

- Optimize your vitamin D levels.
- Sodium ascorbate - take 4,000 mg, daily.
- Nordic Naturals fish oil - take 4,000 mg, daily.
- Thorne Curcumin - take once daily.
- Magnesium glycinate - take 400 mg, daily before bed.
- L-Glutamine – 15,000 mg total – take in divided doses, three times daily with food (use with caution if you have a sensitivity to glutamic acid, deficiency in GABA, or severe leaky gut and brain).
- Florastor probiotic – take while you have an active *Clostridium difficile* infection.
- Upgraded™ Activated Charcoal – follow the general supplement bottle recommendations.

If symptoms have not improved on antibiotic, or for extra help: add a natural antimicrobial.

- Nature's Way enteric coated peppermint oil - thirty to sixty minutes before meals, twice daily.

Or choose one strong antimicrobial:

- Colloidal silver (Mesosilver, Sovereign Silver).
- Zane Hellas Oil of Oregano - oil of oregano is a broad spectrum, systemic antimicrobial agent; do not use first in a protocol.
- Thorne Research Berberine – take 500 mg, twice daily.
- Allicin-C.

If *Clostridium difficile* infection continues to get worse even after the protocol, consider fecal matter transplant.

- Follow the severe gut rebuilding protocol (Ch. 9) after *Clostridium difficile* infection is cleared. Add Florastor probiotic to protocol.

EDTA or NAC is used to destroy biofilm made by *Clostridium difficile.*

Vitamin D is to bolster the immune system, and the vitamin C is to help detoxification and reduce inflammation.

Fish oil and curcumin are recommended to help reduce inflammation.

Magnesium glycinate and L-glutamine are for general bowel health.

Florastor has been shown to help improve intestinal health greatly by reducing *Clostridium difficile.*

Activated charcoal will help with diarrhea and absorb toxins.

Clostridium perfringens

Clostridium perfringens is a Gram-positive, spore-forming bacterium that is normal intestinal flora in humans. *Clostridium perfringens* produces enterotoxins that cause foodborne illness from poorly prepared food, mainly meat, and poultry, or from ingestion of excess bacterial spores from food that is not properly stored or refrigerated. Most *Clostridium perfringens* infections come from cafeterias where food is prepared in large quantities and may be kept warm unsafely for long periods.

Clostridium perfringens infection has an incubation period of six to twenty-four hours and is usually self-limiting. Symptoms of a *Clostridium perfringens* illness include abdominal cramping, diarrhea, vomiting, and mild fever. Most cases of foodborne illness last at most a day or two and are resolved very quickly.

Escherichia Genus

The *Escherichia* genus is Gram-negative, rod-shaped bacteria that are either probiotic or opportunistic bacteria depending on the strain. Many different strains of *Escherichia* cause foodborne illnesses including O157:H7, O154:H4, O121, and O104:H21. Most *Escherichia coli* infections come from contaminated beef, dairy products, and the contaminated fecal matter left on vegetables and fruit.

Escherichia coli infections range from being self-limiting to severe medical emergencies depending on the strain of bacteria. The strains mentioned above are extremely virulent, and some cause serious medical conditions including bloody diarrhea, excessive vomiting, kidney failure, high fever, and sepsis. If you have any of the above symptoms during your bout of food poisoning, immediately go to your nearest emergency room for treatment.

Escherichia coli produce biofilms so combine anti-biofilm protocols (Ch. 9) with antibiotic therapy for maximum effectiveness. Antibiotic treatment with certain *Escherichia coli* infections (O157:H7), have been linked to increased kidney issues, so caution may be needed in the use of antibiotics if you have that strain.

Klebsiella Genus

Different strains of *Klebsiella* are normal flora in our body. The bacteria is ubiquitous in nature and is found almost everywhere. As long as this Gram-negative, rod-shaped bacteria is kept in check by our immune system it lives as a commensal with us. *Klebsiella* colonizes a lot of the human body, from our nasal passages, mouth, to our digestive tracts. The bacteria's colonization occasionally benefits us; it breaks down and ferments lactose in the intestinal tract. *Klebsiella* can break down resistant starch type two and three (corn starch, potato starch, rice starch) easily using its enzymes. When *Klebsiella* is probiotic flora, it can help to break down occasional ingestion of resistant starch for better digestion by helping to feed our microbiome. *Klebsiella* is also able to break down and ferment the prebiotic FOS (inulin), fructose, and mannose. *Klebsiella* uses some of the carbohydrates for fuel and what is left over, it breaks down for us or other microorganisms that can digest them.

Klebsiella serves niche purposes in strengthening our overall digestive health when it is commensal by helping us assimilate carbohydrates.

Klebsiella species list:

- *K. granulomatis*
- *K. michiganensis*
- *K. oxytoca* – human colonizer.
- *K. pneumoniae* – human colonizer.
- *K. quasipneumoniae* – human colonizer.
- *K. variicola*

What Medical Conditions Does Opportunistic *Klebsiella* Cause?

I guess we should not blame *Klebsiella* for its breaking bad ways, most microorganisms if given the chance become opportunistic. What are known infection areas of the bacteria?

Conventional acute infection areas of opportunistic *Klebsiella:*

- Blood – a cause of septicemia.
- Brain – a cause of meningitis.
- Joints – a cause of rheumatoid arthritis.
- Lungs – a cause of pneumonia.

- Mouth – a cause of dental caries.
- Small intestine – a cause of SIBO-D.
- Spine – a cause of ankylosing spondylitis.
- Urinary tract – a cause of infections.

Opportunistic *Klebsiella* infects different parts of the body and causes many medical conditions. So what about *Klebsiella* colonizing and causing chronic inflammation in the joints or spine? Is it possible that *Klebsiella* produced endotoxins leak out of the gut and trigger certain immune responses that cause issues with collagen production and increased inflammation in the joints or spine? Why is it so hard for mainstream medicine to believe that chronic infections or immune reactions stemming from *Klebsiella* leaky gut can cause two different "autoimmune conditions (RA and AS)"?

Listeria monocytogenes

Listeria monocytogenes is a Gram-positive bacterium that is implicated in the cause of listeriosis. *Listeria monocytogenes* infection can range from being asymptomatic / self-limited in healthy people to causing severe central nervous system and brain infections in immunocompromised people. Infection of the bacteria is known as the disease listeriosis.

Symptoms of a *Listeria monocytogenes* infection in healthy people are usually asymptomatic. An infection may rarely cause self-limiting fever, vomiting, and diarrhea. *Listeria monocytogenes* infections in immunocompromised people, elderly, pregnant women, or infants on the other hand, may cause a serious infection known as listeriosis. Symptoms of listeriosis in high-risk people are fever, muscle aches, headache, stiff neck, confusion, neurological issues, loss of balance, and convulsions. Listeriosis can spread to the brain and spinal cord if left untreated or if the person has a poor immune system, and may cause meningitis and brain abscesses. If a pregnant woman has listeriosis, her symptoms on the other hand, are very mild and are akin to having the stomach flu. However, an infection of the bacteria can lead to miscarriage, stillbirth, premature delivery, or a life-threatening infection in the newborn or fetus.

The main causes of *Listeria monocytogenes* ingestion are contaminated food products, uncooked or raw meat, contaminated dairy products, vegetables, fruits, and seafood. Pregnant women should limit ingestion of soft cheeses, unpasteurized milk, and pâté because of the potential danger of self-inoculation.

Listeriosis is treated with antibiotic therapy and requires hospitalizations ranging from two – six weeks depending on the severity of the disease and if it spread to the brain and spinal cord. *Listeria monocytogenes* produces biofilms; therefore, anti-biofilm protocols (Ch. 9) combined with antibiotic therapy may improve recovery outcomes.

Helicobacter pylori

Helicobacter pylori are Gram-negative bacteria that can be found residing in the human stomach. *H. pylori* infections are a common cause of stomach ulcers, gastritis, GERD, and stomach cancer. Symptoms of an *H. pylori* infection include gastritis, abdominal pain, nausea, bloating, GERD, and occasional vomiting in a severe infection.

H. pylori may be part of a normal stomach microbiome. In some people, though, *H. pylori* may become opportunistic, and cause numerous health issues. If you have a normal stomach acid level, *H. pylori* populations are usually kept in balance by the acid. Opportunistic *H. pylori* infection is the cause of most ulcers. Signs of an opportunistic *H. pylori* infection are ulcers, gastritis, stomach pain, or unrelenting heartburn because the stomach increases gastrin levels and acid (that is propelled through the esophagus by the excess gas that *H. pylori* produce) in an attempt to rid the stomach of *H. pylori*.

Some research suggests *H. pylori* might be probiotic stomach bacteria and only becomes opportunistic after proper digestive conditions change in the stomach. When the stomach has normal levels of stomach acid, *H. pylori* populations are kept under control. Children that were studied having normal *H. pylori* populations in their gut were found to have a lesser chance of developing asthma. In addition, even though research links prolonged opportunistic infections of *H. pylori* to stomach cancer, it also links probiotic colonization of the bacteria to lower levels of esophageal cancer. More data that is scientific needs to be published before *H. pylori* will be considered natural flora of the stomach. Most doctors recommend eradicating the bacteria from the stomach if infected.

The best diagnostic tests to determine if you have an *H. pylori* infection are either a stool sample or a urea breath test. Blood tests are ineffective at determining if you have a current *H. pylori* infection or have had an infection in the past. Follow my eradication of *H. pylori* protocols (Ch. 4) if you have an active infection.

Mycobacterium avium paratuberculosis

Mycobacteria is a genus of bacteria that causes serious diseases in mammals (tuberculosis and leprosy are examples of *Mycobacteria*). A type of *Mycobacteria* called *Mycobacterium avium paratuberculosis* is a pathogenic bacteria found in the gut of ruminant animals like cows and causes Johne's disease (*paratuberculosis*) in cattle.

Paratuberculosis causes diarrhea and wasting in the cattle and also causes the cows to develop inflammatory bowel disease. Treatment of *paratuberculosis* in cattle is limited because of the cost of using human treatments for *Mycobacterial* infection. Usually, the most cost effective measure is to destroy the infected herd.

MAP is the primary cause of ulcerative colitis and Crohn's disease in humans. One of the deciding factors in whether anyone succumbs to ulcerative colitis or Crohn's disease seems to be the amount of *MAP* that that person is exposed to. Lesser exposure to *MAP* leads to ulcerative colitis, where greater exposure to *MAP* causes Crohn's disease.

MAP has recently been discovered as a zoological disease (a disease that can be transferred from animals to humans or vice versa). *MAP* can be transferred to humans when contact with infected cattle feces occurs, drinking improperly treated farm runoff water, ingesting beef, or ingesting milk and dairy products from infected cows. There are case studies identifying farmers with *MAP* after contact with aerosolized cow feces. *MAP* infections also originate from cattle farm runoff coming into contact with municipal drinking water. *MAP* is a very resistant bacterium that can survive up to nine months in mud, a year in cow manure, and up to two years in water. Standard industrial water treatment such as filtration systems and chlorination may prove to be an ineffective treatment against eliminating *MAP*.

MAP also has been discovered in beef, but the levels are lower than other infection routes if the meat is prepared properly. Cow muscle tissue does not naturally contain many bacteria, but if the meat is not processed and prepared properly, feces can encounter the meat and infect it with *MAP*. *MAP* can also survive standard cooking temperatures, but it can be eliminated at prolonged temperatures around 165F. *MAP* also appears to be resistant to nitrates and smoke as well.

Scientific literature indicates that humans are commonly exposed to *MAP* from the ingestion of milk and other dairy products. The proposed reason is that the bacteria in milk are more invasive and populous than other routes of exposure. *MAP* is protected by the higher fat content of some dairy products. Fat globules protect *MAP* from stomach acid so that it can survive in greater numbers allowing it reaches the intestines. Raw dairy has a greater concentration of *MAP* bacteria than properly pasteurized dairy. The correlation between this data is unknown though because *MAP* can survive pasteurization. Research is mixed about if pasteurized milk and dairy products are safer and contain less *MAP* than if they are raw. I suggest anyone who is drinking dairy to consume pasture raised, vat pasteurized milk, for the healthiest way possible of trying to avoid *MAP*. Finally, *MAP* can also survive freezing (ice cream) for up to a year.

Salmonella enterica

Salmonella enterica are Gram-negative bacteria that are implicated as the main cause of salmonellosis. *Salmonella enterica* is commonly found on contaminated improperly prepared or undercooked beef, chicken, and pork, contaminated egg products (most *Salmonella enterica* contamination of egg dishes comes from the eggshell, not from the egg yolk or whites), and fecal matter contaminated fruit or vegetables. Cooking contaminated food thoroughly eliminates most *Salmonella enterica* bacteria, but any toxins and bacteria that may survive cooking may be able to cause salmonellosis. Salmonellosis mainly occurs if enough live *Salmonella enterica* survive ingestion / stomach acid, and can multiply and produce toxins in the small intestine. Even though proper cooking eliminates *Salmonella enterica* if you believe any food is contaminated with elevated amounts of bacteria, (chicken that looks and smells off) toss it.

Salmonellosis is usually a self-limited infection; most people develop diarrhea, vomiting, fever, and abdominal cramps 12 -72 hours after infection. Salmonellosis usually lasts for one to three days, but may last for up to a week. People with a severe infection might need to be hospitalized. Most hospitalizations from salmonellosis are due to dehydration from excessive vomiting and diarrhea. Reactive arthritis may also develop after a severe salmonella infection in some people. Salmonellosis may be treated with antibiotics in people hospitalized with the infection and if they have compromised immune systems to prevent further infection complications.

If someone with salmonellosis has a compromised immune system, the bacteria may enter the bloodstream and become a systemic infection. This serious infection is known as typhoid fever. Symptoms of typhoid fever worsen over a period of weeks as the bacteria spreads to different organ systems and include slowly rising body temperature, malaise, headache, cough, abdominal pain, bloody nose, delirium, hemorrhages, septicemia, encephalitis, coma, and possibly death. Typhoid fever is a serious medical condition and needs to be treated with antibiotics promptly.

Shigella Genus

Shigella is a genus of Gram-negative bacteria that are the cause of the infection shigellosis. Very few *Shigella* bacteria are needed to be ingested for infection (few hundred) compared to other bacteria. *Shigella* also produces toxins that can cause acute kidney failure and other issues.

Most *Shigella* infections come from the improper washing of hands in food preparation (fecal / oral route). *Shigella* infections can also occur from the ingestion of improperly prepared or washed fruits and vegetables contaminated with fecal matter. Symptoms of a *Shigella* infection usually develop within two to four days of ingestion, but sometimes may take as long as a week to develop.

Symptoms of shigellosis include diarrhea, fever, nausea, vomiting, stomach cramps, and blood and mucus in the stool. *Shigella* infection may also cause dysentery (a worse version of shigellosis), a condition where the bacteria begin to destroy the intestinal mucosa, causing further issues.

Most cases of the disease resolve themselves within a week. Severe cases of the disease (dysentery) may require hospitalization for fluids / electrolyte replacement, and possible treatment with antibiotics. Anti-diarrheal medications should never be used during an active infection because they have been shown to prolong the infection.

Staphylococcus aureus

Staphylococcus aureus is a Gram-positive bacterium that is the cause of the dreaded staph and MRSA infections. *Staphylococcus aureus* is natural flora bacteria on the skin and inside the nose for about 25% of the population. Ingestion of *Staphylococcus aureus* toxins can cause a food poisoning illness known as *Staphylococcal* enteritis.

Staphylococcus aureus routes of poisoning include ingestion of improperly cooked meats, contaminated fruits and vegetables, cross-contamination from food preparation, contamination from food preparers not wearing gloves on their hands with a *Staphylococcal aureus* infection, and improperly stored food.

Ingestion of the toxin causes inflammation and swelling of the intestines. Manifestations of symptoms usually appear quickly after ingestion of *Staphylococcus aureus* toxin and appear between one to eight hours. Symptoms of *Staphylococcus aureus* food poisoning include nausea, violent vomiting, abdominal cramps, headache, weakness, diarrhea, and a slightly elevated body temperature that usually lasts for twenty-four hours and up to two days.

Treatment for *Staphylococcus aureus* usually is supportive (rest, fluid, and electrolyte replacement), but hospitalization may be needed if dehydration becomes severe.

Streptococcus pyogenes

Streptococcus pyogenes are Gram-positive opportunistic bacteria that make up the natural skin, throat, and respiratory system flora. *Streptococcus pyogenes* can cause many different infections within the body, but we are going to focus on only strep throat.

Strep throat is a type of pharyngitis that is caused by *Streptococcus pyogenes*. The incubation period of a *Streptococcus pyogenes* infection is one to three days after infection. Symptoms of strep throat include fever, sore throat, headache, and enlarged lymph nodes. Strep throat is a highly contagious infection, and most diagnosis of the illness is made with a throat culture of the bacteria at your doctor's office.

Treatment usually consists of pain relievers and antibiotics. Young children should be treated with antibiotics because they have a greater risk of the bacteria getting into the bloodstream and cause heart issues. The risk of complications in most healthy adults and older children are mild, and the illness is mainly self-limiting for a few days. It is possible in some immunocompromised individuals for the bacteria to spread systemically and cause further issues that require antibiotic therapy and hospitalization, but this is rare.

Strep Throat Natural Protocol for Adults

- Manuka honey – one tbsp, two – three times daily.
- Symbiotics lactoferrin – two – four capsules daily with food.
- Swish and gargle with colloidal silver (Mesosilver), three times daily.

Sore Throat Relief

- Seagate olive leaf throat spray raspberry spearmint – follow supplement recommendations for dosage.

OR

- Traditional Medicinals Organic Throat Coat – follow tea recommendations for general usage. Do not use if you suffer from high blood pressure because the licorice extract in the tea may cause water retention and raise blood pressure.

Manuka honey, lactoferrin, and colloidal silver are strong antimicrobial agents that can help eliminate *Streptococcus pyogenes.*

Vibrio cholerae

Vibrio cholerae is a Gram-negative bacterium; some strains are implicated as the cause of cholera. Cholera is an infection of the small intestine by the bacteria. Cholera is transmitted by the ingestion of either fecal matter contaminated water or food.

The main symptoms of the infection are vomiting and extreme amounts of diarrhea within one to five days after ingestion of contaminated food or water. A rapid dipstick test exists to determine the presence of a *Vibrio cholerae* infection. An untreated cholera infection will cause a person to produce up to three to five gallons of diarrhea a day. Dehydration is the main medical concern of someone infected with cholera; rehydration therapy is almost always necessary.

Most people infected with cholera are hospitalized and are treated with antibiotics and rehydration therapy for a few days. I would recommend adding anti-biofilm protocols (Ch. 9) to help speed up recovery.

Yersinia enterocolitica

Yersinia enterocolitica is a Gram-negative bacterium that is the cause of the disease yersiniosis. Yersiniosis is an infectious disease that comes from the ingestion of undercooked meat, unpasteurized milk, or water contaminated with *Yersinia enterocolitica.* Symptoms of the disease manifest themselves four to seven days after infection and usually last one to three weeks.

Yersiniosis symptoms mimic many different medical conditions, and different symptoms depend on an infected person's age. Infected infants usually get the brunt of the disease; they suffer from fever and diarrhea. Yersiniosis in infants might turn into bacteremia and is more than likely to be treated in the hospital with antibiotics than an infection in adults. Infected children usually suffer from fever, abdominal pain, and diarrhea that may become bloody. Adults, on the other hand, might only have right-sided abdominal pain (sometimes confused with appendicitis) and fever. Yersiniosis in an adult is mainly self-limiting.

Antibiotic therapy and hospitalization may be required in severe cases of the disease. I would also recommend adding anti-biofilm protocols (Ch. 9) to help speed up recovery.

Chapter 15

Diets

For the diet section of this book, I am going to list specific diets, their pro and cons, suggestions of their use, and information about where you can learn more about these diets. Most people, sadly, do not change their diet until they are already diagnosed with a disease and are forced to change their lifestyle. For a diet to work, someone has to make a complete lifestyle change. Diets are listed in specific protocols if needed to help the protocol succeed.

Bulletproof® Diet

http://www.bulletproofexec.com/the-complete-illustrated-one-page-bulletproof-diet/

Pros

The Bulletproof® Diet is a cyclic ketogenic diet that helps you lose weight quickly. It improves the whole body experience (life, brain function, exercise, and sleep). It also detoxifies the body and helps the body regenerate from diseases, eliminates gluten, is a low lactose, low fructose, mostly organic, non-GMO diet, and limits mycotoxin exposure.

Cons

The Bulletproof® Diet is contraindicated in people with adrenal fatigue or people who cannot regulate cortisol easily. It does not address some antinutrients. There is a lot of exposure to dioxins from excessive meat consumption.

Summary

The Bulletproof® Diet is a great diet that originated from Silicon Valley genius Dave Asprey. He was extremely overweight and with much research modified the Paleo diet so that it would eliminate mycotoxins and help speed up weight loss and increase mental clarity. He also teaches a complete lifestyle change that can help you sleep better, exercise more efficiently, and achieve greater health.

The Bulletproof® Diet shows great results in people who are sensitive to mycotoxins and in people with active yeast infections. The average person might not see a great difference in mental clarity and performance in limiting mycotoxins. Any ketogenic diet should be avoided by people suffering from adrenal fatigue until their adrenal glands repair themselves.

Elemental Diet

http://www.siboinfo.com/elemental-formula.html

http://www.siboinfo.com/uploads/5/4/8/4/5484269/homemade_elemental_diet_options.pdf

Pros

The Elemental Diet is indigestible by bacteria and can be used to eliminate SIBO and ulcerative colitis / Crohn's disease. It is a gluten-free, lactose-free diet, and helps eliminate excess yeast from the body.

Cons

Fructose is added to the elemental diet, it is an extremely rigid, bland tasting diet, and is expensive.

Summary

The elemental diets have been around for a long time but were usually supplemented by readymade products ripe with hydrogenated oils, preservatives, and GMO byproducts.

This homemade elemental diet by Dr. Allison Siebecker, on the other hand, is a perfect alternative for traditional elemental diets. This diet is extremely useful in eliminating opportunistic bacteria in the colon like SIBO and ulcerative colitis /Crohn's disease.

FODMAP DIET

http://www.ibsdiets.org/wp-content/uploads/2016/03/IBSDiets-FODMAP-chart.pdf

Pros

The FODMAP diet greatly eliminates SIBO and IBS symptoms by starving the opportunistic bacteria. It is a gluten-free, lactose-free, fructose limiting, and GMO limiting diet.

Cons

It is non-ketogenic, does not recommend limiting all GMOs, does not limit mycotoxins, and does not encourage consumption of organic foods.

Summary

The low FODMAP diet was developed at the Monash University in Melbourne Australia. It is a great diet for treating SIBO and IBS and is easier to adopt than an elemental or semi-elemental diet. It helps decrease some opportunistic bacteria in the small and large intestine by starving them of the fermentable FODMAP carbohydrates that they need to survive. Sadly, the low FODMAP diet also decreases probiotic flora as well over time.

FODMAP stands for fermentable, oligo, di, monosaccharides, and polyols. Mono-di-oligosaccharides are different types of carbohydrates. A polyol is a sugar alcohol which has lower caloric content than most other carbohydrates. The goal of the diet is to restrict the amounts of FODMAPS you consume in your diet to a bare minimum. The low FODMAP diet will hopefully reduce your symptoms if you suffer from SIBO.

The low FODMAP diet is to help reduce opportunistic bacteria in your small intestine to a lower population. During this time, you might have some symptoms of a herx reaction. You might either develop constipation or have diarrhea briefly as your gut microbiome becomes more acclimated.

The moderate FODMAP diet adds a few increased FODMAP foods into the diet as a test to see if your gut can now handle FODMAP. FODMAPS need to be added back slowly into the diet. I would add more fruit in first, and increase the servings to about two to three daily. If you can tolerate an increase of fructose in your diet, then slowly add in lactose and high FODMAP foods like onions and garlic. I would still avoid wheat, polyols, and most FOS's if possible.

Different Foods That Are Restricted on a Low FODMAP Diet

Foods with Elevated Amounts of Fructans(FOS):

Artichoke, Spelt, Freekeh, Cous Cous, Cho Cho, Bourghal, Garlic, Leek, Onion, Spring Onion (White Part), Shallots, Wheat, Rye, Barley, Inulin, FOS Prebiotic Supplements, Watermelon, Cashews, Pistachios, Asparagus, Broccoli, Peaches, Almonds, Hazelnuts (twenty plus nuts), Persimmon, Tamarillo, Choko, Nectarines, Pomegranates, Chicory Root, Snow Peas, Okra, Brussel Sprouts, Butternut Pumpkin, Amaranth, Savoy Cabbage, Grapefruit, and Beetroot

Foods with Elevated Amounts of Fructose:

Apples, Cherries, Figs, Pears, Peaches, Mango, Watermelon, Guava (Unripe), High Fructose Corn Syrup

Foods with Elevated Amounts of Galactans:

Legumes, Soy Milk, Cashews, Cassava, Pulses, Snow Peas, Hazelnuts (twenty plus nuts), Peas, Taro, Yucca Root, Custard Apple

Foods with Elevated Amounts of Lactose:

Milk, Fresh Cheese, Ice Cream, and Custard

Foods with Elevated Amounts of Polyols:

Apples, Apricots, Avocado, Blackberries, Cherries, Lychees, Pears, Nectarines, Plums, Prunes, Watermelon, Cauliflower, Celery, Mushrooms, Snow Peas, Sweet Corn, Sweet Potato, and Sugar Alcohols / Sweeteners (Xylitol, Sorbitol, Mannitol, Isomalt, Maltitol)

What Foods Can I Eat on a Low FODMAP Diet?

The low FODMAP diet limits several different foods you can eat daily. Even though, your choices are limited you can still cook a lot of different meals on a low FODMAP diet. It might be difficult to eat at restaurants, but most Americans need to eat healthier home cooked meals more often.

There is some conflict about what foods are allowed on the low FODMAP diet and what foods should be avoided. My safe food list is a list of foods that have the lowest amounts of FODMAPS, if any. That way you do not have to worry if you are sticking to the low FODMAP diet or not.

Low FODMAP – Low Fermentation Diet Safe Food List

Carbs – Must be consumed hot after preparation (NO RESISTANT STARCH)

Arrowroot, Buckwheat Groats, Buckwheat Flour, Millet, Jasmine Rice, Sushi Rice, Corn (non-GMO), Potatoes (red, russet, yellow), Quinoa, Plantain, Tapioca Flour, Sorghum Flour, White Rice Flour, Rutabaga, Butternut Squash (1/4 cup), Spaghetti Squash, Yam

Condiments

Hot Sauce (check for added FODMAPS), Organic Mustard, Organic Tamari Soy Sauce, Apple Cider Vinegar, Tomato Paste (no added FODMAP ingredients Like garlic and onions), Homemade Broth (no FODMAPS), Homemade Mayo (no FODMAPS, good recipe: http://whole30.com/2014/05/mayo/)

Dairy

Hard Cheeses

Fats

Ghee, Lard, Macadamia Nut Oil, XCT Oil, Brain Octane Oil, Organic Extra Virgin Olive Oil, Extra Virgin Sesame Oil, High Oleic Sunflower Oil, Organic High Oleic Peanut Oil, Tallow

Fruit

Limit to Two Servings Daily, Must be Fresh, Not Canned Fruit:

Blueberries, Breadfruit, Clementine, Cumquat, Dragon Fruit, Mangosteen, Paw Paw, Starfruit, Cantaloupe, Grapefruit, Honeydew Melon, Kiwi, Lemons, Limes, Oranges, Papaya, Passion Fruit, Pineapple, Raspberries, Rhubarb, Strawberries

Fish / Meat / Seafood / Eggs

Most fish / seafood / meat / eggs are permitted except processed meat with added FODMAPS.

Nuts / Seeds / Nut Butters

Limit to One Serving Daily:

Chia Seeds, Brazil Nuts, Pumpkin Seeds, Hazelnuts, Macadamia Nuts, Sesame Seeds, Sunflower Seeds, Pecans, Pumpkin Seeds, Walnuts, Nut Butters (made with listed low-FODMAP nuts or ingredients)

Seasoning / Spices

Most are fine except for spices obtained from FODMAPS (for example, no, onion and garlic powder.)

Sweeteners

Dextrose (non-GMO), Maple Syrup (one tablespoon daily), Stevia

Vegetables

Alfalfa, Bamboo Shoots, Bean Sprouts, Bok Choy, Carrot, Chives, Choko, Choy Sum, Collard Greens, Green Beans, Cucumber, Kale, Lettuce, Mustard Greens, Olive, Parsnip, Radish, Red Bell Pepper, Spinach, Squash, Swiss Chard, Tomatoes, Turnip, Turnip Greens, Zucchini, Arugula, Aubergine, Eggplant, Fennel, Okra, Nori, Celeriac

Moderate FODMAP Diet – Moderate Fermentation Safe Food List

Carbs – Must be consumed hot after preparation (NO RESISTANT STARCH)

Arrowroot, Buckwheat Groats, Buckwheat Flour, Millet, Jasmine Rice, Sushi Rice, Corn (non-GMO), Potatoes (red, russet, yellow, no sweet), Quinoa, Plantain, Sorghum Flour, Tapioca Flour, White Rice Flour, Rutabaga, Butternut Squash (1/2 cup), Spaghetti Squash, Yam

Condiments

Hot Sauce (check for added FODMAPS), Organic Mustard, Organic Tamari Soy Sauce, Apple Cider Vinegar, Tomato Paste (no Added FODMAP Ingredients like garlic and onions), Homemade Broth (no FODMAPS), Homemade Mayo (no FODMAPS, good recipes: http://whole30.com/2014/05/mayo, http://nomnompaleo.com/post/3440774534/paleo-mayonnaise)

Dairy / Fats

Avocado Oil, Butter (two tablespoons daily), Extra Virgin Coconut Oil, Ghee, Hard Cheeses (cheddar, parmesan), Lard, Macadamia Nut Oil, XCT Oil, Brain Octane Oil, Organic Extra Virgin Olive Oil, Extra Virgin Sesame Oil, Sour Cream (one tablespoon daily), High Oleic Sunflower Oil, Organic High Oleic Peanut Oil, Tallow

Fruit

Limit to Three Servings Daily, Must be Fresh, Not Canned Fruit:

Avocado (1/4 daily), Bananas (ripe only), Blueberries, Breadfruit, Clementine, Cumquat, Dragon Fruit, Mangosteen, Paw Paw, Grapes, Starfruit, Cantaloupe, Grapefruit, Honeydew Melon, Kiwi, Lemons, Limes, Oranges, Papaya, Passion Fruit, Pineapple, Raspberries, Rhubarb, Strawberries

Fish / Meat / Seafood / Eggs

Most fish / seafood / meat / eggs are permitted except processed meat with added FODMAPS.

Nuts / Seeds / Nut Butters

Limit to Two Servings Daily:

Chia Seeds, Brazil Nuts, Hazelnuts, Macadamia Nuts, Sesame Seeds, Sunflower Seeds, Pecans, Pumpkin Seeds, Walnuts, Nut Butters (made with listed low-FODMAP Nuts or ingredients)

Seasoning / Spices

Most are fine except for spices obtained from FODMAPS (for example, no, onion and garlic powder.)

Sweeteners

Limit to Two Servings Daily, Except Stevia:

Dextrose (non-GMO), Maple Syrup, Stevia

Vegetables

Alfalfa, Bamboo Shoots, Bean Sprouts, Bok Choy, Carrot, Celery (two stalks MAX), Chives, Choko, Choy Sum, Collard Greens, Eggplant, Green Beans, Green Onion (green part only), Kale, Lettuce, Mustard Greens, Parsnip, Radish, Red Bell Pepper, Spinach, Squash, Swiss Chard, Tomatoes, Turnip, Turnip Greens, Zucchini, Arugula, Aubergine, Eggplant, Fennel, Okra, Nori, Celeriac, Cabbage, Red Cabbage

How to Improve the Low FODMAP Diet So It Works for You!

Some people have great results with the low FODMAP diet and others not so much. Is there any way to optimize the low FODMAP diet so that it can help more people achieve symptom relief from overgrowth in the gut while addressing its drawbacks? The low FODMAP diet mainly should be used for symptom reduction so if you have overgrowth you can hopefully find some relief and try to reduce it through antimicrobial protocols. The low FODMAP diet does have issues, and long-term use of the diet may increase the time it takes for the gut to heal and recover from overgrowth. Those issues include:

1. It may reduce probiotic bacteria in the gut as well including *Bifidobacteria* and *Lactobacillus*.
2. It may reduce diversity in the gut. Studies have shown the more diverse your gut, the more likely they will have fewer digestive issues.
3. It may reduce SCFA production in the gut.
4. May slow motility because of reduction of fiber and probiotic bacteria in the diet.
5. Increases intestinal pH leading to a greater chance in overgrowth.

So how can these issues be addressed so that the low FODMAP diet can work for you? Supplementation of specific prebiotics, fibers, and foods rich in SCFA's may help make up the gut health deficits in the low FODMAP diet and improve your outcome when using the diet.

Ways to Reduce the Amount Of Probiotic Bacteria Lost on the Low FODMAP Diet

Most probiotic bacteria require FODMAPS in our diet to ferment so that they can thrive and improve our microbiome. Well-fed probiotic bacteria keep our digestive system happy, helping to maintain our immune system, motility, mental health, and sleep. Even though FODMAPS keep our probiotic flora happy, they also feed some of the opportunistic bacteria as well, like *Clostridia* and *Klebsiella*. The low FODMAP diet works well in reducing hydrogen-producing bacterial overgrowth.

What can be done so that the loss of probiotic bacteria is reduced when on the low FODMAP diet? Increased intake of low fermentable fiber like acacia fiber may help. Using the prebiotic GOS (which is a FODMAP) may help as well. GOS, even though it is a FODMAP, seems to feed the opportunistic bacteria less, and increases probiotic bacteria in the gut. Cellulose fiber is a low fermenting bulking agent that might increase *Bifidobacteria* in the colon. Even though it is not well known as a prebiotic, ingestion of collagen has been found to increase *Bifidobacteria*. Start with small amounts of any of the low FODMAP fibers or prebiotics, mixed well in filtered water in the morning to see if it improves your gut health. Too much of any of these recommendations may still create digestive issues in people with overgrowth.

Increasing Fiber in the Low FODMAP Diet to Help Motility

Any of the above recommendations may help increase motility in the gut. One of the biggest complaints of the low FODMAP diet is that it seems to worsen constipation. The clean fiber in our diet helps keep our probiotic bacteria happy, and in doing so they accomplish important tasks, including the production of serotonin to help move our food along in our digestive system.

Just because you are on a low FODMAP diet does not mean you cannot get plenty of fiber in your diet to feed your microbiome and improve digestion. The starches on this list must be consumed hot; resistant starch, when cooled, may cause digestive problems in people that have overgrowth in their digestive systems. Finally, try to purchase organic or locally grown food whenever possible. Some of these foods include:

- Certified gluten free oatmeal (some people might have issues with the opioid peptide avenin in oats if they have issues with gluten. Avoid if you have celiac disease).
- Chia seeds
- Berries
- Melons (cantaloupe, honeydew)
- Oranges

- Spinach
- Rutabaga
- Organic potatoes with skin (avoid if you have issues with nightshades)
- Quinoa (avoid if you have issue with saponins)
- Brown rice
- Yam
- Buckwheat
- Carrots
- Parsnips
- Plantains
- Low FODMAP nuts
- Butternut squash (1/4 cup)
- Spaghetti squash
- Millet
- Okra
- Eggplant (avoid if you have issues with nightshades)

In addition, maintaining proper hydration, using a squatty potty, and magnesium intake may help improve sluggish motility.

Obtaining SCFA's From Your Diet to Improve the Gut While on the Low FODMAP Diet

Reduction in probiotic bacteria including *Bifidobacteria* and *Lactobacillus* from long-term diet changes may reduce SCFA production in the gut. Short chain fatty acid metabolism by the bacteria in our intestinal tract does a lot to improve our health. The production of acetate for example by *Lactobacillus* creates many beneficial actions in the gut. Acetate has antimicrobial properties, enhances lipogenesis and cholesterol synthesis, improves gluconeogenesis, and reduces intestinal pH. The production of butyrate by some *Clostridium* strains and *Bifidobacteria* also improves our digestive health. Butyrate improves the health of our enterocytes, has antimicrobial properties, improves mucosal integrity, reduces the formation of colon cancer cells, and increases energy levels.

You can take supplemental acetate and butyrate, but these supplements are highly concentrated, and most people seem not to tolerate them as well as obtaining these SCFA's in the diet.

The easiest way to increase acetate is just to ingest organic, raw, unfiltered apple cider vinegar. You may need to avoid this if you have histamine issues because apple cider vinegar does contain histamine. Increasing butyrate ingestion is just as easy. Organic grass fed butter, organic or raw European hard cheese, and organic pastured ghee are sources of dietary butyrate. Most people with digestive issues can tolerate at least one of these foods. Finally, taking a prebiotic supplement if needed like GOS has been shown to increase SCFA acid production in the gut and increase concentrations of probiotic bacteria in the gut. Sadly, if you are suffering from an overgrowth of *MAP*, dairy consumption, arabinogalactans, and GOS should be restricted. Supplemental butyrate or GOS intake through the diet (small amounts of beans) may be needed in people with *MAP* overgrowth.

GAPS Diet

http://www.gapsdiet.com/

Pros

The GAPS Diet greatly eliminates SIBO and IBS symptoms by starving the opportunistic bacteria. It is a gluten-free, lactose-free, fructose limiting, GMO-free, organic, anti-nutrient limiting diet, and can completely rebuild and realign the entire gastrointestinal tract. It encourages the consumption of homemade probiotic culture within the diet.

Cons

A severely limiting diet that lasts for almost a year. There is no discussion of mycotoxin and dioxin exposure.

Summary

Dr. Campbell McBride developed this diet so that all digestive problems can be solved with the use of one complete diet. This diet has the chance to help with rebuilding the digestive system from the ground up in most people. The main problem with the GAPS diet is that it is a highly restrictive diet, and it may make adrenal fatigue worse from the lack of carbohydrate sources in the diet.

Standard Ketogenic Diet (Atkins® Diet)

http://www.atkins.com/home.aspx

Pros

This diet helps you lose weight, and is easier to adopt than most ketogenic diets (Bulletproof®, Primal®, and Paleo). It is gluten-free (for the first two phases).

Cons

It does not talk about GMOs or organic foods. It is not a cyclic ketogenic diet. It is not gluten-free after the second phase. The standard ketogenic diet is contraindicated in people with adrenal fatigue or people who cannot regulate cortisol easily because it will make those disorders worse. It does not discuss mycotoxin exposure and does not discuss increased dioxins from meat.

Summary

The Atkins® diet is just an example of your average ketogenic diet. Ketogenic diets are excellent for weight loss potential. The Atkins® diet has more flaws than most ketogenic diets. The Atkins® diet does not discuss food quality, it allows gluten in the later phases, and like all ketogenic diets, it can be harmful in people with adrenal fatigue.

Low Acid Diet

http://www.voiceinstituteofnewyork.com/

Pros

It is excellent for the relieving the symptoms of LERD and GERD, and helps alkalize the body.

Cons

It just focuses on lowering acid ingestion in the body.

Summary

ENT doctor Jamie Koufman developed this diet for specifically treating LERD. The diet works by lowering or eliminating the amount of acidic foods that one ingests during the day. I hope that if you ingest less acidic foods, less acid and pepsin will be silently refluxed into the lower and upper esophagi and airways.

Low Residue Diet

http://www.mayoclinic.com/health/low-fiber-diet/MY00744

Pros

The Low Residue diet is a good diet for anyone suffering from diverticular disease.

Cons

It is not gluten-free. It does not discuss GMOs, organic foods, gluten, mycotoxins, dioxins, or antinutrients in the diet. It also lacks some nutrients, and is a limited diet.

Summary

This diet was developed by the Mayo clinic for people before intestinal surgeries or who are suffering from diverticular disease. The diet consists of less than 7-10 grams of fiber a day and is supposed to prolong intestinal transit time. If you are on this diet, you should take a multivitamin because the diet is deficient in a lot of essential vitamins and minerals.

Foods that are okay to eat on the diet:

- White bread, refined pasta, cereal, and white rice
- Limited servings of canned or well-cooked vegetables that do not include skins
- Moderate fresh fruits without peels or seeds, certain canned or well-cooked fruits
- Tender, ground, and well-cooked meat, fish, eggs, and poultry
- Milk and yogurt (usually limited), mild cheeses, ricotta
- Butter, mayonnaise, vegetable oils, margarine, plain gravies and dressings
- Broth and strained soups from allowed foods
- Pulp-free, strained, or clear juices

Foods to avoid:

- Whole grain bread and pasta
- Whole grain food products
- Hard cheeses, yogurt containing fruit skins or seeds
- Raw vegetables, except lettuce
- Tough meat
- Peanut butter
- Millet, buckwheat, flax, oatmeal
- Dried beans, peas, and legumes
- Dried fruits, berries, other fruits with skin or seeds
- Chocolate with cocoa powder
- Coconut
- Juices with pulp
- Highly spiced food and dressings, pepper, hot sauce
- Coffee and other foods with caffeine
- Popcorn
- Nuts and Seeds

Paleo Diet

http://thepaleodiet.com/

Pros

The Paleo Diet helps you lose weight. It is a ketogenic, gluten-free, lactose-free, GMO-free, and mostly organic diet.

Cons

It does not address mycotoxins or dioxin exposure. It is contraindicated in people with adrenal fatigue or people who cannot regulate cortisol easily. It does not limit specific high fructose fruits and does not address antinutrients like phytic acid.

Summary

The Paleo diet is one of the first diets to modify the ketogenic diet so that it is more down to earth and more organic. Loren Cordain developed the concept for the modern "Paleo diet". Credit however, should go to ancient man for inventing the diet.

Perfect Health Diet®

http://perfecthealthdiet.com/

Pros

This diet helps you lose weight, it limits carbohydrate intake compared to the SAD, includes organic and non-GMO, gluten-free, no lactose, less dioxin exposure, is not contraindicated in people with adrenal fatigue, and includes a high intake of vegetables.

Cons

This diet does not address mycotoxins. It is not ketogenic (unless modified) and does not limit fructose.

Summary

The Perfect Health® Diet was invented by Paul Jaminet. This diet is a great way to balance a Paleo diet with a non-ketogenic diet. It allows "safer" carbs than your average ketogenic diet, while eliminating gluten. Compared to the Bulletproof® Diet, The Perfect Health® Diet does not limit mycotoxin exposure in food. Because of this, I do not recommend the Perfect Health® Diet for people with yeast issues. Even though the diet is not a ketogenic diet, it could be modified to be a ketogenic diet if needed. The Perfect Health® Diet is the diet I follow.

Primal® Diet

http://www.marksdailyapple.com/definitive-guide-to-the-primal-eating-plan/

Pros

The Primal® Diet helps you lose weight fast! It is a cyclic ketogenic diet, gluten-free, lactose-free, GMO-free, mostly organic, and limits antinutrients and fructose.

Cons

It does not address mycotoxins or dioxin exposure, and is contraindicated in people with adrenal fatigue or people who cannot regulate cortisol easily.

Summary

Health enthusiast Mark Sisson invented The Primal® Diet. Mark wanted to address some of the problems with the basic Paleo diet like anti-nutrient exposure and excess fructose. He consistently aand frequently modifies the diet with new research.

Semi-Elemental Diet

Pros

This diet incorporates food that is indigestible by bacteria and can be used to eliminate SIBO and ulcerative colitis / Crohn's disease. It uses ingredients that are easy to digest, is a gluten-free, lactose-free, GMO-free diet, reduces yeast overgrowth, and is less expensive than the elemental diet. Many people find that the foods on the semi-elemental diet taste better than elemental diet.

Cons

Digestion of fructose is not good for the gut. It is also extremely rigid and expensive.

Summary

Semi-elemental diets have always been around but were usually supplemented by readymade products ripe with hydrogenated oils, preservatives, and GMO byproducts. This diet is extremely useful in eliminating opportunistic bacteria in the colon and can help people with SIBO, ulcerative colitis, and Crohn's disease. It is different from the elemental diet in that the amino acids are partially broken down, instead of being completely in their elemental forms.

My Version of a Semi-Elemental Diet

One month supply list, $350 or less (not bad for a month's worth of food):

- Two containers of nutrabio 5lbs. hydrolyzed whey protein unflavored
- One jar of 10lb. Now dextrose
- Three bottles of XCT Oil
- One large bottle of organic extra virgin olive oil
- One large bottle of extra virgin avocado oil
- One large bottle of Carlson Norwegian cod liver oil lemon
- Two jars of Klaire Labs Vitaspectrum powder
- One container of Real Salt
- One jar of Now potassium gluconate powder
- One satchel of Upgraded™ VanillaMax

Per meal dose (three meals a day):

- Two cups of filtered water
- One scoop of Nutrabio whey protein
- Five tablespoons of Now dextrose
- Two tablespoons of Upgraded™ MCT oil
- ¼ teaspoon of Real Salt
- ½ a scoop of Klaire Labs Vitaspectrum powder
- One teaspoon now potassium gluconate powder
- Sprinkle Upgraded™ Vanilla for taste

Instructions for Meals:

Mix all ingredients in a blender on the lowest speed possible until blended. Ice may be added after all ingredients have been blended if needed.

Once a day:

You are going to have to drink the oils down the best you can; the lemon in the cod liver oil should mask the taste of the other oils.

In a small glass mix and consume:

- One tablespoon extra-virgin olive oil
- One tablespoon extra-virgin avocado oil
- Two teaspoons Carlson Norwegian cod liver oil

If you have constant loose stools:

- Galactomune – one scoop daily, mixed well in filtered water. Use with caution if you have Th2 elevation or yeast sensitivity.

Start with one tablespoon daily with a meal to see if that helps eliminate loose stools. You may increase to three tablespoons a day, one tablespoon each day daily if needed.

Cellulose is not supposed to contribute to SIBO issues for most people, but be aware that if symptoms worsen during the protocol, you should discontinue consuming cellulose.

General Instructions:

You are able to take capsule supplements (as long as you break open the capsule, and the supplement ingredients contain no FODMAPS) and softgels (as long as the formulation contains no FODMAPS) if needed.

In addition, drink one – two liters of water during the day as needed to maintain hydrated during the diet.

SCD Diet

http://www.breakingtheviciouscycle.info/

Pros

This diet helps to dramatically decrease opportunistic bacteria in the colon, limits carbohydrates, incorporates homemade yogurt, is gluten-free, GMO-free, and limits some FODMAPS.

Cons

It does not limit all FODMAPS, is not ketogenic, does not discuss mycotoxins, antinutrients, or dioxin exposure. Aspartame is allowed on this diet.

Summary

Elaine Gottschall developed this diet with the help of Dr. Sidney Haas. SCD diet is an excellent diet for those suffering from opportunistic bacteria and is one of the easiest of the limiting "healthy" diets to follow.

Wheat Belly Diet

http://www.wheatbellyblog.com/

Pros

This diet eliminates gluten, is ketogenic, reduces fructose, eliminates lactose and GMOs, and is mostly organic.

Cons

There is no discussion of mycotoxins, dioxins, or antinutrients (except for gluten and some carbohydrates).

Summary

Cardiologist William Davis developed this diet after he discovered that he could eliminate his patient's heart conditions by placing them on a gluten-free diet. After his patients had been put on a gluten-free diet for at least three months, they were totally off their heart medications and diabetic medications during his study.

Chapter 16

Colon Cleansing

Periodically, colon cleaning is extremely important for digestive health. It is done so that you can eliminate opportunistic bacteria, toxins, undigested fecal matter, and restore proper intestinal function. Proper fiber and water intake should be all the average person needs to keep their bowels regulated. Some alternative medicine experts recommend colonics or even coffee enemas for colon cleansing. I believe that both of these types of colon cleansings should be used sparingly if used at all. Both of these commonly recommended forms of colon cleansing can cause electrolyte imbalances and imbalances of gut flora, as well.

I believe that everyone should do one of my colon cleansing protocols at least once a year to keep the digestive system running smoothly. I also would do the protocol no more than six times a year, because too much cleansing can destroy the body's natural flora and limit the body's natural elimination.

Fiber

Fiber's biggest job in the body is to help the intestinal tract bulk up stools and clean toxins from the intestinal tract by absorbing toxins and regulating the digestive system. Not all fiber is great for the digestive tract, and some fiber should be limited to certain digestive conditions and situations. There are two different types of fiber soluble and insoluble.

Soluble Fiber

Sources: oatmeal, lentils, apples, oranges, pears, oat bran, strawberries, nuts, beans, peas, blueberries, psyllium, cucumbers, carrots, sweet potatoes, and chia seeds

Indicated: Average amounts needed for intestinal health, and to be used by people suffering from diarrhea.

Contraindicated: SIBO, IBS, GERD

Soluble fiber attracts water and forms a gel that can slow down digestion, delays the emptying of the stomach, and can help you feel full. Soluble fiber has also been indicated to help reduce the absorption of oxidized cholesterol in the intestine.

Soluble fiber is fermented in the colon and can be pre-biotic. It is fermented into short chain fatty acids that can help rebuild a healthy colon by nourishing colonocytes, lower colonic pH, and improving the mucus barrier. If someone has an increased unhealthy opportunistic bacteria count in their small intestine (SIBO), soluble fiber causes opportunistic bacteria to flourish. For the average person, soluble fiber intake is important. For conditions in which the intestinal tract is filled with opportunistic bacteria, it should then be limited.

Insoluble Fiber

Sources: legumes, nuts, seeds, potato skins, vegetable fiber (green beans, cauliflower, zucchini, and celery), avocado, unripe bananas, kiwi, grapes, tomatoes, cellulose. Whole grain foods are high in insoluble fiber but other than brown rice, wheat, corn and oat bran are not worth eating.

Indicated: Constipation, better form of fiber for most people, ingest to help regulate the digestive tract.

Contraindicated: diverticulosis, SIBO (non-FODMAP insoluble fiber)

Insoluble fiber does not dissolve in water and is used to absorb water in the intestines to bulk the stool. It also helps the intestines eliminate the waste faster and more efficiently. It also controls and balances the pH of the intestines. Unlike, soluble fiber, insoluble fiber usually does not ferment in the intestines, or feed opportunistic bacteria. Insoluble fiber helps promote regular bowel movements and prevents constipation.

Is Fiber Even Needed?

Some people argue that fiber is not important to ingest for digestive health. I do believe that there is merit to this for some people. Fiber should be limited in those with SIBO and diverticulitis. For the average person, some fiber is good for regulating the digestive health. It all depends on the source of the fiber. Is it from whole wheat bread (which is bad), nuts, vegetables, or fruits? If you want to see, the arguments against the intake of fiber visit this website (http://www.gutsense.org/reports/myth.html).

Colon Cleansing Protocol

Support and Restore Your Gut Health:

- Two tsp of organic extra virgin coconut oil – three times daily with meals.
- Thorne Research L-glutamine or NOW Foods L-glutamine – take 4,000 – 10,000 mg in divided doses, daily with meals (use with caution if you have a sensitivity to glutamic acid, deficiency in GABA, upper gut overgrowth [*H. pylori*], or severe leaky gut and brain).
- Galactomune – one scoop daily mixed well with water at breakfast. Use with caution if you have yeast overgrowth or Th2 elevated issues.
- Allergy Research Group – N-Acetyl glucosamine – (do not use if allergic to shellfish or have yeast overgrowth) – follow the general supplement bottle recommendations.
- Collagen supplementation is very important in restoring your digestive health.
- I would follow the Perfect Health® Diet and proper ingestion of omega 3 fatty acids.

Binding and Reduction of Toxins and Heavy Metals

- Sonne's No. 7 Detoxification – follow supplement recommendations.
- Sun chlorella – chew ten tablets daily with meals, do not use if you have Th1 dominance.
- Unifiber – one tablespoon, three times daily, mixed well with a glass of filtered water before consuming.
- Glutathione Force – follow supplement recommendations.
- Ingest a raw carrot salad to help reduce estrogen and endotoxin build up in the gut. Grate one raw organic carrot, and mix with one tablespoon of extra virgin olive oil, one tablespoon of extra virgin coconut oil, and one tsp of apple cider vinegar. Use with caution if you have histamine or fat malabsorption issues.

Facilitate Proper MMC Function

- Himalaya triphala – take one capsule twice daily, right before meals.
- Drink a cup of organic ginger tea with breakfast daily.
- Proper magnesium supplementation, use magnesium malate or peroxide.
- Drink up to ten glasses of filtered water, each with 1/8 tsp of Real Salt to help speed up elimination.

- Use a squatty potty and exercise daily.

Coconut oil ingestion will help reduce any yeast overgrowth.

L-glutamine and NAG are important for GALT (gut associated lymphatic tissue) health and preventing leaky gut.

GOS and collagen will act as prebiotics to help increase endogenous probiotic growth including *Bifidobacteria* and *Lactobacillus*.

Carrots, unifiber, and bentonite clay will help bind to excess endotoxins produced in the gut and eliminate them.

Glutathione is a powerful antioxidant that helps increase liver function and detoxification.

Ginger increases bile production, which aids in digestion and elimination of toxins.

Bentonite clay and chlorella will bind to heavy metals that are released from bile and eliminate them.

Triphala, magnesium, salt, and proper hydration increases motility and MMC function.

Chapter 17

Supplements Used for Digestive Ailments

5-HTP

Uses: LES strengthening, intestinal spasms, depression.

Brand: Jarrow Formulas 5-HTP

Side effects: RARE: systemic allergic reaction, EXTREMELY RARE: serotonin syndrome

5-HTP is a naturally occurring amino acid and is used by the body for the biosynthesis of serotonin and melatonin. Serotonin is a neurotransmitter that is used to regulate intestinal movements, muscle contractions, for the regulation of appetite, mood, and sleep.

Correcting serotonin levels in the body might help with depression and also with regulating intestinal contractions. Ninety-five percent of the serotonin the body produces is found in the intestinal system. An underutilization of serotonin in the gut causes constipation from the lack of muscle contractions in the gut.

An over production or high circulating cellular level of serotonin can be one of the causes of intestinal problems like IBS. A high level of serotonin causes the bowels to spasm and constantly contract causing cramps and diarrhea. This is the reason one of the main side effects of SSRIs is IBS. It is important for you to get your neurotransmitters tested before supplementing with 5-HTP for a long period.

5-HTP supplementation also increases melatonin levels in the body.

Activated Charcoal

Uses: absorbs toxins from meals that we eat and reduces herx reactions that occur in the digestive tract

Brand: Upgraded™ Activated Charcoal

Side effects: RARE: systemic allergic reaction, constipation

Activated charcoal comes from burning a carbon source that yields a blackish porous material. There are many different grades of activated charcoal that differ in their absorption, Fix Your Gut, however, is going to focus on standard food grade or medical grade activated charcoal.

Activated charcoal is more than just for "detoxing"; it serves a medical purpose. There is medical grade activated charcoal that is used for accidental oral overdose and poisoning (depending on the substance) in hospitals across the world.

Activated charcoal only binds to larger molecules, non-polar molecules, or molecules that have a negative charge since activated charcoal itself has a slight positive charge. Some things that activated charcoal cannot bind to include:

- Alcohol (activated charcoal, however, can bind to some impurities found in alcohol)
- Glycols
- Strong acids or bases
- Some heavy metals like lithium and iron

We are lucky, though; activated charcoal can bind to endotoxins produced in the gut when ingested. Binding of endotoxins in our digestive tract reduces inflammation, improves liver / kidney function, and helps reduce symptoms of a Herxheimer reaction.

Activated charcoal can also absorb excess gas as well produced by overgrowth that might reduce bloating and abdominal pain.

Finally, it can bind with some of the toxins in the food we ingest including mycotoxins.

How Much Activated Charcoal Should Be Supplemented and Drawbacks of Activated Charcoal Supplementation

This depends on the severity of your Herxheimer reaction.

I suggest one to two activated charcoal capsules an hour after taking your antimicrobial supplements so that it does not interfere with their use if you are having a Herxheimer reaction.

In addition, I suggest one to two capsules if you are having strong reactions to food as well if you have overgrowth even if the food does not come from a questionable source.

Do not be surprised if your stool darkens when ingesting activated charcoal; this is normal.

There are drawbacks to supplementing with activated charcoal, though. Activated charcoal can interfere with your intake from food, medications, or supplements. I would take it a few hours away from supplements, medications, and meals if possible.

If you take too much, there is also a possibility that it can cause gastrointestinal blockages, but most of the time this is only seen in medical emergencies where too much might be accidentally given to try to help someone who overdosed. If you have severe abdominal pains from ingesting normal amounts of activated charcoal, you might want to notify you doctor or go to the emergency room because you might have an intestinal blockage.

Allicin-C

Uses: antimicrobial

Brand: Allicin-C

Side effects: RARE: systemic allergic reaction

Allicin is an antimicrobial organosulfur compound that is well studied and found in garlic. Allicin is very unstable and very little survives from ingestion of garlic because of the rapid chemical breakdown of allicin when exposed to heat, or low pH. Allicin-C is a supplement where the allicin is stabilized so that it can survive stomach acid and be absorbed into the bloodstream. Allicin cream has been shown to be extremely effective in eliminating MRSA.

It is also possible that allicin will exhibit antiviral properties. Multiple studies have indicated that allicin can be used in the elimination of viral infections, but the results yet are still inconclusive.

Bioperine

Uses: eliminate parasites, increases absorption of minerals and supplements

Brand: Bio-Perine Source Naturals

Side effects: RARE: systemic allergic reaction

Bioperine is a natural alkaloid extract from piperidine. Piperidine is an alkaloid extract that is harvested from black pepper. Bioperine can increase absorption of supplements and medications and should be taken two hours before or after ingestion of medicines and supplements to decrease the chance of hyper-concentration of the medication or supplement in the blood.

Piperidine is used in both the treatment of parasites and worms in animals and is also used in the treatment of schizophrenia in humans. Researchers propose that schizophrenia may sometimes result from a parasite infection like *T. gondii*.

The mechanism behind piperine is currently unknown. It may cause paralysis in parasites by increasing the permeability of schistosome cell membranes causing an influx of calcium ions. This could dislodge the parasites from the site of action and eliminate them by phagocytosis (engulfment by white blood cells of the immune system). Piperine also decreases adenosine uptake by the parasites causing mitochondrial disruption causing them to tire to death.

If this correlation is based on truth, then a simple bio-piperine extract in supplement form could prove to be effective in eliminating parasitic infections. Piperine is a natural alkaloid of piperidine. Piperine is known to eliminate parasites with fewer side effects than piperidine drugs. Piperine can increase absorption of supplements and medications and should be taken two hours before or after ingestion of medicines and supplements to decrease the chance of too much concentration of the medication or supplement in the blood.

Chlorella

Uses: heavy metal binding agent, has a full amino acid spectrum, high in protein, and is a food source

Brands: Clean Chlorella

Side effects: RARE: Systemic Allergic Reaction

Chlorella is a genus of single-cell algae that grow in fresh water. Chlorella was originally grown in mass quantities in the 50's and 60's as a potential food source. It was later discovered that chlorella's cell walls were not broken down and assimilated by the human digestive system very well, so the nutrient content was considered worthless. Later, methods were developed so that the digestive system absorbs the nutrients in chlorella by breaking the cell wall (pressure, steam, and mechanical).

Ways chlorella might be able to improve your health:

- Chlorella is high in protein, omega 3 fatty acid (ALA), a source of saturated fats, antioxidants, vitamins, and contains all of the essential amino acids.
- Chlorella binds to some metals (mostly mercury, hexavalent chromium, arsenic, lead, and cadmium) in the gut making it easier to eliminate.
- Chlorella also reduces the neurotoxin dioxin load (binds with it in the gastrointestinal tract to eliminate it) and seems to be one of the only available nutritional routes of doing so.
- Chlorella may help increase SIgA (secretory immunoglobulin a) and help improve gut immune function in people with leaky gut.
- Chlorella may also reduce Bisphenol-A accumulation in the body and support healthy estrogen metabolism (in vitro studies).
- Chlorella ingestion has been studied in pregnant women to help boost their and their fetuses immunity, prevent anemia, reduce dioxin exposure through breast milk for the infant, and reduce edema.
- Chlorella decreases Th2.

Chlorella contains endotoxins within their cell wall just like Gram-negative bacteria. Yes, you read that right, chlorella contains endotoxins. We have written a lot about endotoxins on our website. I believe that they are one cause of elevated Th1 inflammation and many health conditions stemming from it (heart disease, liver disease, diabetes, rheumatoid arthritis, psoriasis, rosacea, multiple sclerosis, and alkalizing spondylosis, to name a few).

Ingestion of chlorella should be fine in people with balanced immune systems, people with histamine intolerance (Th2 dominance), or if you have a good gut barrier and microbiome. The Gram-negative bacteria in our body produce endotoxins constantly; your detox and immune system can keep it in check if it is not overwhelmed. Gram-negative bacteria are natural flora in your gut; the endotoxins they produce are eliminated through stool and proper immune reactions unless you have leaky gut. They should not be absorbed into the bloodstream causing inflammatory issues if you have a healthy gut.

Now the big question is, are all endotoxins similar and do they provoke similar responses in the human body? If they are all the same and elicit the same response, the endotoxins in chlorella should cause Th1 inflammation in people with leaky gut. It appears in what limited studies that we have on chlorella, its endotoxins seem to be weaker in the damage they may cause to cells and the increase of inflammation in the body compared to most Gram-negative produced endotoxins. The effects of chlorella may be less, but it is unknown what may occur if you have a Th1 elevated immune system, and what part of the body has issues with their exposure. For example, immune reactions from endotoxins produced by *Campylobacter* in the gut seem to damage the MMC causing motility issues where immune responses from endotoxins by *Klebsiella* seem to attack the formation of collagen and harm the spine and joints.

Nevertheless, there are studies that cast doubt that chlorella increases Th1 reactions and may decrease them even though they contain endotoxins. A few studies also show that chlorella may protect the body from Gram-negative endotoxins. That being said, I believe people with Th1 dominance should still avoid the ingestion of chlorella until we have more studies. In an overwhelmed immune system, the body's reaction to the endotoxins in chlorella may be upregulated, and if you have leaky gut, the endotoxins could get into the bloodstream and trigger systemic inflammation from the immune imbalance. There are different supplements that one can take to modulate their immune system or get the benefits that each performs; there is no strong need to take either to improve one's health if you have Th1 dominance issues.

Chlorella ingestion can improve one's health, but I believe it should be avoided if you are suffering from strong Gram-negative overgrowth or extreme Th1 dominance.

Collagen

Uses: improve skin, joint, and intestinal / LES integrity, prebiotic

Side effects: RARE: systemic allergic reaction

Most people take collagen supplements to improve the health of their joints and skin. Many athletes use collagen as a source of protein and to improve the recovery and health of their overused joints. Collagen peptides are utilized in the cosmetic industry to reduce wrinkles, rejuvenate skin, and give you that coveted glow, but did you know that the ingestion of the different types of collagen might improve your digestive health and can even affect the probiotic growth of your microbiome?

So What Is Collagen?

Collagen is a naturally occurring protein that is found the most in flesh and connective tissues. Collagen also contains many different amino acids, and most collagen supplements are high in glycine and proline. Glycine is used by the body as an inhibitory neurotransmitter, protects against glutamate hyperexcitability, and promotes relaxation and sleep. Glycine also helps improve insulin insensitivity, reduces inflammation, and improves liver function. We use proline to complete protein synthesis, for proper metabolism, to reduce atherosclerosis, and to regulate immune responses. Glycine and proline can both be produced by our body from other amino acids, but only if you take in enough clean protein in your diet. Ingestion of collagen would provide both amino acids and more like glutamine, lysine, and arginine to improve your health.

These are three types of collagen that you can mainly supplement with:

- **Type 1 collagen** – most abundant collagen in the human body. It is present in scar tissue, tendons, skin, arterial walls, cornea, surrounds muscle fibers, fibrocartilage, intervertebral disks, and bones and teeth. Its use is important in improving muscle, eye, skin, cardiovascular, bone, wound, and back health.
- **Type 2 collagen** – found in joint cartilage, intervertebral disks, and the vitreous body of the eye. Its use is important in improving joint, back, and eye health.
- **Type 3 collagen** – the second most abundant type of collagen in the human body. It is found in the intestinal walls, reticular fibers, uterus, muscles, blood vessels, and combined with type 1 collagen. Its use is important in improving digestive, uterine, muscle, and cardiovascular health.

The digestion of collagen begins in the stomach. The first step in digestion consists of the breakdown of collagen to form dipeptides and tripeptides or free amino acids in the stomach. Several proteases (proteases produced by the pancreas, small intestinal brush-border proteases, peptidase) further break down the collagen into amino acids, some of which are used in the gastrointestinal tract and the rest enter into systemic circulation. Finally, some of the collagen peptides are fermented by *Bifidobacteria* and act as a prebiotic, increasing both probiotic colonies and motility.

Here are the recommended types of collagen to be used with different health issues:

- **Cardiovascular** – if you want healthier cardiovascular health, a type 1 and 3 supplement and Biocell or alternating ingestion of chicken and beef bone broth should be supplemented.
- **Eyes** – type 1 and type 2 should be supplemented for proper health.
- **Joints** – if you are having joint issues, a type 2 collagen supplement like Biocell may help improve your joint health. Biocell collagen is a collagen supplement that is made from the hyaline cartilage of chicken sternum. The supplement itself has type II collagen, hyaluronic acid, and chondroitin sulfate. The body to lubricate joints uses hyaluronic acid. Chondroitin is a chain of alternating sugars that help make up the structure of cartilage. Biocell contains all three and might be the best to improve the health of your joints. Ingestion of chicken bone broth can also be used.
- **Intestinal** – for intestinal health, all three collagen types should be supplemented. A type 1 and 3 supplement and Biocell or alternating ingestion of chicken and beef bone broth.
- **Skin** – if you want healthier skin, a product with type 1 and type 3 collagen or hydrolyzed collagen peptides should be used.

- **Spine** – for spinal health, all three collagen types should be supplemented. A type 1 and 3 supplement and Biocell or alternating ingestion of chicken and beef bone broth should be supplemented.
- **Uterus** – type 3 collagen should be a supplement for proper uterine health.

How Does the Ingestion of Collagen Improve Digestive Health?

Ingesting collagen has many different positive effects on our digestive health. As I wrote earlier, collagen is high in the amino acid glycine, which improves digestive health, regulates inflammation, protects the mucosal barrier, and improves enterocyte function in the intestinal tract. It protects against systemic endotoxin damage from leaky gut. Glycine also protects the liver and aids in detoxification and bile acid production. Finally, glycine improves fructose malabsorption.

Collagen can also be used as a prebiotic to increase *Bifidobacteria* growth and increase motility. Collagen increases all necessary amino acids to facilitate proper *Bifidobacteria* growth. The amino acids that are in collagen can be broken down by *Bifidobacteria* and used for energy and growth just like carbohydrate sourced prebiotics like GOS.

If you are on a low carb, very low carb, or no carb diet, it is paramount that you ingest collagen supplements or beef and chicken bone broth regularly. The ingestion of collagen would help you maintain the integrity of your mucosal barrier, improve mucus membrane health in the entire body, protect microbiome diversity and population, and keep proper energy production by the bacteria in our microbiome.

If you have ulcerative colitis and Crohn's disease or other forms of *MAP* overgrowth, you might want to avoid bovine sourced collagen and stick with poultry and marine sources. Granted, *MAP* contamination of collagen or bone broth should be very limited; it is still advised for most people to prevent flareups.

Finally, collagen derived from marine sources might be the best in improving leaky gut. Collagen derived from fish has been shown to close the tight junctions of the intestinal tract reducing permeability.

How to Increase Collagen Ingestion and Endogenous Synthesis to Improve Health

There are many different ways you can increase collagen intake in your daily life.

You can take type 1, type 2, and type 3 collagen supplements. The collagen supplements I recommend are:

- Type 1: Bulletproof® Upgraded™ Collagen, Great Lakes collagen
- Type 2: Biocell (poultry source), Vital Proteins (beef source)
- Type 3: Ancient Nutrition Bone Broth Collagen
- Collagen peptides: Vital Proteins Collagen Peptides
- Marine: Seacure, Vital Proteins Marine Collagen

Ingestion of chicken (type 2 collagen) and beef bone broth (type 1 and 3 collagen) would also provide collagen to improve your health.

Supplementation of vitamin C and copper (if you are deficient) are both important in encouraging proper endogenous synthesis and utilization of collagen. I suggest if you are using a collagen supplement or increasing it in your diet to take a low dose of a few grams of ascorbic acid daily to increase the potential of collagen helping your issues. For copper, most people may have too much copper in their bodies; that being said, ingestion of beef liver once or twice weekly should provide enough ceruloplasmin bound copper to help improve collagen synthesis and utilization.

Colloidal Silver

Uses: antimicrobial

Brands: MesoSilver, Super Natural Silver

Side effects: RARE: Systemic allergic reaction, EXTREMELY RARE: Argyria (a condition in which the skin turns blue from excess Silver deposits)

Colloidal silver (particles of silver that are suspended in a medium) is a very strong antimicrobial agent. This silver ion chelates sulfur and iron from bacteria that causes reactive oxygen species to build up (oxidative stress) in the bacteria and destroy it. Silver also pokes small holes in the bacteria's cell wall that both makes it easier for antimicrobials and Immune cells to destroy it as well as cause more oxidative stress damage to the bacteria.

The problem with advocating silver is that there are not many in vivo studies in humans. There are plenty of studies that show that silver is an effective antimicrobial on skin, but the internal intake of silver having antimicrobial effects is lacking in studies currently. Internal silver consumption should bolster the immune system nonetheless. The main reason I suggest silver for gastrointestinal distress is that it will be exposed to pathogenic bacteria through the ingestion of silver.

Diatomaceous Earth

Uses: anti-parasitic

Brand: Food Grade diatomaceous earth

Side effects: RARE: systemic allergic reaction

Diatomaceous earth is a naturally occurring rock made from the skeletons of fossilized algae. When the food grade diatomaceous earth is grounded into a fine powder and ingested, it is used to eliminate parasites in the human body. When the razor-sharp edges of the diatoms come in contact with the parasites, it punctures their cellular walls. It is recommended that the earth is mixed with water when taken so that the risk of inhalation is very low. Diatomaceous earth is irritating to the lungs; try not to breathe in the dust when pouring or mixing.

I would suggest mixing a half teaspoon in a glass of water twice a day (upon waking and before bed) for a week and slowly working up to one teaspoon twice a day. Do not use the diatomaceous earth drink more than three times a day. The diatomaceous earth should be taken for at least a month but no more than three months. Mix the diatomaceous earth with purified water.

Diatomaceous earth may degrade the mucus membrane in the stomach and intestines if used over a long period. People with ulcers may need to limit the amount of diatomaceous earth they consume until their ulcers have healed.

Digestive Enzymes

Uses: helps breakdown and digest food in the stomach, helps to improve fructose malabsorption, lactose intolerance, and gluten insensitivity digestion issues

Brand: Enzymedica Digestive Enzyme

Side effects: RARE: systemic allergic reaction

Digestive enzyme supplements usually consist of different enzymes that are used by the gastrointestinal system to break down foodstuffs. The main enzymes used are proteases (for protein), lipases (for fat), and carbohydrates (for carbohydrates).

Different Digestive Enzymes Used in Supplements

- **Protease** - A digestive enzyme that is useful in digesting protein. Look for a good digestive enzyme that includes different proteases.
- **Lipase** - A digestive enzyme that is useful in digesting fat. Look for a good digestive enzyme that includes different lipases. There are some concerns that long-term lipase supplementation may degrade the stomach lining.
- **Amylase** - A digestive enzyme that is produced by the saliva glands in humans, and in small amounts, produced by the pancreas. Amylase is a digestive enzyme that catalyzes the breakdown of starches into simple sugars. If you are diabetic, you might want to use a digestive enzyme that has low amounts of amylase, or none at all. Amylase use in a diabetic might cause a major increase in blood glucose levels because of the rapid breakdown of starches into glucose in the stomach. Look for a good digestive enzyme that uses different amylases.
- **Cellulase** - A digestive enzyme that breaks down cellulose. Cellulose is mostly indigestible by the body and is a form of plant cell wall fiber.
- **Glucoamylase** - A digestive enzyme that breaks down maltose, a disaccharide sugar.
- **Lactase** - A digestive enzyme that breaks down lactose, a disaccharide sugar that is found in milk. Most people who are lactose intolerant, lack in the production of lactase; that is the source of their digestive issues when consuming dairy products. Supplementing with lactase when consuming those products might help prevent digestive issues.
- **Beta-Glucanase** - A digestive enzyme that breaks down beta-glucans, a polysaccharide. Beta-glucans are found in oats, cereal grains, and mushrooms. Beta-glucans might also occur as some part of the cell wall of fungi and bacteria.
- **Invertase** - A digestive enzyme that breaks down inverted sugar. Inverted sugar is a combination of fructose and glucose.
- **Pectinase** -A digestive enzyme that breaks down pectin, a polysaccharide found in plant cell walls, mostly in fruit.
- **Hemicellulase** -A digestive enzyme that breaks down hemicellulose, one of the major components of plant and fungi cell walls.
- **Xylanase** - A digestive enzyme that breaks down the polysaccharide, beta-1 4-xylan into xylose. Xylose is a building block of hemicellulose in some plants, one of the major components of the plant cell walls.
- **DPP-IV Enzyme** - A proteolytic / digestive enzyme that may degrade the immunodominant, proline-containing epitope of gliadin, the primary allergenic protein in gluten. In studies, DPP-IV has been shown to lessen or eliminate allergic reactions to gluten. That being said, it should only be used for people sensitive to gluten or someone with Celiac disease when the source of the food might be contaminated with gluten. The enzyme should NEVER be used

for people with gluten digestive issues to consume gluten because damage may still be done in the body, even when the enzyme is used.

- **Bromelain** - Bromelain is a proteolytic / digestive enzyme found in the stem and fruit of the pineapple. Bromelain works as a natural digestive enzyme that helps to break down proteins. Bromelain also increases stomach-emptying time, which is helpful in the reduction of symptoms of Gastroparesis. It has also been implicated in relieving the symptoms of gastrointestinal upset, aids in healing gastric ulcers by reducing inflammation, and helps with pancreatic insufficiency. It has also been shown to lower inflammation in people with IBD. Bromelain should also be limited to two weeks of use; it can be used longer, but the use must be warranted. It is possible for bromelain to degrade the stomach lining over a long period.
- **Papain** - Papain is a proteolytic / digestive enzyme that is found in papaya fruit. Papain works as a natural digestive enzyme to help break down proteins. Papain should also be limited to two weeks of use; it can be used longer, but the use must be warranted. It is possible for Papain to degrade the stomach lining over a long period.
- **Pepsin** - Pepsin is the main enzyme used by the stomach to digest protein. Pepsinogen activates and converts into the enzyme pepsin in the presence of stomach acid. Pepsin helps break down protein into amino acids the body can absorb and then becomes inactivated, by turning back into pepsinogen when it is mixed with bicarbonate released from the pancreas in the small intestine. This transformation protects the rest of the intestinal system from the pepsin and stomach acid. Pepsin should rarely be supplemented in people with silent reflux since it is the main cause of their issues. I recommend for most people to use a digestive enzyme or betaine supplement without pepsin if all possible.

Digestive enzymes should be used in people who have problems breaking down and assimilating foods. It is extremely beneficial for people with Celiac disease, gallbladder disorders, heartburn, and people that are suffering from SIBO.

To evaluate the quality of your digestive enzyme supplement, break open two capsules in a bowl of cooked oatmeal (let it cool to about 98 F first) and stir it with a fork for one minute. The oatmeal should break down into a liquid after a few minutes if you have a quality supplement. Finally, I would suggest supplementing with a digestive enzyme that uses as little fillers as possible.

Digestive enzymes should be used sparingly, and during certain protocols, if needed. Digestive enzymes should not be used for a very long period. Long term use of digestive enzymes has been theorized to cause the body to make less digestive enzymes and can lead to a dependency. If you take them for an extremely long period, your digestive system might need a boost by taking Swedish bitters to encourage endogenous production of enzymes again. This period where your digestive system produces fewer enzymes might cause some digestive problems to flair back up. You should just try to wait it out if at all possible; eventually, your body will catch back up. If you need to take digestive enzymes indefinitely, you should cycle off one week every month. During the off week, you should take Swedish bitters every day.

Fish Oil

Uses: important to increase omega-3 levels and overall health, Crohn's disease, ulcerative colitis, reduces excess inflammation

Brand: Nordic Naturals Ultimate Omega

Side effects: RARE: systemic allergic reaction

Fish Oil is high in omega 3 fatty acids, of which most Americans are deficient. Most Americans have a higher omega 6 fatty acid intake in their diet than omega 3's, which causes an increase in inflammation and heart disease. A fatty acid is a chain of lipids bound to a carboxy backbone. The chain is either saturated or unsaturated because of the types of bonds in the attached triglycerides. Your average American has an omega 6 to omega 3 ratio of at least 25:1.

Omega 6 is necessary for the body for cell membrane integrity, inflammation, and pain responses, but an excess of omega 6 causes systemic inflammation. Omega 3 helps to curb excess inflammation in the body. The optimal ratio of omega 3 to omega 6 is debatable, but I believe a 4:1 ratio is fine for most people.

You can get healthy amounts of omega 3 from eating fish two to three times per week. There are plant-based forms of omega 3, but they are made of longer chains of lipids. The octadecatrienoic acids from plants oxidize quickly and cause additional inflammation. The omega 3's that are most beneficial are other long-chained fatty acids like EPA and DHA, which are found in fish oil. ALA, a long chain fatty acid, has to be converted into EPA and DHA, and sadly, most of it is oxidized in the process. The best source of ALA that one can take is through the ingestion of chia seeds.

One of the most important things one can do for their health is to take a high-quality fish oil supplement. You do not want to take a cheap or poor quality fish oil supplement because the oil is rancid and can do more harm than good. One of the easiest ways to tell that you are taking a good quality fish oil is that the oil's omega 3 content is at least 80% or greater of the total oil. Out of 2,000 mg of fish oil, at least 1,600 mg of it should be omega 3's. In addition, you want fish oil that is guaranteed to be free of heavy metals and toxins, in a triglyceride form and is not ethyl ester, has been molecularly distilled, and is pharmaceutical grade. Finally, make sure the fish oil is in the sn/2 position or known as the triglyceride form, which is better absorbed than ethyl ester.

Fish oil is great for inflammatory bowel disease because it lowers systemic inflammation. The amount of fish oil taken might need to be limited in people taking blood thinners.

Humic Acid

Uses: ulcerative colitis, Crohn's disease, gallstones

Brands: Allergy Research humic acid, food grade humic acid

Side effects: RARE: systemic allergic reaction

Humic Acid is a competent of our soil that is produced by the degradation of plant material and is full of micronutrients. Humic acid helps supplement absorption and detoxifies heavy metals in the body. Humic acid also works as a chelating agent on gallstones, loosening and dissolving them. Humic Acid reduces systemic inflammation by regulating the immune system through anti-oxidation.

Humic acid is also rich in zinc, magnesium, and other minerals. Finally, some studies have also shown that humic acid has the potential to increase oxygen levels in the red blood cells, and might increase recovery time as well.

EDTA

Uses: SIBO, bacterial infections

Brand: Metabolic Response Modifier Cardio-Chelate with EDTA

Ethylenediaminetetraacetic acid is often used in the medical industry for chelation therapy or the removal of heavy metals from the body. In alternative medicine, taking EDTA bonds with the iron that fortifies biofilm. Like kicking an ant hill, EDTA destroys the structures that microorganisms dwell within so that they can be exposed to antimicrobial agents and killed. Without first destroying the biofilms, many bacteria are impervious to even the strongest antibiotics.

Lactoferrin

Uses: SIBO, bacterial and viral infections, yeast overgrowth, hepatitis C

Brand: Symbiotics

Side effects: RARE: systemic allergic reaction

Lactoferrin is a multifunctional protein that is one of the many components of an animal's innate immune system. Lactoferrin exhibits strong antimicrobial activity and can easily be extracted from most mammals' milk (mainly from cows, goats, and sheep). Lactoferrin may also help improve bone strength and function. Finally, lactoferrin supplementation also might help increase tear production in people afflicted with Sjogren's syndrome.

Lactoferrin has strong antibacterial properties; it can destroy both opportunistic bacteria itself and the biofilm that some bacteria love to use as armor from antibacterials. Lactoferrin scavenges extra free iron in the body and binds to lipopolysaccharides in the bacterial cell walls. These reactions cause bacteria not to be able to use iron for respiration, which is necessary for bacteria growth and function. When lactoferrin binds to lipopolysaccharides in bacterial cell walls, the oxidized bonded iron scavenged by the lactoferrin creates excessive oxidative damage. Lactoferrin also damages the bacterial cell membranes causing them to lose permeability. Finally, lactoferrin stimulates the immune system by increasing the phagocytic ability of white blood cells.

Some bacteria produce protective biofilms (one of the most common examples of a biofilm is the "film" on your teeth when you have not brushed for a while) that make eradication sometimes with antibacterial agents very difficult. Biofilm protects the bacteria from elimination by antibiotic treatments, natural antibacterial agents, bactericides, and probiotics. To eliminate the opportunistic bacteria, you have to destroy the biofilm that it is hiding behind. Lactoferrin breaks down bacterial biofilm by chelating iron out of the biofilm cell walls so that the biofilm breaks down and dissolves. The immune system and antibacterial agents are now free to eliminate the opportunistic bacteria.

Finally, lactoferrin may help prevent the attachment of *H. pylori* to the stomach lining, leading to its eventual elimination from the body.

Lactoferrin is used in the treatment of Hepatitis C and other viral infections because it also processes strong antiviral properties. Lactoferrin binds to lipoproteins in vitro and prevents viruses from entering a cell for replication. Lactoferrin may also bind to viruses, directly blocking them from being able to bind to host cells in the body for replication. Viruses without a proper cell host are eventually eliminated by the body's innate immune system. Finally, lactoferrin may also suppress cellular viral replication once a cell has been infected to hinder a viral infection further.

Iron-free apolactoferrin might be the best form of lactoferrin to eliminate viruses because the iron binding action of lactoferrin is useless in combating viral infections. Research apolactoferrin to see if it applies to your condition.

Lactoferrin has been shown to have anti-fungal and yeast activity, but the mechanism is not yet known. There is a theory proposed that lactoferrin can destroy the cell walls and bind to the plasma membrane of *Candida albicans*. Lactoferrin has been shown to help control yeast infections in a few in vivo / in vitro studies.

Lactoferrin might be able to be supplemented on a low dose of 100 mg on a daily basis long term safely if needed. Honestly though, I would only supplement lactoferrin if I had an infection or believed that I might be getting an infection. The average dosage that would be taken if you were ill ranges from 250 mg - 1,000 mg a day, depending on the severity of the infection. Always take lactoferrin in divided doses throughout the day with food.

I believe the only known side effect of lactoferrin supplementation is that a rare systemic allergic reaction may occur (you may be more susceptible to a reaction if you are allergic to cow's milk, which most lactoferrin is produced from).

Lauricidin

Uses: SIYO, *Candida* opportunistic infection, yeast overgrowth, viral infections

Brand: Lauricidin

Side effects: RARE: systemic allergic Reaction

Lauricidin is a supplement that contains a high concentration of purified monolaurin.

Lauric acid (a fatty acid found in coconuts and breast milk) is converted into monolaurin in the human body that has strong antibacterial and anti-yeast properties. There is some anecdotal evidence that the monolaurin content of breast milk is why it cures thrush in infants.

Monolaurin has been theorized to be able to keep yeast cells from being able to attach to the cell walls in your body so that they are destroyed by the immune system or eliminated from the body. Finally, monolaurin has been shown in studies to have possible antiviral properties as well.

Monolaurin is non-toxic to humans and should not cause any major reactions except for the occasional rare systemic allergic reaction. Monolaurin might cause a strong herx reaction with large amounts. Therefore, it is always best to start with a small dose when beginning to supplement.

Limonene

Uses: GERD, heartburn

Brands: Jarrow Formulas D-limonene, Heartburn Free Enzymatic Therapy D-limonene

Side effects: RARE: systemic allergic reaction

D-limonene is lighter than water, so it floats to the surface of gastric juices in the stomach. When someone has reflux, the D-limonene coats the esophagus, protects the esophagus from acid and gastrin, and helps heal erosions. D-limonene also increases gastric emptying and helps improve the flow of bile.

Joe S. Wilkins, the Houston-area scientist who developed this natural approach to heartburn relief, believes that the minor burping that occurs with D-limonene causes this orange peel extract to be directly carried into the esophagus. By coating the esophagus, D-limonene may protect the esophagus against caustic contents that would have otherwise been regurgitated from the stomach. D-limonene may promote quicker gastric emptying of food and gastric juices out of the stomach so that these esophageal irritants do not promote as much reflux. Finally, D-limonene might inhibit *H. pylori*, help the stomach produce extra mucus, and heal.

I recommend that you either use the Jarrow D-limonene or the Enzymatic Therapy D-limonene supplement. Be sure to follow the supplement instructions.

L-glutamine

Uses: Gut rebuilding, general gut health, supplementation after surgery

Brands: Now L-glutamine powder, Thorne Research L-glutamine powder

Side effects: RARE: systemic allergic reaction

L-glutamine is an amino acid that is used by the body for protein synthesis, regulation of pH balance in the kidneys, cellular energy, nitrogen donation, and a nontoxic transporter of ammonia in the blood. Intestinal cells consume more L-glutamine than anywhere else in the body does. This is why it is important for gut healing. L-glutamine maintains the gut barrier and helps with the mucus barrier. It reduces hospital recovery time after surgery because it increases white blood cell activity at the site of injury.

People with cancer should use L-glutamine with caution because it can accelerate tumor growth theoretically in some forms of tumors. L-glutamine may also be used by upper gut overgrowth like *H.*

pylori, to increase metabolism, replication, and endotoxin production. In people with leaky gut and leaky brain, L-glutamine supplementation may increase inflammation in the brain and reduce GABA. If you get an increase in brain fog, headaches, increased anxiety, or herx symptoms with the use of L-glutamine, discontinue its use.

How to Make Fresh Homemade Cabbage Juice - Full of Natural L-glutamine

1. Boil the water in a small pot for thirty minutes if you are using tap water. Boiling will rid the water of most unwanted elements, but you can also use filtered water that you do not have to boil if you want.
2. Wash and chop up the cabbage.
3. Put the chopped cabbage and the water into a blender. Use a large blender so that the blender is only about 2/3 full if possible. Do not fill the blender completely because the cabbage and the water will not blend well if you do!
4. Blend the cabbage and water together at low speed. Stop when the water is green-tinted, with noticeable chunks of cabbage still floating around. This should only take one or two minutes. The reason you spend most of the blending time at low speed is to prevent oxidization of the cabbage phytochemicals.
5. Then blend the mixture on high for about ten seconds. Do not blend the mixture for much longer than that on high speed. You do not want to create a paste or a puree.
6. Place a mesh strainer over a clean, empty jar (boil the jar first to sanitize the jar). Use a strainer, to separate, as much of the cabbage liquid from the solid cabbage parts as possible. Make sure that the strainer you use is also smaller than the mouth of the jar to avoid any spillage.
7. Pour the leftover solid liquid through the strainer and into the second jar. Strain the liquid slowly to avoid accidentally spilling the juice or causing the strainer to become clogged with pulp.
8. Pour the extra juice from the second jar into the first jar.
9. Cap the jar. Store your cabbage juice inside the refrigerator until ready to use and serve it chilled.
10. Pour four ounces in a glass mixed with four ounces of filtered water and drink twice daily on an empty stomach for maximum effect and enjoy!

Fermented Cabbage Juice - Probiotic Goodness!

Only drink the fermented cabbage juice for one week every two months for great probiotic health! One batch should keep in the refrigerator for up to two months.

1. Boil the water in a small pot for thirty minutes if you are using tap water. Boiling will rid the water of most unwanted elements, but you can also use filtered water that you do not have to boil if you want.
2. Wash (only in chlorine-free tap water) and chop up the cabbage.
3. Put the chopped cabbage and the water into a blender. Use a large blender so that the blender is only about 2/3 full if possible. Do not fill the blender completely because the cabbage and the water will not blend well if you do!
4. Blend the cabbage and water together at low speed. Stop when the water is green-tinted, with noticeable chunks of cabbage still floating around. This should only take one or two minutes. The reason you spend most of the blending time at low speed is to prevent oxidization of the cabbage phytochemicals.
5. Then blend the mixture on high for about ten seconds. Do not blend the mixture for much longer than that on high speed. You do not want to create a paste or a puree.
6. Pour the mixture into one-quart sterilized jar. Also, add one tsp. of Real Salt, or toxin free sea salt to the mixture in a jar. Make sure that there is at least one full inch (2.5 centimeters) between the surface level of the cabbage mixture and the rim of the jar. The liquid will likely expand as it ferments, so give the liquid extra room.
7. Tightly seal the jar with plastic wrap. If the jar you have came with a lid, that will also work well. For an even tighter seal, stretch plastic wrap over the mouth of the jar and screw the cap onto the jar over the wrap. Shake the jar to mix the salt with the cabbage juice.
8. Allow the cabbage mixture to sit undisturbed at room temperature. Avoid allowing the temperature to drop below 68 degrees Fahrenheit or to rise above 78 degrees Fahrenheit. Keep the jar out of the sun as much as possible and in a dark cabinet away from the stove would be best if all possible.
9. Let the cabbage mixture sit for at least six weeks. The juice is fermenting and growing cultures that will help your digestive health.
10. Place a mesh strainer over a clean, empty jar (boil the jar first to sanitize the jar). Use a strainer, to separate, as much of the cabbage liquid from the solid cabbage parts as possible. Make sure that the strainer you use is also smaller than the mouth of the jar to avoid any spillage.
11. Pour the leftover solid liquid through a strainer and into the second jar. Strain the liquid slowly to avoid accidentally spilling the juice or causing the strainer to become clogged with pulp.
12. Pour the extra juice from the second jar into the first jar.
13. Cap the jar. Store your cabbage juice inside the refrigerator until ready to use and serve it chilled.
14. Repeat this process when your original supply gets low, reserving 1/2 cup of your original batch of cabbage juice. This new 1/2 cup should be added to your new batch prior to the fermentation process.
15. Allow your new batch to sit at room temperature for twenty-four hours before straining. By adding cultured juice from a previous batch, you sped up the time it took for your new batch to ferment.

Manuka Honey

Uses: Extremely antimicrobial, helps heal and sooth the digestive tract, anti *H. pylori*, anti-opportunistic bacteria

Brand: Look for a brand that might be organic, the honey should have a high active count, and one might look for pharmaceutical grade Manuka honey if it is available.

Side effects: RARE: systemic allergic reaction

Manuka honey is a type of honey that is produced in New Zealand. The honey that is collected is made from tea tree nectar that is concentrated into the honey. Tea tree oil is widely known for its antibacterial properties. Methylglyoxal is the major antibacterial component of manuka honey and has been shown effective against MRSA.

Manuka honey also has a high, natural hydrogen peroxide bioavailability that might also explain its antimicrobial properties.

Melatonin

Uses: Strengthens the LES, helps with sleep disorders, may help relieve GERD symptoms

Brands: Thorne Research melatonin, Pure Encapsulations melatonin

Side effects: RARE: systemic allergic reaction

Melatonin is a hormone that is produced by the pineal gland that causes drowsiness to prepare the body to sleep. Melatonin is also a very strong antioxidant and immune system regulator. Melatonin is made from 5-HTP in the brain by the pineal gland.

Melatonin is important in the natural circadian rhythm of human beings. It is produced by the pineal gland when no blue light is visible by the human eye. There are some studies that show that light shined on the skin can also decrease melatonin production but not to the extent of visual interaction. I would suggest making your bedroom as dark as possible at night and wearing blue light blocking glasses an hour before bedtime.

Melatonin as a hormone has been shown to strengthen the LES and lower the chance of gallstones. It has also been shown to protect the gastrointestinal integrity and strengthen mucus barriers. Finally, it might protect the esophagus from erosion by increasing blood flow to the esophagus reducing inflammation.

Mitochondrial Support Supplements (Ubiquinol [CoQ10,] PQQ, and L-carnitine)

Uses: heart Issues, chronic fatigue syndrome, cyclic vomiting syndrome, mitochondrial syndromes

Brands: Ubiquinol: Kaneka QH, PQQ: Life Extension, Jarrow

Side effects: RARE: systemic allergic reaction

Ubiquinol

Ubiquinol is a lipid-soluble form of CoQ10 that is found in nearly every cell, tissue, and organ in mammals. Your body synthesizes ubiquinol from the CoQ10 taken in from your diet. Ubiquinol is a potent antioxidant capable of recycling other antioxidants such as vitamin E, and vitamin C. The highest concentration of ubiquinol in your body is your heart! Ubiquinol is not very stable outside of the body, but recently scientists in Japan have found a way to stabilize it and have made it available to people around the world. Ubiquinol is only available by prescription in Japan, but in America it is available as a supplement.

Ubiquinol lowers inflammation, strengthens the heart, provides the heart more energy, and regulates blood pressure with relatively no side effects. The only side effect to my knowledge (other than the few systemic allergic reactions that can happen with any medication or supplement) is that ubiquinol may have a rebound effect if discontinued suddenly. A rebound effect of the lack of CoQ10 makes you feel tired, weak, and your blood pressure might increase a little. These symptoms may last for about a week. Your body synthesizes less CoQ10 when you are supplementing with it, so it begins to make fewer enzymes. Over time, there will not be enough enzymes to produce significant quantities of CoQ10, and there may be a temporary disparagement if it is suddenly discontinued. In time, genes will be activated due to the low concentrations of CoQ10 in the cells, and you will begin to produce it on your own once again.

Ubiquinol also helps restore the gum line in people with gum disease and will stop gum bleeding. Anyone over thirty should take ubiquinol instead of CoQ10 because the body produces insufficient CoQ10 as we age. Organic red palm oil has one of the highest concentrations of CoQ10 in food.

PQQ

PQQ is a quinoprotein and is used by the body to produce new mitochondria for your cells. PQQ also protects current mitochondria from oxidative stress. PQQ is a neuroprotectant, promotes memory, attention, and boosts cognition.

PQQ protects the heart from further damage after a heart attack and is a potent antioxidant. This might be the mechanism of action behind its functions because it protects against and reverses oxidative stress.

L-carnitine

L-carnitine is a derivative of the amino acid, lysine. L-carnitine can be synthesized in the body from the amino acids lysine and methionine. L-carnitine can also be obtained through the diet as well. The reason is that they are vulnerable to an L-carnitine deficiency. L-carnitine also has an important relation to CoQ10, because both are primarily concentrated in heart muscle, and both are also found in large numbers in skeletal muscle. L-carnitine also plays an important role in energy production within the mitochondria. Carnitine conjugates fatty acids for transport into the mitochondria so that the fatty acids can then be metabolized for energy.

Long-chain fatty acids have to become esters of L-carnitine first before they can be used by the mitochondria. This conversion occurs so that the acids can enter the mitochondrial matrix and provide source material for the production of energy. L-carnitine serves in a number of different ways in increasing the capacity of the mitochondria by helping in the generation of ATP. Carnitine also works synergistically with coenzyme A to metabolize fatty acids and transport them within the individual cells.

Different Forms of L-carnitine:

There are six recognized forms of L-carnitine currently, and each form serves its unique purpose. The six forms of L-carnitine are:

Standard L-carnitine and its Chelations

L-carnitine - This is the standard L-carnitine. L-carnitine supplementation is used in the body to increase energy production. L-carnitine should be used in people who are sensitive to Acetyl L-carnitine, which can over stimulate some people and cause racing thoughts.

The daily-recommended dose of L-carnitine for most people is 2,000 mg. I would not take more than 4,000 mg daily if possible because the excess L-carnitine might cause a fishy body odor and skin sensitivities at this large of a dose.

When you should take the supplement: to help facilitate weight loss L-carnitine should be taken on an empty stomach, for everyone else L-carnitine should be taken with your largest meal.

- Recommended Brands: Jarrow Formulas L-carnitine, Life Extension - L-carnitine Powder

L-carnitine-L-tartrate - L-carnitine L-tartrate is a chelation of L-carnitine and tartaric acid. Tartaric acid is a natural acid found in grapes. Tartaric acid is supposed to help with the stability and absorption of the L-carnitine in the body. This form of L-carnitine has been discovered in one study to decrease the recovery time for athletes after workouts.

The daily-recommended dose of L-carnitine L-tartrate for most people is 2,000 mg. I would not take more than 4,000 mg daily if possible because the excess L-carnitine L-tartrate might cause a fishy body odor and skin sensitivities at this large of a dose.

When you should take the supplement: to help facilitate weight loss L-carnitine L-tartrate should be taken on an empty stomach, for everyone else L-carnitine-L-tartrate should be taken with your largest meal.

- Recommended Brand: Jarrow Formulas L-carnitine tartrate

L-carnitine fumarate - L-carnitine fumarate is a chelation of L-carnitine and fumaric acid. Fumaric acid is an acid found in some mosses and mushrooms. Fumaric acid is also supposed to help with the stability and absorption of the L-carnitine. Fumarate can help activate the NrF2 antioxidant response pathway, the primary cellular defense against cytotoxic effects of oxidative stress. L-carnitine chelated with fumarate might provide some mitochondrial defense, compared to the other forms of L-carnitine that may perform no known defense.

The daily-recommended dose of L-carnitine fumarate for most people is 2,000 mg. I would not take more than 4,000 mg daily if possible because the excess L-carnitine fumarate may create fishy body odor and skin sensitivities at this large of a dose.

When you should take the supplement: To help facilitate weight loss L-carnitine fumarate should be taken on an empty stomach, for everyone else L-carnitine fumarate should be taken with your largest meal.

- Recommended Brands: Doctor's Best L-carnitine fumarate, Pure Encapsulations L-carnitine fumarate

Specialized L-Carnitine Chelations

Acetyl L-carnitine - L-carnitine often does not cross the blood-brain barrier very well on its own. Scientists discovered that by acetylating L-carnitine, carnitine was able to cross the blood-brain barrier more effectively. Acetyl L-carnitine makes the transport of fatty acids to the brain easier by allowing the acids to cross the blood-brain barrier easily and nourish the brain. In addition, the acetyl part of the chelation helps create more acetylcholine in the brain by donating an acetyl group. Acetyl L-carnitine has been shown in studies to improve memory and brain function, especially in people who are suffering from type 2 diabetes. It has been theorized that this increase of brain function occurs because acetyl L-carnitine nourishes the brain with essential fatty acids for optimal functioning.

One of the only drawbacks that I know with acetyl L-carnitine supplementation is that for some people it can stimulate the brain so much that they develop racing thoughts. If that occurs, switch to a standard L-carnitine chelation and receive some of the benefits of supplementation with carnitine.

The daily-recommended dose of acetyl L-carnitine for most people is 2,000 mg. I would not take more than 4,000 mg daily if possible because the excess acetyl L-carnitine might cause a fishy body odor and skin sensitivities at this large of a dose.

When you should take the supplement: it should be taken with your largest meal.

- Recommended Brands: Jarrow Formulas acetyl L-carnitine, Life Extension acetyl L-carnitine, Pure Encapsulations – acetyl L-carnitine

Acetyl L-carnitine arginate - This special chelated form of acetyl L-carnitine is acetyl L-carnitine bonded with the amino acid L-arginine. It is believed that the extra arginine in which the carnitine is bounded to crosses the blood-brain barrier and may increase blood flow to the brain. Acetyl L-carnitine arginate is also an excellent form of carnitine for bodybuilders. This is because the extra arginine increases nitric oxide production in the body and acts as a vasodilator. Increased arginine supplementation has been theorized to increase blood flow to the muscles as well.

The daily-recommended dose of acetyl L-carnitine arginate for most people is 2,000 mg. I would not take more than 4,000 mg daily if possible because the excess acetyl L-carnitine arginate might cause a fishy body odor and skin sensitivities at this large of a dose.

When you should take the supplement: it should be taken with your largest meal.

- Recommended Brand: Life Extension acetyl L-carnitine arginate

Glycine propionyl L-carnitine - Propionyl L-carnitine is the main recommended form of L-carnitine for people with arterial blood flow problems and heart disease. The propionyl is also an extra donator to the coenzyme A cycle. Since L-carnitine works synergistically with coenzyme A, taking a propionyl L-carnitine supplement is a great way to increase natural coenzyme A production in the body.

Propionyl L-carnitine has been shown in studies to increase nitrate / nitrite production in the body, as well. Extra nitrates / nitrites in the body have been known to increase nitric oxide production theoretically. This is why propionyl L-carnitine promotes proper arterial blood flow because the extra nitric oxide production is a potent vasodilator. This is also the preferred form of L-carnitine for people with poor blood flow in their extremities, people that suffer from intermittent claudication, and most athletes, as well.

The daily-recommended dose of propionyl L-carnitine for most people is 2,000 mg. I would not take more than 4,000 mg daily if possible because the excess propionyl L-carnitine might cause a fishy body odor and skin sensitivities at this large of a dose.

When you should take the supplement: it should be taken with your largest meal.

- Recommended Brand: Jarrow Formulas glycine propionyl L-carnitine

L-carnitine Supplementation Side Effects

L-carnitine is safe for most people to supplement with daily and has very few known side effects. In some people, L-carnitine can cause upset stomach and indigestion, which can be relieved when the L-carnitine supplement is taken with a meal instead of on an empty stomach. L-carnitine supplementation may also rarely cause nausea, vomiting, diarrhea, and seizures. L-carnitine can cause some people to develop a fishy body odor if taken in quantities greater than 4,000 mg daily. There are also extremely rare systemic allergic reactions caused by L-carnitine supplementation in some people.

L-carnitine should be used in caution with people who have an underactive thyroid or people who have a history of seizures. Carnitine can make the symptoms of hypothyroid worse and may increase the frequency of seizures in people with seizure disorders.

NAC

Uses: Destroys biofilm, increases glutathione in the body, and thins mucus secretions

Brands: Jarrow Bi-Layer NAC

Side effects: RARE: systemic allergic reaction

NAC is a supplement and pharmaceutical drug that is made from the amino acid cysteine. As a drug, it is used to increase glutathione and protect the liver from acetaminophen (Tylenol) overdose. It is also used as a mucolytic (thin mucus) agent in the lungs in the use of treating cystic fibrosis. NAC has also been used as a treatment regimen for mental disorders including schizophrenia and bipolar. Finally, NAC is also used as a nephroprotective agent in people with kidney failure who receive radiocontrast dyes for imaging procedures.

NAC breaks down and detaches bacterial biofilms that help eliminate bacteria from the body. Its mechanism of action is not yet known. One possible theory of how NAC breaks down biofilm is that it might interfere with the mucus production needed to produce the biofilm by the bacteria.

N-Acetylglucosamine

Uses: Reinforces the integrity of the intestinal wall, reduces autoimmune overreactions

Brands: Jarrow Formulas NAG, Designs for Health GI-Revive, Allergy Research Group NAG, DaVinci G.I. Benefits

Side effects: RARE: systemic allergic reaction (shellfish allergy)

NAG is a monosaccharide derivative of glucose (may feed yeast overgrowth, use with caution if you suspect you have overgrowth). NAG can correct an overactive immune system so that autoimmune reactions occur less often. The mechanism of action believed to be behind this action is that NAG controls immune T-cell over activity.

NAG is also involved in the repair of mucous membranes throughout the body. NAG can be supplemented to help repair the extracellular tissue and barrier of the gastrointestinal system. It can also decrease the binding of some lectins (proteins that can damage the intestines) from food ingestion. Use with caution if you are suffering from yeast overgrowth, NAG can be a source of food for yeast overgrowth. Finally, NAG has also been shown in a recent study to reduce inflammation in the digestive tract in people suffering from IBD, leading to remission.

Nu-Nefarious

Uses: hiatal hernia

Brand: Thaumaturge Nu Nefarious

Side effects: RARE: systemic allergic reaction

Nu-Nefarious is a homeopathic supplement that can help relieve some of the complications due to a hiatal hernia.

It contains:

- **Spleen extract** - an extract of cow spleen that can help the spleen and immune system function better because of pressure that is put on the spleen by a hernia.
- **Milk Thistle** - a herb that is used to detoxify the liver and the body.
- **Red Raspberry** – a fruit that can protect the esophagus.
- **Manganese** - a mineral that can help with muscle toning and fat metabolism.
- **Quercetin** - an antioxidant that can help reduce inflammation and allergic responses.
- **Black Currant Oil** - oil that is high in GLA that can protect the pancreas.

Ox bile

Uses: Prevention of gallstones, elimination of gallstones, improves gallbladder function

Brand: Jarrow Formulas Bile Acid Factors, Thorne Research Bio-Gest, Allergy Research Group ox bile

Side effects: May cause diarrhea in some people with bile acid malabsorption if so discontinue OX bile. RARE: Systemic allergic reaction.

Ox bile supplements are used to replace bile in the human body. Bile is important for digestion and regulation of food metabolism. People with liver, gallbladder problems, or have had their gallbladder removed might need ox bile to help supplement the natural bile that they lack. The extra bile is used by the body to break down fats by lowering the PH to change the shape of proteins so that they are properly assimilated into the body by the intestines.

Ox bile supplements have been known to cause diarrhea in people with bile acid reabsorption problems, supplement with caution.

Oxaloacetate

Uses: Eliminates brain fog, reduces oxidative stress from systemic endotoxins that inflame the brain, and increases energy

Brand: Advanced Orthomolecular Research

Side effects: RARE: systemic allergic reaction

Oxaloacetate is a metabolic intermediate that occurs during many processes in our body (gluconeogenesis, citric acid cycle, and urea cycle to name a few). Oxaloacetate can protect our brain neurons from endotoxins and reduce glutamate hyperexcitability. Oxaloacetate also increases brain mitochondrial biogenesis, enhances the body's use of insulin, stimulates neurogenesis and reduces brain inflammation. Finally, it may help improve sleep, increase energy levels, reduce tinnitus, and eliminate brain fog.

R-lipoic Acid

Uses: LES / nerve problems, diabetes

Brands: Geronova R-lipoic acid, Life Extension R-lipoic acid, Jarrow Formulas R-lipoic acid

Side effects: RARE: systemic allergic reaction, rash, and foul smelling urine, lowers blood sugar so use with caution if you have blood glucose control issues

R-lipoic acid is probably one of the most important supplements when it comes to relieving complications caused by nerve damage and diabetes. R-lipoic acid reverses diabetic neuropathy restores proper liver function and reverses insulin resistance. Lipoic acid is produced in the body as antioxidant and has many functions. One of its primary functions is to transport insulin into cells that have been overloaded with glucose. Lipoic acid also helps reverse the excitability of nerves leading to less neuropathy.

Taking R-lipoic acid supplements also increases glutathione levels in the body. This improves liver function and fights against cancer. Finally, lipoic acid helps the body recycle and retain vitamins C and E preventing cellular damage.

The only known side effects of lipoic acid supplementation are odd-smelling urine, paresthesia, skin rash, and muscle cramps. This is more commonly seen in the less expensive, synthetic alpha lipoic acid instead of the natural R-lipoic acid. Lipoic acid is also a powerful chelator so do not take it with mineral supplements. If you are mercury toxic, it can cause side effects like tingling, brain fog, and changes in mood. The lipoic acid binds to the mercury, and it is removed from the body.

Take lipoic acid with food because the supplement may lower blood glucose levels.

Seacure

Uses: reinforces the integrity of the intestinal wall

Brand: Seacure

Side effects: RARE: systemic allergic reaction

Seacure is a supplement that is made from pre-digested fish peptides. The proteins in the supplement are broken down into peptides for maximum absorption from fermentation instead of normal heat processes. Heat can denature many beneficial proteins that would otherwise help with recovery and repair in the production of most other protein supplements; using fermentation instead is what makes Seacure better!

When ingested, the stomach easily assimilates these proteins. The peptides work locally in the gut lining and increase healing and protein synthesis.

Undecylenic Acid

Uses: Reduces yeast overgrowth, prevents fungal virulence

Brand: SF722

Side effects: RARE: systemic allergic reaction

Undecylenic acid is an eleven-carbon monounsaturated fatty acid, which is found naturally in our sweat and is produced from castor bean oil for supplemental form.

Undecylenic acid is used to reduce yeast overgrowth and to help prevent yeast from becoming more virulent and become fungal (a process known as morphogenesis). Undecylenic acid disrupts the pH of yeast cell cytoplasm, interfering with its ability to form hyphae (fungal biofilm) and become more virulent.

Zeaxanthin

Uses: Helps increase eye function, helps protect eyes from damage

Brand: Life Extension Super Zeaxanthin

Side effects: RARE: systemic allergic reaction

Zeaxanthin is one of the most common carotenoids found in nature. The pigment gives corn, paprika, and saffron their color.

This pigment is found in high concentrations in the macula of the eye. Zeaxanthin has been shown in studies to protect the eye against damage from degenerative diseases (macular degeneration) and free radicals.

Zinc Carnosine

Uses: Heal ulcers, relieves gastritis, and helps stomach disorders

Brands: Pure Encapsulations zinc carnosine, Doctor's Best zinc carnosine

Side effects: RARE: systemic allergic reaction

Zinc carnosine is a supplement that is the combination of the mineral zinc and the amino acid carnosine. Zinc is beneficial in decreasing wound healing time and also increases immune functions. Carnosine is an amino acid that is highly concentrated in muscle tissue and has been shown to protect organs from oxidative stress.

Zinc binds quickly to stomach tissue if taken on an empty stomach. If zinc is taken on an empty stomach, it causes severe stomach pain and gastritis. It has been theorized that zinc ions are highly soluble in stomach acid and have corrosive, antimicrobial, and immune stimulating properties that irritate the stomach tissue because of the direct absorption of the zinc ions. If you chelate zinc with carnosine, the chelation slows down the absorption and elimination of zinc from the stomach. Zinc is then able to repair the stomach and intestinal tissue directly without irritating it so zinc carnosine may be taken on an empty stomach as needed. Zinc carnosine also protects the stomach lining for opportunistic *H. pylori* infection, and NSAID damage that cause ulcers that develop from long-term use of the medication.

High doses of zinc carnosine may cause zinc toxicity and reduce immune function. Take no more than 45 mg of zinc carnosine each day or 100 mg of elemental zinc daily.

Chapter 18

Herbs / Foods That Are Helpful for Digestive Ailments

I believe that herbs, if used in the right situations, are very beneficial in helping with any medical condition, especially digestive issues. Most herbs should only be reserved for certain diseases for most people and should only be taken when needed. Herbs that are used in cooking may be used with regularity. This is because these herbs have been used in the human diet for thousands of years, and we have adapted to them. Herbs are very powerful and should only be used when they are utmost necessary.

Aloe Vera

Uses: General relief of heartburn, GERD, esophagus issues, constipation (if the aloe contains aloin)

Brands: George's Always Active aloe vera, Lily of the Desert organic aloe vera

Side Effects: diarrhea (if aloin is left in), RARE: hypersensitive allergic reaction

Aloe vera is a plant that is native to northern Africa. Aloe vera can be used to soothe heartburn by coating the esophagus (protecting it) and also settles the stomach. It has also been shown to help heal tissue damage done to the esophagus and stomach.

Try to use aloe vera that has the aloin distilled out of it so that diarrhea does not occur. Aloe vera with aloin should only be used sparingly with someone who is constipated, and rehydration therapy should be given afterward as needed.

Astragalus

Uses: helps improve liver and intestinal function

Brands: Gaia Astragalus Supreme, Now astragalus, Douglas Labs Astragalus Max-V

Side Effects: RARE: hypersensitive allergic reaction

Astragalus is a bushy member of the legume family native to the northern hemisphere. Astragalus strengthens the movement and muscle tone of the intestines increasing the movement of food through the gastrointestinal tract. It has also been shown to protect the liver in in vitro studies.

People taking blood thinners should be careful when using astragalus because it contains natural coumarins causing blood-clotting issues. Beta-blockers have also been shown to be less effective when someone is taking an astragalus supplement. Astragalus supplementation should be avoided if you are taking a beta-blocker.

Black Cumin Seed Oil

Uses: SIBO, dyspepsia, has antibacterial properties, reduces an elevated Th1 / Th2 immune system

Brand: Black cumin seed oil

Side Effects: RARE: hypersensitive allergic reaction

Black cumin seed oil is sourced from the flowering plant Nigella sativa. Its seeds are used in Indian and Middle Eastern culinary dishes and have a pungent, peppery taste. Black cumin seed oil in studies has antibacterial properties and relieves dyspepsia. Thymoquinone that is extracted from black cumin seeds is cardio, hepatic, and nephroprotective. Thymoquinone ingestion may help prevent the development of colon cancer. Black cumin seed oil calms an overactive immune system; it reduces both Th1 and Th2 dominance.

Black Raspberry Powder

Uses: protection from Barrett's Esophagus

Brand: Virgin Extracts

Side Effects: RARE: hypersensitive allergic reaction

Black raspberries are native to North America. When the black raspberry powder is mixed with water and consumed, the powder might help by coating and protect the esophagus from stomach acid and pepsin.

Black raspberries may even reverse Barrett's esophagus by protecting the esophagus and by helping combat free radical damage caused by stomach acid reflux and pepsin.

Black Walnut Hulls

Uses: Can be used to eliminate parasites, and as an astringent, it can help relieve canker sores, as well

Brand: Dr. Hula Clark's black walnut tincture

Side Effects: diarrhea, RARE: hypersensitive allergic reaction

Juglone is a phytochemical in black walnuts making them toxic to parasites and even other plants. Juglone is believed to be harmless to humans as long as they are not allergic to black walnuts.

Black walnut tinctures might also be helpful in eliminating painful canker sores if swished in the mouth for thirty seconds.

Boswellia

Uses: Reduces inflammation in people with IBD, has been shown to help in people with asthma

Brands: Himalaya boswellia, Pure Encapsulations boswellia

Side Effects: RARE: hypersensitive allergic reaction, possible hepatotoxicity with large doses (in vivo in rats only, no in vivo human studies)

Boswellia is a tree native to India. The incense, frankincense, is obtained from the resin of the Boswellia tree. More importantly, boswellic acids have been shown to produce anti-inflammatory effects by inhibiting leukotriene synthesis. Boswellia may also help with inflammation in IBD sufferers.

Butcher's Broom

Uses: hemorrhoids

Brands: Now butcher's broom

Side Effects: RARE: hypersensitive allergic reaction

Butcher's broom is an evergreen bush native to Europe. Butcher's broom supports circulation and tightens dilated blood vessels that form from hemorrhoids. It also relieves the burning and itching associated with hemorrhoids.

Cardamom

Uses: dyspepsia (upset stomach)

Side Effects: RARE: hypersensitive allergic reaction

Cardamom is medicinal herb native to China and Vietnam. According to the German Herbal Commission E, it has been shown to help relieve an upset stomach by stimulating bile flow. Cardamom stimulates the production of bile and digestive enzymes in the body.

Carnivora

Uses: regulates the natural immune system

Brand: Carnivora

Side Effects: RARE: hypersensitive allergic reaction

Carnivora is made from the Venus flytrap native to the west coast of North Carolina. The compounds in carnivora have been shown to regulate the body's immune system so that it can return to normal function.

Cayenne

Uses: Reduces inflammation, can help repair ulcers, helps regulate bowels and relieves constipation, hemorrhoids, colon cleanser, stimulate bile release from the gallbladder, decreases gastric and intestinal transit time

Brands: Organic cayenne pepper powder, Solaray Cool Cayenne

Side Effects: RARE: hypersensitive allergic reaction and cayenne can irritate esophagus and intestinal tract in some people

Consumption of cayenne pepper is very important for overall health, and especially for digestive health. Cayenne pepper contains capsaicin (which is responsible for the peppers "heat,") which is a very strong anti-inflammatory compound. Cayenne pepper repairs stomach ulcers by reducing inflammation and stimulating the stomach to produce more mucus to protect the lining. It also reduces hemorrhoids in the same way by reducing swelling and inflammation at the rectum.

Spicy food does not cause heartburn, as most people believe that it does. Spicy food irritates the esophagus in someone who already has GERD because of the lack of a proper protective mucus barrier in the esophageal lining. This is why consumption of spicy food causes throat pain in the sufferers of GERD. The spicy food is not the actual cause of acid reflux.

Capsaicin binds to receptor TRPV1 in the intestines, preventing endotoxins released by *E. coli* from binding and causing issues. These endotoxins cause food poisoning. This binding irritates nerves in the intestines and causes diarrhea in people who are not used to eating spicy food. The body eventually adapts to capsaicin consumption if you eat spicy food frequently. Furthermore, studies have shown that people who consume capsaicin have a less chance of developing gastrointestinal cancer.

One of the best ways to clean your gallbladder is to make cayenne pepper drink. People without a gallbladder should limit the use of cayenne pepper.

Cayenne Pepper Protocol

1. Boil cold distilled water.
2. Put your designated or acclimated amount of cayenne pepper powder in a small glass. Start with 1/8 of a teaspoon and work up to ½ of a teaspoon.
3. Pour the very warm water over the cayenne pepper powder. Squeeze half a lemon into the glass.
4. Let it steep for a minute, and then mix thoroughly.
5. Drink it as fast as you can and feel the burn!

Cinnamon

Uses: very potent antimicrobial agent, used in SIBO protocols (Ch. 9), facilitates proper blood glucose regulation

Brands: Ceylon cinnamon oil

Side Effects: RARE: hypersensitive allergic reaction, use with caution if you have hypoglycemia

Cinnamon is a culinary spice that is sourced from the inner bark of trees from the *Cinnamomum* genus. Most of the cinnamon that is sourced is either Ceylon (true) cinnamon or cassia cinnamon.

If you ingest cinnamon as a spice or take it in supplement form, you want to make sure that it is produced from Ceylon cinnamon. Both forms of cinnamon contain coumarin, which is a natural blood-thinning agent but is hepatotoxic. Ceylon contains minute amounts of coumarin compared to cassia cinnamon. Cinnamon has been shown in studies to help improve blood glucose metabolism and help improve insulin sensitivity.

Cinnamon in studies seems to have many very potent antimicrobial properties. In studies against pathogenic bacteria, cinnamon showed the highest antibacterial properties, out of many different natural essential oils (including limonene, carvacrol, and thymol). The main antibacterial agent in cinnamon oil seems to be cinnamaldehyde. Cinnamon oil contains anti-yeast properties as well, but because it elevates Th2 immune reactions and people with yeast issues have trouble detoxing aldehydes, I cannot recommend its use. I recommend using Ceylon cinnamon essential oil to help reduce bacterial overgrowth in the gut. I recommend consuming one drop in at least six oz. of filtered water with a meal; it can be very potent.

Chamomile

Uses: good for people suffering from IBS and peptic ulcers

Brands: Organic chamomile tea, Herb Pharm chamomile tincture

Side Effects: systemic allergic reaction for people allergic to ragweed RARE: hypersensitive allergic reaction

Chamomile is an aromatic annual plant native to Europe. It has been shown to have antispasmodic properties in the colon and helps people with IBS. Chamomile also has anti-inflammatory and antihistamine properties that may help relieve peptic ulcers.

Chamomile contains natural coumarins and should be avoided in people taking blood thinners.

Echinacea

Uses: Stimulates appetite, anti-yeast, stimulates proper immune system functioning

Brands: Gaia Echinacea Supreme, Planetary Herbals Echinacea extract

Side Effects: RARE: hypersensitive allergic reaction

Echinacea is a group of North American prairie perennials that produce purple flowers and leaves. Echinacea stimulates cannabinoid receptors, which stimulate both the immune system and appetite. Marijuana is another herb that stimulates cannabinoid receptors and stimulates the immune system and appetite. In German studies, echinacea has been shown to stimulate macrophages to engulf yeast cells through phagocytosis in animals. Use *Echinacea purpurea* for yeast-related disorders.

Echinacea modifies drug metabolism in drugs that use the CYP3A4 enzyme for breakdown (Viagra, immunosuppressive drugs, and calcium-channel blockers to name a few) and should be avoided in people using medications that rely on this enzyme for metabolism. Echinacea should also be avoided in people that are allergic to ragweed.

Fennel

Uses: fennel seeds relieve stomach gas buildup

Side effects: RARE: hypersensitive allergic reaction

Fennel is a vegetable that originated in the Mediterranean. Chewing on fennel seeds suppress appetite, relieve stomach gas pressure, and helps you burp. Fennel relaxes the smooth muscle in the digestive system, which is beneficial for people suffering from achalasia.

If you suffer from decreased LES tone, taking fennel might be a bad idea because of the smooth muscle relaxing mechanism. Finally, fennel may help stimulate appetite in some people.

Ginger

Uses: Strongly anti-inflammatory, stimulates digestion and bile flow from gallbladder, soothe an upset stomach, ginger can help with morning sickness and general nausea, and can help with gastric emptying

Brands: Reed's Ginger Beer, Gin Gin ginger chews, New Chapter Ginger Force, Jarrow Formulas ginger

Side effects: RARE: hypersensitive allergic reaction. You need to limit ginger intake if you are missing your gallbladder, also should be limited in people taking anticoagulants

Ginger is a plant from South Asia. Most people use the rhizome or root for cooking and medicine. Ginger has a very strong odor, taste, and the root itself can be spicy.

Ginger helps with nausea and stomach sickness. Components in the ginger bind to the serotonin receptors in the gastrointestinal tract and might work the same way as the popular emetic drug Zofran. Ginger also has strong anti-inflammatory properties in the gastrointestinal tract when digested. Zingerone is one of the main components of ginger's essential oils and might have some antimicrobial activity against opportunistic *E. coli* in the colon.

Goldenseal

Uses: antibacterial properties

Brands: Thorne Research Berbercap

Side effects: RARE: systemic allergic reaction, Berberine should only be used as a last resort herbal antibacterial because of possible toxicity

Goldenseal is a plant native to the northeastern United States. It has a component called berberine and has been shown to be antibacterial. Berberine is not a systemic antibacterial, but it is known to have strong antibacterial properties when it comes into direct contact with the bacteria. Goldenseal supports healthy mucous flow and increases IgA antibodies in the mucous to eliminate the bacteria.

Berberine interferes with any medication that uses the cytochrome p450 pathway. Goldenseal has been known to interfere with anticoagulants (heparin and warfarin), as well. Berberine can also reduce blood glucose levels so take with food. It also inhibits the aldose reductase pathway so avoid sorbitol and other sugar alcohols while taking it to protect your vision. Large doses of berberine can be harsh on the stomach mucosa, so discontinue if it causes gastritis or worsens it. Check with your doctor if you are on any medication before you use goldenseal to make sure it is safe.

Horse Chestnut

Uses: hemorrhoids

Brand: Planetary Herbals horse chestnut, Now horse chestnut

Side effects: RARE: hypersensitive allergic reaction, kidney damage

Horse chestnut comes from a tree that is native to the Caucasus Mountains. Aescin, a compound found in horse chestnut, increases circulation. In a study, people who took aescin (standardized extract of 40 mg, three times daily) had a reduction in pain and hemorrhoids.

Licorice

Uses: Strongly anti-inflammatory, helps heal the mucus lining in the stomach, has been shown to repair ulcers and is an actual prescription medication for ulcers in Germany, inhibits *H. pylori*, lessens abdominal spasms

Brand: Enzymatic DGL ULTRA chewable licorice

Side effects: Non-DGL Licorice can cause water retention and elevation of blood pressure. DGL should only be used for a short period, because of the possibility that small amounts of glycyrrhizic acid still might be left in the supplement. RARE: Hypersensitive Allergic Reaction.

Licorice is a plant native to southern Europe. The root of the plant is used in food and supplement preparation. Licorice has a huge medicinal potential, but the main problem is the glycyrrhizic acid found in the licorice that causes most of its side effects.

Glycyrrhizic acid protects liver cells against injury in people with hepatitis and has antiviral properties. Glycyrrhizic acid is also used as a sweetener in food products. Glycyrrhizic acid causes water retention at high doses, and this can increase blood pressure and volume. In some cases, this can become fatal.

Glycyrrhizic acid depletes potassium in the body causing a blood pressure spike. In addition, the enzyme 11B-hydroxysteroid dehydrogenase is inhibited by glycyrrhizic acid causing a spike in cortisol. This sharp increase of cortisol can produce a dump of potassium extracellular. The dump of potassium outside the cell increase potassium in the blood plasma.

DGL Licorice lacks glycyrrhizic acid and is still theorized to have most of the anti-inflammatory processes of regular licorice. DGL is great in repairing ulcers, gastritis of the stomach, and can inhibit *H. pylori*. DGL tablets must be chewed thoroughly, and saliva must mix well with it for it to work efficiently.

Marijuana

Uses: Extremely anti-inflammatory, anticancer, stimulates appetite and digestion, IBD

Drawbacks: Not legal in some areas and countries, its use may worsen adrenal fatigue

Side effects: Extremely Rare: systemic allergic reactions

Marijuana is a plant that originated in central Asia. Marijuana has very strong anti-inflammatory properties and can be used to help people with IBD disease and in people who have a poor appetite.

Marshmallow Root

Uses: Helps protect the stomach mucous lining; helps protect the esophagus lining, good for a sore throat

Brand: Solaray marshmallow root

Side effects: RARE: hypersensitive allergic reaction

Marshmallow is a flower native to Europe and was originally used in the production of meringue. It is used to increase mucus production and protects the stomach and esophageal lining. Supplements of marshmallow are rich in complex polysaccharides that swell to fifteen times their volume, coating the stomach lining and protecting it, as well. Marshmallow is also known to stimulate the immune process in the esophagus and the stomach by increasing phagocytosis. Marshmallow blocks the absorption of many medications and should be taken two hours before or after medication.

Mastic Gum

Uses: Strongly inhibits *H. pylori*, soothes the stomach

Brands: Jarrow Formulas mastic gum, ARG Mastica

Side effects: RARE: hypersensitive allergic reaction

Mastic gum is an evergreen shrub closely related the pistachio and is native to Greece. It is used in a lot of Greek food. In medicine, it has been shown greatly to inhibit *H. pylori* infections in the stomach because of its isomasticadienolic acid content. Mastic gum, which is a mucilage, may coat and help protect the stomach lining and reduce gastritis.

Olive Leaf

Uses: Inhibits *H. pylori*, strongly antibacterial, anti-yeast, lowers an elevated Th1 immune response

Brand: Gaia olive leaf

Side effects: RARE: hypersensitive allergic reaction

Olive leaf extract is produced from the leaf of the olive tree. Olive leaf extract contains a concentrated amount of the compound oleuropein. Oleuropein in studies has shown antimicrobial properties, has anti-tumor properties, is cardioprotective, neuroprotective, anti-inflammatory, and reduces an elevated Th1 response. Olive leaf extract in studies has also shown to reduce pathogenic *H. pylori* load. Oleuropein also protects the body from endotoxins by reducing the body's exaggerated inflammatory response to them, reducing Th1 responses and inflammation. Finally, if you have yeast issues or an elevated Th2 response, I would avoid the use of olive leaf extract; it has been shown to increase Th2.

Oregano Oil

Uses: Inhibits *H. pylori*, strongly antibacterial, anti-yeast

Brand: Zane Hellas Oil of Oregano

Side effects: RARE: hypersensitive allergic reaction, stomach upset from oil ingestion

Oregano is a plant from the mint family and is native to the Mediterranean region. Oregano has a high amount of antioxidant activity because of the increased amount of phenolic acids and flavonoids found in the oil. Carvacrol and thymol are the main components of oregano oil that have the antibacterial and anti-yeast properties.

Thymol is a monoterpene phenol that has been shown in studies to inhibit the opportunistic growth of *E. coli* and *S. aureus*. Thymol inhibits the bacterial growth and lactate production in bacteria causing decreased cellular glucose uptake.

Carvacrol is a monoterpenoid phenol that has been shown to inhibit opportunistic growth of *E. coli*, *S. aureus*, and *Bacillus cereus*. The mechanism of action of the antibacterial properties of carvacrol is that carvacrol disrupts bacterial membranes.

Peppermint Oil

Uses: Strongly antibacterial, relaxes the LES, stops spasms of the intestines, relieves constipation, important to sufferers of IBS and SIBO, and helps relieve abdominal pain

Side effects: RARE: hypersensitive allergic reaction. Acid reflux from relaxation of LES (Enteric Coated Peppermint Oil should be used in those with acid reflux), diarrhea (usually for a few days at first, but will taper off later)

Peppermint is a hybrid mint plant. It is a cross between watermint and spearmint. Peppermint is native to Europe, but the herb has now grown widespread throughout the world. People everywhere value peppermint for its strong cooling scent, its cooling sensation on the skin, and it is flavoring capabilities in baking, candy making, and drink preparation.

Peppermint has a long tradition of herbal use and is used by the Egyptians, Greeks, and the Europeans for medicinal purposes. Peppermint has been studied intensively for its use in reducing the symptoms of IBS and other intestinal disorders. Peppermint is known to have high natural menthol content, contributing to its use throughout history to soothe sore throats. Menthol vapors that are produced from peppermint oil can be inhaled to relax bronchial passages and relieve congestion.

On the Importance of Menthol

Menthol is an organic compound that can be obtained from peppermint oil. Menthol has quite a few known medicinal properties, including:

- Pain relief - Menthol weakly activates the k-opioid receptors, which can be beneficial for pain relief. Different substances can activate the Kappa-opioid receptors in the brain. When the receptors are activated by these different substances (including menthol), they change both the perception of pain by the brain and reduce inflammatory pain nerve signaling pathways in the body, therefore, increasing the pain threshold.
- Muscle relaxant - Menthol's mechanism of action as a muscle relaxant is by blocking voltage-sensitive sodium channels in the neuromuscular junction. This blockage reduces neural activity in the muscles, which in turn relaxes the muscles and reduces muscle spasms.
- Vasodilatation - Menthol is a known vasodilator when it is applied to the skin. It increases blood flow to capillaries in the skin by dilating veins that are close to the dermis, or the top layer of the skin.
- Activating TRPM8 receptors - Menthol can chemically activate the TRPM8 receptors in the skin. These receptors are responsible for the cooling sensation that menthol is known for when menthol is inhaled, eaten, or applied topically to the skin. Activating the TRPM8 receptors has also been theorized to be a potential protocol for eliminating prostate cancer. Finally, TRPM8 receptors that are activated in the intestinal tract correctly modulate inflammatory responses and can help to correct an overactive immune system in people suffering from inflammatory bowel diseases.
- Relieving congestion and pain from sore throats - Menthol has been used for centuries to help relieve bronchial/nasal congestion and sore throat pain by reducing inflammation and relaxing nasal, bronchial, and throat passageways.

Uses of Peppermint Oil for Digestive Purposes

- Peppermint oil has strong antibacterial properties.
- Relaxes the lower esophageal sphincter (LES), which can be beneficial in people suffering from achalasia. It can worsen heartburn symptoms in people with GERD by relaxing the LES. People with GERD should only use enteric-coated peppermint oil.
- Peppermint oil reduces spasms of the intestines.
- Peppermint oil can help relieve constipation.
- Peppermint oil may help relieve abdominal pain.
- Peppermint oil is used to help relieve the symptoms of IBS and SIBO.
- Topical peppermint oil cream can be used to help reduce hemorrhoids.

Enteric-Coated Peppermint Oil: Magic Bullet for Intestinal Issues?

Enteric-coated peppermint oil (ECPO) is extremely versatile in the relieving of intestinal issues. ECPO can be used in eliminating intestinal infections, SIBO, IBS, chronic functional abdominal pain (CFAP), inflammatory bowel diseases, and hemorrhoids. It even helps in the relief of chronic constipation.

In a 2007 study, 75% of the people in the study took enteric-coated peppermint oil for four weeks and had a major reduction of IBS symptoms. Some people even went into remission during the study (compared to the 38% that took a placebo). Another study using ECPO was conducted in Iran in 2009 and produced similar results. Results from the study concluded enteric-coated peppermint oil greatly reduced symptoms of IBS and can be theoretically used in relieving symptoms of chronic functional abdominal pain.

It has been theorized that ECPO is very effective in the treatment of both IBS and CFAP. The proposed mechanism of action is that the oil both reduce intestinal spasms and increase the pain threshold by activating k-opioid and TRPM8 receptors. Peppermint oil eliminates opportunistic bacteria in the colon and / or small intestine that has been linked to one of the possible causes of IBS and the main cause of SIBO.

Supplementation of peppermint oil for a short period may produce loose stools and help relieve constipation. The mechanism of action for the loosening of stools may be that menthol is a mild irritant to the intestines and causes the intestines to draw in more water, causing it to act as an osmotic laxative to loosen stools. A reverse reaction may occur in people who have IBS-D the peppermint oil may calm intestinal spasms and regulate bowel movements so that their diarrhea is instead relieved.

Lastly, peppermint oil has even been used as an ingredient in a few natural hemorrhoid creams to help both reduce and alleviate pain that is caused by hemorrhoids. The peppermint oil in the cream acts as a vasodilator to the hemorrhoid tissue and helps increase blood flow to the afflicted area. Increasing blood flow to the tissue promotes healing by reducing swelling and the size of the hemorrhoid. The peppermint oil would also activate the k-opioid and TRPM8 receptors on the hemorrhoid tissue and would reduce pain.

Recommended Forms of Peppermint Oil

- Recommended forms of enteric-coated peppermint oil (known non-phthalate coating): Enzymatic therapy peppermint plus, Colpermin peppermint oil capsules (does contain peanut oil)
- Other recommendation (possible phthalate coating): Pepogest peppermint oil

- Liquid peppermint oil (use very little, follow bottle instructions): "Country Gent" peppermint oil
- Peppermint oil hemorrhoid cream: http://www.alleviatehemorrhoids.com/

Sangre de Drago

Uses: diarrhea

Brands: Rainforest Pharmacy Sangre de Drago

Side effects: RARE: hypersensitive allergic reaction

Sangre de Drago “blood of the dragon” is a tree native to the Amazon rainforest. The sap of the tree has medicinal properties. The locals have used the latex of the tree as liquid bandages. Sangre de Drago has also been studied for the healing of gastric ulcers. The herb also displays antimicrobial and anti-inflammatory properties, as well.

An active compound extracted from the tree; SP-303 (a mixture of proanthocyanidin oligomers), has been shown beneficial in stopping diarrhea, specifically in people with AIDS. It has also been shown to help with traveler’s diarrhea and people infected with the rotavirus. Crofelemer is an FDA approved drug with the same active ingredient that is in Sangre de Drago.

Slippery Elm Bark

Uses: Helps soothe and protect the digestive tract; helps protect the mucous lining of the intestine and stomach.

Brands: Now slippery elm

Side effects: RARE: hypersensitive allergic reaction, decreases absorption of some medications

Slippery elm is a tree native to North America. The inner bark of the tree has been used traditionally to help soothe digestive problems. The mucilage is made up of complex carbohydrates that soothe inflammation and relieves irritation of the mucus membrane. The high mucilage makeup of slippery elm bark can make it hard for the stomach to absorb medicines, so they should be taken separately. Slippery elm can also block the absorption of an iron supplement, so iron should be taken two hours before or after someone takes slippery elm.

Swedish Bitters (Gentian)

Uses: Helps to stimulate digestion, improves gallbladder issues, and increases digestive enzyme production

Brand: Nature Works Swedish bitters

Side effects: RARE: hypersensitive allergic reaction

Swedish bitters are mixtures of herbs that vary by brand. Your average Swedish bitter tonic can be used to help stimulate digestion and help the body make natural digestive enzymes.

Gentian is a bitter herb from a plant native to China and is used in most digestive bitter formulas. Gentian has been shown to ease gallbladder issues and indigestion. It increases appetite, stimulates the production of digestive juices, increases pancreatic activity, and boosts blood supply to the digestive organs. It also stimulates the flow of bile. Do not use gentian if you have a stomach ulcer.

Triphala

Uses: Clean the colon, return proper digestion function to the colon

Brand: Himalaya triphala

Side effects: RARE: hypersensitive allergic reaction

Triphala is an Ayurvedic herb mixture of amla, bihara, and harada fruits. Triphala is high in vitamin C, is a mild laxative, and it cleanses and tones up the digestive tract. Triphala acts as a lubricating laxative and stimulates bile flow and peristalsis. This lubrication might stem from the linoleic acid content in triphala.

Amla has a sweet flavor and is the highest known natural source of vitamin C by weight, having more than twenty times the vitamin C of an orange. Even when amla is subjected to prolonged heat, the vitamin C stored in the amla fruit is left intact. This is because tannins found in the fruit protect the vitamin C from degradation. Amla is also known to have anti-platelet coagulation properties, as well.

Bihara has a bittersweet flavor that is known for having astringent, digestive, and intestinal antispasmodic properties. It acts as a demulcent by thinning excess mucus.

Harada has a bitter flavor that also has been shown to have antispasmodic properties. Harada also has laxative, astringent, and anti-parasitic properties.

Turmeric (Curcumin)

Uses: Strongly anti-inflammatory, helps repair intestinal integrity, anti-cancer, helps relieve symptoms of IBD

Brands: Thorne Curcumin

Side effects: RARE: hypersensitive allergic reaction, people on blood thinners, should use caution

Turmeric is a plant native to South Asia and is related to ginger. Turmeric is a rich source of the curcuminoid, curcumin, which is being studied immensely for its health properties. Curcumin is a strong anti-inflammatory and is being used to relieve symptoms of arthritis and to help with people suffering from IBD. Curcumin also has some anti-tumor properties, as well.

Curcumin has also been shown to increase glutathione levels in the body by up-regulating the transcription of genes that encode GCL (the enzyme that converts L-glutamine and cysteine into glutathione). Curcumin thins the blood by inhibiting platelet aggregation; because of this, it increases the bleeding risk of people who are taking anticoagulants. In high doses, curcumin lowers iron levels in the blood by suppressing hepcidin (a hormone that regulates iron usage and storage in the body).

Witch Hazel

Uses: hemorrhoids

Side effects: RARE: hypersensitive allergic reaction

A shrub that is native to North America whose leaves and bark have astringent properties. An astringent is a chemical compound that can shrink or constrict body tissues. Witch hazel reduces hemorrhoids because it shrinks the blood vessels that surround them. Witch hazel tincture can also be used on sores and bruises because it reduces swelling and inflammation. It can also be used in eliminating symptoms of acne because it is a strong antioxidant and astringent.

Wormwood

Uses: parasites

Brand: Gaia Herbs wormwood / black walnut

Side effects: RARE: hypersensitive allergic reaction

Sweet Wormwood is a plant that is native to Asia. Wormwood has been used for malaria and parasite elimination protocols for ages. Artemisinin (an essential oil in wormwood) destroys parasites. This mechanism involves the cleavage of endoperoxide bridges of iron in parasites. It produces free radicals and causes oxidative stress in cells on contact eliminating them.

Chapter 19

Antibiotic Information Guide

Antibiotics, if used properly, are very effective in treating severe infections. Even though most natural antimicrobial agents are great at treating infections, occasionally an antibiotic is needed to treat the infection. This is a brief guide to the different types of antibiotics, the safety of, and which antibiotics should only be used if needed. The ranking scale used in this guide will be from 1-10. Number one on the scale being one of the safest antibiotics on the scale and number ten being an antibiotic that should only be used as a last resort.

Furthermore, during any antibiotic treatment regimen, a basic probiotic regimen (Ch. 13) should be followed to discourage *C. difficile* infection. I will also suggest you follow the average probiotic protocol (Ch. 13) if you have taken an antibiotic for less than a month. If you have taken an antibiotic for more than a month, then the severe probiotic regimen (Ch. 13) should be considered.

Aminoglycoside Class (Tobramycin, Neomycin, and Gentamicin)

RANK 10: DRUG OF LAST RESORT / IV, RANK 6: POSSIBLY SAFE / ORAL, RANK 4: POSSIBLY SAFE / SKIN

The aminoglycoside class of antibiotics is highly ototoxic and can cause hearing loss. This class of antibiotics should only be used in the direst implications and should be closely monitored. They are also nephrotoxic and cause irreversible kidney damage. These drugs are usually safe topically and are absorbed poorly through the skin. There are some documented instances in which toxicity of the drugs increases and new side effects were discovered in people after cessation of the antibiotic.

Neomycin is now given orally to help treat SIBO-C or methane dominant archaea. It is claimed that it is not absorbed in the gastrointestinal tract, but early studies show that it is possible in those with leaky gut to be absorbed systemically and may cause ototoxicity.

Carbapenem Class (Imipenem, Meropenem, Doripenem)

RANK 4: POSSIBLY SAFE / Imipenem RANK 6: INCREASED CAUTION

The carbapenem families of antibiotics have typical side effects, including hypersensitivity allergic reaction, *C. difficile* opportunistic infection, and diarrhea.

Imipenem must be given with the medication cilastatin, or it will be metabolized by the renal enzyme dehydropeptidase into a nephrotoxic metabolite that causes kidney damage.

Cephalosporin Class (Keflex, Rocephin)

RANK 2: SAFE

If I was to take an antibiotic, and a cephalosporin happened to be effective against the bacteria I was infected with, I would try to take an antibiotic from this class.

Cephalosporin antibiotics have been around a very long time and have a great safety record. If you are taking a cephalosporin, the most common side effects are systemic allergic reactions, *C. difficile* opportunistic infection, and diarrhea.

Glycopeptide Class (Vancomycin)

RANK 10: DRUG OF LAST RESORT

Vancomycin has been around for a long time, but because of its side effects, it is listed as a drug of last resort. Vancomycin should only be used if all other antibiotic treatments have failed and need to be closely monitored when used.

Vancomycin causes some of the same side effects standard to antibiotics like hypersensitivity reactions, *C. difficile* opportunistic infection, nausea, and diarrhea. Vancomycin is highly nephrotoxic to the kidneys, ototoxic, and renal function must be monitored while the person is taking the drug. Blood levels of Vancomycin also have to be monitored during its use. Vancomycin is also ototoxic, which means it damages hearing.

Ketolide Class (Telithromycin)

RANK 9: EXERCISE EXTREME CAUTION

Telithromycin is the only antibiotic that has been approved out of the ketolide antibiotic class and has been approved fairly recently. Telithromycin is a semi-synthetic derivative of erythromycin. There were safety concerns and even accusations of fraud with the producer of the antibiotic, Ketek, by the FDA because of the increased frequency of side effects that developed after clinical trials.

These proposed side effects include prolonged QT syndrome, liver failure, and hepatitis. In some people, this antibiotic has additional side effects, including gastrointestinal upset, systemic allergic reactions, and headaches. It has also been known to cause blurred vision and rashes. Avoid if all possible.

Lincosamide Class (Clindamycin)

RANK 5: POSSIBLY SAFE

Clindamycin is an antibiotic that has been around for a long time. The safety rank of clindamycin would be lower, but it has been recently linked to an increase of *C. difficile* opportunistic infection, more than the other antibiotics. Severe heartburn may occur in people taking clindamycin and people should sit up for at least thirty minutes after taking it.

Clindamycin has side effects similar to other antibiotics like hypersensitivity reactions, nausea, and diarrhea. Clindamycin does have an increased risk of causing a *C. difficile* infection.

Lipopeptide Class (Daptomycin)

RANK 9: EXERCISE EXTREME CAUTION

Daptomycin is mainly used in the U.S. to treat MRSA infections. Daptomycin has strong multiple side effect profiles that affect all organ systems (including possible heart, lungs, kidneys, endocrine, liver, and intestinal) in the body. If you are on a statin, make sure you discontinue it while using this antibiotic because both have been possibly implicating in causing myopathy and rhabdomyolysis if they are taken together. In 2010, the FDA issued a warning that daptomycin has been implicated in causing multiple cases of eosinophilic pneumonia.

Macrolide Class (Azithromycin, Clarithromycin)

RANK 6: INCREASED CAUTION

The macrolide class of antibiotics contains azithromycin, one of the best-selling and most widely used antibiotics. Azithromycin used to be considered relatively safe, until recently, where it has been implicated in causing permanent heart arrhythmia issues.

Azithromycin has an average rate of antibiotic adverse reactions, including hypersensitivity reactions, nausea, and diarrhea. It has also been shown to cause hepatitis and delirium in rare cases.

Monobactam Class

RANK 5: POSSIBLY SAFE

The monobactam class of antibiotics has an average rate of adverse reactions hypersensitivity allergic reactions, *C. difficile* opportunistic infection, and diarrhea. Monobactams have also been linked to increasing TEN (Toxic Epidermal Necrolysis) complications and liver damage in rare cases.

Nitrofuran Class (Macrobid)

Rank 8: INCREASED CAUTION

Macrobid is mainly used to treat UTI infections. The most common side effects associated with Macrobid use are nausea, vomiting, diarrhea, and rarely systemic allergic reactions. Its use may turn your urine brown, but it is harmless.

Macrobid has been linked to pulmonary fibrosis, drug-induced autoimmune hepatitis, and tingling and numbness have been reported after a few days use that rarely is irreversible.

Nitroimidazole Class (Flagyl)

RANK: 9: EXERCISE EXTREME CAUTION

Flagyl is an antibiotic that is mostly used in the treatment of opportunistic *C. difficile* infection. It is also used to eliminate other bacterial infections like *H. pylori* infection and anaerobic bacteria infections. It can also be used to eliminate protozoan.

Flagyl has an average rate of adverse effects like systemic allergic reactions, diarrhea, and nausea. High doses and prolonged use have been linked to the development of leukopenia, neutropenia, and CNS toxicity. Flagyl has also been listed as a possible carcinogen. Steven-Johnson syndrome and serotonin syndrome have been linked to Flagyl, as well.

Flagyl is a recognized human carcinogen. Flagyl does, however, have its uses as medication, but its side effects should be more widely known. One of the lesser known side effects of the antibiotic is its possible aldehyde breakdown enzyme down-regulation which increases mold sensitivity.

What Are Aldehyde Breakdown Enzymes and Why Do They Matter?

The body to breakdown aldehydes produces aldehyde oxidase and aldehyde dehydrogenase. Aldehydes are many different compounds, including formaldehyde and acetaldehyde. We encounter many different aldehydes throughout our daily life and they differ in their toxicity.

Alcohol, for example, is a frequent human exposure to aldehydes that our body needs to process correctly. If we consume alcohol and the body is not able to detoxify it, consumption of alcohol becomes deadly.

Consumption of alcohol requires ample amounts of aldehyde oxidase and aldehyde dehydrogenase to convert acetaldehydes produced from ethanol detoxification by the liver into carboxylic acids that can be used by the body. Without theses enzymes, alcohol consumption becomes quite toxic. The medication disulfiram was developed to help treat alcoholism by depleting alcohol and aldehyde detoxification enzymes (mainly ALDH1A1 and ALDH2 somewhat). When a person consumes alcohol on the drug, they develop symptoms similar to mold sensitivity, including, headaches, brain fog, visual disturbances, elevated heart rate, face flushing, allergic reactions, digestive issues, and shortness of breath. If enough alcohol is consumed the symptoms intensify from a severe hangover to coma and eventually death from untreated aldehyde poisoning.

Some people have gene mutations sadly that cause the body to produce less of these enzymes or none at all. ALDH2 is one of these genes and is tested if you get a 23andMe test. Mold and yeast also produce many aldehydes that require these enzymes to help us detoxify them.

Does Flagyl Increase Mold Sensitivity?

Flagyl like the medication disulfiram may reduce the body's ability to produce aldehyde detoxification enzymes. The inhibition of these enzymes is the reason why alcohol is strongly discouraged in people who are taking Flagyl for infections. The same can be said for individuals who have mold sensitivity issues, yeast overgrowth, or live in moldy environments.

Flagyl supposedly inhibits the production of aldehyde detoxification enzymes within our cells and affects our mitochondria and liver function. It is possible that if you needed to take Flagyl and suffer from fungi issues, molybdenum might help increase enzyme production or at the bare minimum help you maintain proper levels of the mineral when you stop the medication so that proper enzyme levels can be up-regulated by the body. The body uses molybdenum to produce aldehyde detoxification enzymes.

There are however a few studies that do cast doubt in Flagyl causing a reduction of aldehyde detoxification enzymes in people who have proper enzyme levels or people that do not have genetic predispositions to lower enzyme potential. One study indicates that the side effects from Flagyl are not from inhibiting aldehyde detoxification enzymes but instead are from the medication producing serotonin syndrome in some people. Another study indicates that the side effects of Flagyl that mimic aldehyde detoxification issues may be from the microbiome shift caused by the antibiotic.

So it would be my recommendation as well that if the serotonin increasing mechanisms of Flagyl are correct that people taking SSRI's, 5-HTP, or anything that increases serotonin to talk with their doctor and use caution when using Flagyl.

Oxazolidinone Class (Linezolid)

SHORT-TERM (LESS THAN ONE MONTH) RANK 4: POSSIBLY SAFE / LONG-TERM RANK 9: EXERCISE EXTREME CAUTION

Linezolid is one of the newest antibiotics on the market and one of the most expensive averaging $100 a pill. This antibiotic can be safely used short-term (less than a month). Side effects include gastrointestinal upset, headache, and systemic allergic reactions.

If linezolid is taken longer than a month, severe side effects may occur. Long-term use causes mitochondrial toxicity, peripheral neuropathy, and optic neuropathy. It can also cause bone marrow suppression, which is a serious side effect. It has also been linked to kidney damage with long-term use. If linezolid is used long-term, it should be closely monitored.

Penicillin Class

RANK: 7 – INCREASED CAUTION FOR FIRST TIME USE ALLERGIC REACTION / RANK: 3 SAFE IF USED BEFORE

The main problem with penicillin antibiotics is that out of all the antibiotics; penicillin is reported the most for causing systemic allergic reactions, including rashes and hypersensitivity reactions.

Penicillin, like all other antibiotics, has side effects like diarrhea, nausea, and possible *C. difficile* opportunistic infection. Penicillin antibiotics have been around the longest and for most people are well tolerated if used before.

Quinolone Class (Ciprofloxacin, Moxifloxacin)

RANK 9: EXERCISE EXTREME CAUTION

Quinolone antibiotics have been used for a long time, but recently more side effects have been reported. Most quinolones are well tolerated, and the average side effects include systemic allergic reactions, diarrhea, and nausea.

If you have to take a quinolone antibiotic, please upregulate your mitochondrial function by asking your doctor if you can take magnesium and ubiquinol with PQQ to see if it can help mitigate the side effects.

The main problem with the use of quinolone antibiotics is that there are more side effects that have been discovered in recent years. CNS toxicity, tendon ruptures, psychosis, cardiac arrhythmias, convulsions, and low blood sugar are newer side effects that have been reported during its clinical use. Moxifloxacin carries a higher chance of long QT syndrome, and gatifloxacin is linked to severely disturbed blood sugar levels. Like some other antibiotics, if *C. difficile* is caused by a quinolone antibiotic it may be harder to treat.

Rifamycin Class (Rifampicin, Rifaximin)

RANK 7: INCREASED CAUTION / RIFAXIMIN RANK 2: SAFE / RIFABUTIN RANK 4: POSSIBLY SAFE

The rifamycin class of antibiotics was discovered in the 1960s and is used in the treatment of *MAP* and MRSA. This drug has an average side effect profile like most other antibiotics, but it also has been associated with hepatotoxicity. This is why the antibiotics rank is not lower on the list. Even though the liver can regenerate itself, it should be used with caution. If you use liver protective agents such as milk thistle and R-lipoic acid while prescribed this antibiotic, it will reduce the risk.

Rifaximin, on the other hand, is poorly absorbed by the gastrointestinal tract and very little, if any, makes it to the liver or systemic circulation. This makes rifaximin a great antibiotic for treating gut disturbances caused by opportunistic bacteria. Its side effects are on par with your average antibiotic profile, including systemic allergic reactions, nausea, and diarrhea.

Rifabutin was discovered by the Italian drug company Achifar in 1975 and received FDA approval in the early 1990s. Rifabutin is used in the U.S. to treat tuberculosis infections. Rifabutin mechanism of action is that it inhibits bacterial DNA-dependent RNA synthesis, which causes bacteria to fail to replicate. Finally, *Mycobacteria* appear to be very sensitive to rifabutin's mechanism of action more than any other antibiotic.

Rifabutin has been found in a few studies including one phase three study, significantly to relieve Crohn's disease symptoms, and complications even in people were an *MAP* infection was unknown.

Rifabutin also seems to lack rifampicin's hepatotoxicity and its major side effects, which mean that it "might" be a safer antibiotic. Rifabutin has similar side effects to other antibiotics like gastrointestinal upset and systemic allergic reactions.

Sulfonamide Class (Sulfamethoxazole)

RANK 7: INCREASED CAUTION FOR FIRST-TIME ALLERGIC REACTION / RANK 5: POSSIBLY SAFE IF USED BEFORE

Sulfonamide drugs were the first antimicrobials and paved the way for the future medical science known as antibiotics. The problem with most sulfonamide drugs is the common systemic allergic reactions that they cause for some people.

Sulfonamide drugs cause gastrointestinal upset in most people and may cause abdominal pain, nausea, heartburn, and diarrhea. Sulfa antibiotics have also been linked to migraines. Sulfur antibiotics have been linked to the increased risk of Stevens – Johnson Syndrome and TEN. Finally, megaloblastic anemia has been linked to sulfa antibiotics because it interferes with B12 and folate metabolism.

Tetracycline Class

RANK 6: POSSIBLY SAFE

Tetracycline antibiotics have been used for a long time, but there are some safety concerns with taking antibiotics from this class. Tetracycline can cause systemic allergic reactions, diarrhea, and nausea.

Tetracycline antibiotics have been shown to stain teeth, cause skin photosensitivity, cause hepatitis and drug-induced lupus, can cause tinnitus, and rarely causes Stevens - Johnson syndrome and TEN. Tetracycline becomes a toxic compound after its expiration date, so toss it in the garbage after it expires.

Chapter 20

Medicine Prescribed for Digestive Ailments

This part of the book is just a reference guide for the drugs that are prescribed for people who have digestive issues. I will rank how safe I feel these medicines are, and general information and side effects of the medicines. All medicines and supplements may have side effects, so it depends on the risk versus benefit analysis in all people receiving medical care. Always talk to your doctor about choosing the safest medication for you to use to treat your condition.

Antacids

Used mainly in people with: GERD, heartburn

SHORT TERM RANK: 1 SAFE / LONG TERM RANK: 7 INCREASED CAUTION / LONG TERM RANK CALCIUM CARBONATE: 9 EXTREME CAUTION

Antacids are drugs that neutralize stomach acid or raise pH levels in the stomach. Antacids are usually free of side effects for most people if they are taken short term. Magnesium is one of the safest antacids most people can use unless you have kidney problems, and then it should only be used in low doses. Sodium bicarbonate is the next safest antacid, but it should be avoided in people with kidney problems and people with extremely high blood pressure. Sodium bicarbonate can cause stomach distension and gas.

Calcium carbonate is not as safe as the other two antacids mentioned prior. Calcium carbonate causes excess calcium to build up in the arteries and causes alkalosis with long-term use, which is a serious medical condition. Aluminum is the worst antacid anyone can take since aluminum is neurotoxic and can cause constipation. People with limited kidney function should limit the use of all antacids.

Azathioprine

Used mainly in people with: ulcerative colitis, Crohn's disease

RANK: 8 INCREASED CAUTION

Azathioprine is an immunosuppressive drug that inhibits the enzyme that is required for the synthesis of DNA. Azathioprine strongly affects proliferating immune cells including T cells and B cells. Azathioprine is used in IBD to stop the autoimmune symptoms in the intestines and to lower inflammation. The most common side effects are nausea and vomiting. Rare side effects include systemic allergic reactions, dizziness, diarrhea, fatigue, rash, suppression of bone marrow, anemia, pancreatitis, and infection. Azathioprine is also listed as a carcinogen and has been linked to increased risk of cancer in people who are taking the drug.

5-ASA

Used mainly in people with: ulcerative colitis, Crohn's disease

RANK: 4 POSSIBLY SAFE

5-ASA is an anti-inflammatory drug that is used to treat inflammation in inflammatory bowel diseases. 5-ASA is a derivative of salicylic acid (aspirin) that acts locally in the gut causing fewer systemic side effects. The most common side effects are diarrhea, headache, cramping, nausea, and flatulence. Rarer side effects include worsening colitis, systemic allergic reactions, hair loss, pancreatitis, hepatitis, fever, and kidney problems.

Biological agents (Infliximab, Adalimumab)

Used mainly in people with: ulcerative colitis, Crohn's disease

RANK: 9 EXTREME CAUTION

Most biological agents are monoclonal antibodies used against tumor necrosis factor alpha, which is a chemical messenger (cytokine), proposed as a factor in causing autoimmune reactions. TNFa has also been implicated as the cytokine that causes systemic inflammation in the body. These biological agents are artificial antibodies, made from mouse antibodies. They attach to the agent TNFa and inactivate it. This drug is usually administered by IV at a clinic or hospital, typically in six to eight week intervals.

The side effects, and risks for biological agents are severe, and they include serious blood disorders, serious infections, lymphoma, severe liver injury, reactivation of hepatitis B and tuberculosis, drug-induced lupus, demyelinating CNS disorders, psoriasis, and even vitiligo.

Bismuth Subsalicylate

Used mainly in people with: *H. pylori* infection, ulcers, heartburn, gastritis

SHORT TERM RANK: 3 SAFE, LONG TERM RANK (GREATER THAN 6 WEEKS): 8 INCREASED CAUTION

Most bismuth medication that you purchase is bismuth subsalicylate. Bismuth subsalicylate is the colloidal compound of the element bismuth and salicylic acid (a known anti-inflammatory agent). Bismuth compounds are used in people who have ulcers, heartburn, gastritis, and diarrhea. It helps coat and protect the esophagus and stomach.

It is also a weak antacid, and the subsalicylate part of the compound has been shown to reduce inflammation in the gastrointestinal tract. It also has been shown to have antibacterial properties. The antibacterial properties might be why bismuth subsalicylate accelerates ulcer healing in people by limiting *H. pylori* overgrowth. Bismuth possibly reduces *H. pylori's* iron uptake (there is one study that casts doubt on its iron deprivation ability, but the study mentions it still hinders *H. pylori*), reducing its ability for biofilm formation and cellular metabolism.

Bismuth also has been found to bind with the endotoxins and enterotoxins that bacteria produce to help eliminate them from the body. Bismuth reduces *E. coli* overgrowth and endotoxin production in the intestines. Bismuth limits symptoms in people who have ulcers, gastritis, infections, diarrhea, or GERD by these various mechanisms of action to help improve their digestive health.

Bismuth is also useful in helping individuals with the lesser-known third type of SIBO known as SIBO with hydrogen sulfide producing overgrowth. Bismuth bonds with hydrogen sulfide and sulfur within the digestive tract to form bismuth sulfide. This bonding reduces the amount that may leak out of the gut and cause fatigue and brain fog if it crosses the blood brain barrier. If your stools become a very dark color when you supplement with bismuth, you may be either suffering from hydrogen sulfide producing overgrowth or your diet is very high in sulfurous foods. It is better to use bismuth supplements or medications that do not contain subsalicylate to determine hydrogen sulfide overgrowth, which can cause bleeding in some people and melena (dark, tarry stools), which creates issues in determining the possible cause of the darkening of your stools.

Minor side effects that bismuth may cause is a darkening of the tongue and stools from sulfur or sulfide bonding. Again, this "side effect" may be a useful diagnostic tool for determining hydrogen sulfide overgrowth within the digestive tract. In addition, bismuth use may cause headaches and nausea.

Bismuth subsalicylate can cause some rare adverse reactions including bleeding and systemic allergic reactions. I would avoid the use of bismuth subsalicylate if you are allergic to salicylates or suffer from digestive disorders that may increase bleeding like severe ulcerations or IBD. Children should not take bismuth subsalicylate, because it increases their chances of developing Reye syndrome, a serious, life-threatening medical condition. Finally, if you take any anticoagulant medication, any medication that increases your chances of bleeding (NSAIDS for example), or anything with salicylic acid (aspirin, white willow bark), you may want to ask your doctor first before you use bismuth subsalicylate. If you cannot tolerate bismuth subsalicylate, I would try to find a supplemental form of bismuth instead.

I recommend that you do not take bismuth longer than six weeks if possible because of the risk of bismuth poisoning. Bismuth poisoning symptoms include neurological issues, anemia, ataxia, myoclonus, and speech issues.

To reduce bismuth concentrations, our body uses glutathione, so it may be a good idea during bismuth use or afterwards to take a glutathione supplement like Glutathione Force to help facilitate clearance of bismuth from the body.

Brands of Bismuth I recommend:

- **Bismuth subsalicylate** – Kaopectate Vanilla (No dyes, but contains some questionable additives including caramel, flavor, sucrose [possible GMO source,] and xanthan gum)
- **Bismuth subgallate** – Devrom (contains xylitol, talc, and starch[possible gmo source])

Calcium Channel Blocker

Used mainly in people with: LES increased pressure regulation problems

RANK: 7 INCREASED CAUTION

Calcium channel blockers are a class of medicine that is used to treat hypertension but have recently been used in achalasia to lower LES pressure. They disrupt the movement of calcium through calcium channels. This works in people with increased LES pressure by relaxing the smooth muscle and causing the pressure to be reduced.

Side effects of calcium channel blockers are numerous including peripheral edema, fatigue, dizziness, headache, dyspepsia, nausea, palpitations, impotence, depression, and insomnia. Edema is the most frequent side effect and occurs in one out of every ten users. Rarely CCB's have been implicated in causing Stevens-Johnson syndrome and systemic allergic reactions.

Cholestyramine

Used mainly in people with: IBS-D, Crohn's disease, *C. diff* infection

RANK: 3 SAFE

Cholestyramine is a bile acid sequestrant drug, which means it binds bile in the gastrointestinal tract preventing its absorption and eliminating it from the body. Cholestyramine also treats high cholesterol and itching due to increased bile from liver failure.

It is used in Crohn's disease, in people who have had their ileum removed. The ileum is where bile acids are reabsorbed back into the body. When the ileum is removed, bile acids are dumped into the large intestine which attracts water and causes diarrhea. It is also used in people infected with *C. diff* because it can help absorb the toxins created by the bacteria.

The most common side effect for cholestyramine is constipation. It causes tooth discoloration and tooth decay from prolonged oral ingestion of the drug. Long-term use of cholestyramine may hinder thyroid function by reducing hormone production. Finally, it increases the risk of gallstones and blood plasma triglycerides.

Cholestyramine prevents the absorption of several of medications and, therefore, caution should be used when taking this with other medicines. Always check drug interactions with this medicine with your doctor and pharmacist. Finally, it also may reduce thyroid function.

Colace

Used mainly in people with: IBS-C, IBS-A, constipation

SHORT TERM RANK: 4 POSSIBLY SAFE, LONG TERM RANK: 6 POSSIBLY SAFE

Colace is a drug that is known as a surfactant. Colace makes stools softer and easier to pass and is used in the treatment of people that have chronic constipation. Most side effects of Colace include stomach pain, diarrhea, cramping, and in rare cases, systemic allergic reactions and rectal bleeding.

Colace should never be used in combination with mineral oil in relieving constipation. This combination can make foreign body granulomas that block intestinal evacuation. If Colace causes an intestinal blockage, it is considered a medical emergency.

Corticosteroids

Used mainly in people with: ulcerative colitis, Crohn's disease

SHORT TERM RANK: 3 SAFE, LONG TERM RANK: 7 INCREASED CAUTION

Corticosteroids are a class of chemicals that include steroid hormones that are produced by the body. These hormones have anti-inflammatory effects and suppress the immune system.

The side effects of short-term steroid use are usually low and include nausea and systemic allergic reactions. The side effects of long-term steroid use are numerous, including, immunodeficiency, hyperglycemia, bruising, hypocalcemia, osteoporosis, weight gain, adrenal insufficiency (if suddenly stopped), muscle breakdown, glaucoma, and cataracts.

Dicycloverine (Bentyl)

Used mainly in people with: IBS

LOW DOSE RANK: 5 POSSIBLY SAFE, LARGE DOSE RANK: 7 INCREASED CAUTION

Dicycloverine is an anticholinergic drug that blocks muscarinic receptors. It relieves muscle spasms, cramps in the colon, and reduces intestinal hypermotility. Dicycloverine works by blocking the action of acetylcholine on cholinergic receptors on the surface of smooth muscle cells relaxing them in the process.

Side effects include dry mouth, tiredness, and nausea. At high doses, dicycloverine can cause delirium in some people. Sometimes, dicycloverine causes systemic allergic reactions.

H2 Antagonist

Used mainly in people with: heartburn, GERD, LERD

SHORT TERM RANK: 3 SAFE, LONG TERM RANK: 6 POSSIBLY SAFE / TAGAMET RANK: 8 INCREASED CAUTION

H2 antagonists are drugs that are clinically used to block histamine reactions on parietal cells in the stomach. This leads to decreased production of acid by the parietal cells. H2 antagonists have a shorter half-life than PPI's, so they should be taken thirty minutes to an hour before each meal. Tagamet has been linked to increased side effects and should be avoided. Pepcid is probably the safest H2 antagonist with the least amount of side effects.

Common side effects of H2 antagonists include a headache, nausea, dizziness, and diarrhea. Long-term H2 antagonist supplementation can cause problems with B12 absorption, magnesium absorption, and lead to the development of SIBO and food allergies.

Laxatives

Used mainly in people with: IBS-A, IBS-C, constipation

SHORT TERM RANK: 3 SAFE, LONG TERM RANK: 7 INCREASED CAUTION

Laxatives are drugs that are used to loosen stools so that the stool can easily pass through the colon and be eliminated from the body. Laxatives are either taken in oral form or taken by a person as a suppository. Laxatives are usually safe for a person if they are used for a short period. If laxatives are used for a longer period of time, more side effects occur, and this can lead to intestinal paralysis, IBS, pancreatitis, or renal failure that can be reversed if caught early. If laxatives are continued to be abused, the gut can be permanently damaged. If you ever become this ill, you might have to have your intestines removed at this point.

Classes of Laxatives

Bulk-producing agents (fiber, Metamucil, Uni-fiber, Citrucel)

Site of action: small and large intestines

Onset: 12-72 hours

Bulk-producing agents are substances that add bulk and water to stools so that they can pass through the intestines and prevent constipation. The fiber in food and supplements is the most commonly known bulk-producing agent. Bulk- producing agents are the safest stool softener/laxative that anyone can take.

Lubricant laxatives (castor oil)

Site of action: colon

Onset: 6-8 hours

The most common lubricant laxative that anyone can take is mineral oil. Mineral oil is a product of petroleum distillation that is safe short-term to use on the skin, but internally should be used with some caution. It makes the feces slippery, and it also retards the colon's ability to absorb water. This makes the stool easier to pass. The main problem with using mineral oil is that it blocks the absorption of fat-soluble vitamins (A, D, E, K) in the colon and leads to malnutrition.

Hyperosmotic laxatives (glycerin, sorbitol, lactulose, PEG)

Site of action: colon

Onset: 0.5-3 hours

Hyperosmotic laxatives work by retaining water in the colon, and they can increase colonic peristalsis. They sometimes cause electrolyte imbalances (glycerin suppositories are usually the cause). Most hyperosmotic laxatives are safe to use long term and have minimal side effects.

Sorbitol, a sugar alcohol, is safe to use. It causes people with IBS and SIBO to have severe abdominal cramps, so caution should be used in people with these conditions. Sorbitol is considered a prebiotic and can cause excess gas in people with SIBO.

Lactulose, a synthetic non-digestible sugar, is the safest to use long term if you choose a hyperosmotic laxative (unless the person has galactosemia, then it should be avoided). Lactulose is also prebiotic, but it has been shown to reduce opportunistic bacteria and increase probiotics in the colon, which most prebiotics (including sorbitol) fail to do. Lactulose causes excessive gas in people with SIBO, and therefore, should be avoided.

PEG, the active ingredient in Miralax, is a synthetic chemical (polyethylene glycol) that is believed to have low toxicity in humans. PEG is generally recognized as safe by the medical community, although it is known to cause bloating, nausea, gas, and diarrhea. PEG seems like a safe chemical, maybe even perfect for long-term laxative use if needed, right? Unfortunately, PEG medications have serious complications linked to their use including:

- Nephrotoxicity
- Neuropsychiatric events
- Urticaria (allergic hives)
- Mallory-Weiss tears
- Fecal incontinence

PEG was originally approved to be used for seven days at most, but it is now used daily for many people (even in children). In 2009, an FDA drug safety board raised more concerns about its long-term use because PEG has not been studied in long-term treatment, or in large doses. I do not believe PEG should be used as often in people because there are better laxatives like lactulose, bulk producing agents, and magnesium. These are much safer for long-term use.

Saline laxatives (sodium phosphate, magnesium)

Site of action: small and large intestines

Onset: .5 - 6 hours

Saline laxatives attract and retain water in the intestines and increase the intestinal intraluminal pressure that softens the stool and produces peristaltic activity. Saline laxatives also increase the release of CCK, which stimulates the digestion of fat and protein in the small intestine. Sodium Phosphates use has been linked to an increased risk of the alteration of fluid and electrolyte balance in people, and should only be used when it is specifically needed. Electrolyte imbalances are why phosphate solutions now require a prescription. Magnesium for the use of colon cleansing is safer and should only be contraindicated in people with poor kidney function. Magnesium supplementation is safe for most people, but if used in high doses, electrolyte replacement should be given. It is very safe to use lower dosages of magnesium (600 mg) daily for the stool softening effects in most people.

Stimulating laxatives

Site of action: small and large intestines

Onset: 2-12 hours

Stimulant Laxatives are one of the most powerful laxatives that one can take, and should be used with caution. They irritate the lining of the large intestine, cause it to spasm, and eliminate feces. They also raise blood pressure and heart rate in some people and should be avoided in these people. Brand names of stimulant laxatives are Ex-lax, Dulcolax, and Senokot. The herbs that have stimulant laxative effects are senna, cascara, castor oil, and aloe vera. Aloe vera is probably the safest stimulant laxative. Aloe will have less of the blood pressure and heart rate stimulant effects that are associated with cascara and senna use.

Linaclotide

Used mainly in people with: IBS-C, IBD

RANK: 5 POSSIBLY SAFE

Linaclotide is a guanylate cyclase 2C agonist that treats constipation. The medication binds to the GC-C receptors in the gut and helps to draw water into the bowel as an osmotive laxative. Bacterial enterotoxins that cause diarrhea during food poisoning also activate the GC-C receptors in the gut to cause a similar effect to Linaclotide. Linaclotide has also shown to promote mucosal hemostasis in the gut and has both local and low bioavailability in the gut.

Side effects of the medication include diarrhea, abdominal pain, flatulence, GERD, headache, fatigue, dizziness, sinus issues, and vomiting. Most of the side effects are low and are self-limiting. Linaclotide should also not be used in children or if you have an intestinal blockage. Linaclotide is a very new medication, and that is why its rank is not lower, more studies need to be done with this medication before I can further recommend it.

Loperamide

Used mainly in people with: IBS-D, gastroenteritis, IBD

RANK: 5 POSSIBLY SAFE / UNDER THE AGE OF 2: 9 EXTREME CAUTION

Loperamide is a piperidine derivative and opioid that protects against diarrhea. Most opioids like codeine and morphine are known to cause constipation in people, and this is the why loperamide was originally proposed to treat people with diarrhea.

Loperamide, unlike other opioids, is blocked by the blood-brain barrier by the P-glycoprotein. The blockage of the drug by the blood-brain barrier causes no pain relieving benefits or any of the neurological side effects of standard opioids; so that it can be used long term without these drawbacks. Some drugs and spices cause the P-glycoprotein to lose its effectiveness like quinine, PPI's, and piperine. Large dosages of the drug can deplete P-glycoprotein production in the brain and are known to cause standard opioid effects. Even with the P-glycoprotein protection in the brain, mild opiate withdrawal has been observed with long-term use of loperamide.

Loperamide works by decreasing the peristaltic activity of the myenteric plexus muscle of the large intestine and decreases muscle tone in the intestinal wall. This increases the amount of time that feces stay in the intestines allowing greater hydration, which bulks up the fecal matter.

Loperamide should not be used in children under two because of the increased risk of a fatal condition paralytic ileus syndrome. It also has a chance to increase the risk of toxic megacolon and in which is why it is not used for treating *C. diff*, *E. coli*, *Shigella*, or *Campylobacter* infection. Loperamide is also not recommended for pregnant or nursing women or people with liver impairment.

Side effects common with Loperamide treatment are abdominal pain and bloating, nausea, vomiting, and constipation. It has rarely been implicated in causing paralytic ileus, dizziness, rashes, and systemic allergic reactions.

Lubiprostone

Used mainly in people with: IBS-C, chronic constipation

RANK: 5 POSSIBLY SAFE

Lubiprostone is a bicyclic fatty acid derived from prostaglandin E1 that acts by specifically activating CIC-2 chloride channels on the gastrointestinal epithelial cells. The activation produces a chloride-rich fluid secretion that softens the stool and increases motility of the feces.

Lubiprostone, unlike other laxatives, shows no signs of tolerance, dependence, and does not alter electrolyte concentration in the body. There also appears to be no rebound constipation if treatment with the medicine is stopped suddenly. Nausea is a side effect in about 31% of people who use lubiprostone. Other side effects include diarrhea, headache, abdominal distension and pain, flatulence, and rarely systemic allergic reactions.

Since the drug has only been on the market since 2008, I have given it a rating of five because it has not been studied for very long. It also has not been studied in people that have liver dysfunction, kidney problems, or pregnant women.

Mebeverine

Used mainly in people with: IBS

RANK: 4 POSSIBLY SAFE

Mebeverine is a drug that has been used since 1965 to treat abdominal cramping and spasms of the colon. An antispasmodic drug does not have anticholinergic side effects. It works by directly relaxing the gut muscles on a cellular level without affecting the motility of feces. People with IBS suffer intestinal spasms that cause pain and occasionally diarrhea.

Side effects, though rare, include heartburn, constipation, dizziness, insomnia, loss of appetite, headache, and slow heartbeat. Systemic allergic reactions and urticaria systemic rash may also occur, but it is unlikely.

Methotrexate

Used mainly in people with: IBD

SHORT TERM ORAL RANK (1-2 TOTAL DOSES): 4 POSSIBLY SAFE, SHORT TERM ORAL RANK (ONCE A WEEK): 7 INCREASED CAUTION, SHORT TERM ORAL RANK (MORE THAN ONCE A WEEK): 9 EXTREME CAUTION, LONG TERM ORAL RANK (ONCE A WEEK): 8 INCREASED CAUTION / IV RANK: 8 INCREASED CAUTION

Methotrexate is a drug that inhibits the metabolism of folate in the human body. It is theorized that methotrexate interferes with interleukin-1, which is used in the body to increase inflammation responses. It also stimulates adenosine release, which is anti-inflammatory.

When folate is reduced by methotrexate, it impairs the immune system, affects the skin, and nerve cells. Side effects include ulcerative stomatitis, CNS toxicity, low white blood cell count, infection, and rare systemic allergic reactions. Methotrexate is an extremely teratogenic drug and should be avoided be used in women who are pregnant and can become pregnant, as well. Creatinine levels should be monitored every two months to make sure kidney function is optimal.

Penicillin and probenecid increase methotrexate concentration in the body and should not be used in people taking the drug. The antiepileptic drugs phenobarbital and carbamazepine have been shown to cause seizures in people taking the drug, as well. Folinic acid is the antidote to methotrexate overdose.

Metoclopramide (Reglan) / Domperidone (Motilium)

Used mainly in people with: GERD, LERD, LES problems, nausea, and vomiting

METOCLOPRAMIDE RANK: 10 DRUG OF LAST RESORT / DOMPERIDONE ORAL RANK: 5 POSSIBLY SAFE / DOMPERIDONE IV RANK: 8 INCREASED CAUTION

Metoclopramide is a drug that is an antiemetic, a gastroprokinetic agent, and it has been shown to increase LES tone. The antiemetic mechanism of action by the drug is a dopamine D2 receptor antagonist in the CNS. D2 receptors are in the area postrema (the part of the brain that controls vomiting) which communicate with the stomach to make it relax the LES, and contract the stomach to make the person vomit. The gastroprokinetic properties of the drug are caused by the 5-HT4 receptor agonist activity of the drug that causes the stomach muscles to contract and propel food through the sphincter into the duodenum.

Common side effects of metoclopramide are restlessness, drowsiness, fatigue and focal dystonia. Rarer side effects include blood pressure regulation issues, tardive dyskinesia, akathisia, neuroleptic malignant syndrome, and systemic allergic reactions. Metoclopramide can cross the blood-brain barrier resulting in CNS side effects. Dystonic reactions can be treated with diphenhydramine in people if needed.

Tardive dyskinesia is one of the most worrying side effects with metoclopramide use and has increased chances of occurring in people under twenty. The more medicine the person takes and they longer they continue to take it add to the risk and severity of the disease. Tardive dyskinesia is a disease in which the body has permanent, involuntary, and repetitive body movements. The FDA issued a black box warning on metoclopramide stating that it can cause tardive dyskinesia in people. Since metoclopramide is known to cause all of these side effects, I believe it should be withdrawn from the U.S. market.

Domperidone has the same mechanism of action that metoclopramide does, blocking the 5-HT4 receptors, but unlike metoclopramide, it does not cross the blood-brain barrier. All of the CNS side effects are absent with domperidone making the drug much safer. Domperidone has not been approved to be used in the U.S. The IV form of domperidone has been linked to increased QT intervals and should rarely be used.

Misoprostol

Used mainly in people with: NSAID gastric ulcers

RANK: 5 POSSIBLY SAFE / PREGNANCY RANK: 10 DRUG OF LAST RESORT

Misoprostol is a synthetic prostaglandin E1. Its mechanism of action is the inhibition of gastric acid production by decreasing proton pumps. It has also been shown to lower cyclic AMP levels. It stimulates the production of the mucus layer of the stomach, protecting against ulcers. PPI's are superior to misoprostol because of the possible risk of diarrhea, and the multiple daily doses required of the medication (typically four).

Diarrhea caused by misoprostol is usually self-limiting and resolves within a week for most people. Other side effects include abdominal pain, nausea, flatulence, and headaches. Fever may occur if multiple doses are given after every four hours. Pregnant women should not be given misoprostol because it can cause miscarriage.

Nystatin

Used mainly in people with: yeast overgrowth

RANK: ORALLY : 3 SAFE, DERMALLY : 5 POSSIBLY SAFE

Nystatin is a very well tolerated anti-yeast medication. Nystatin binds to ergosterol, which is part of the yeast cell-membrane. The destruction of ergosterol leads to a lysis of the yeast cell wall, destroying the yeast.

Nystatin is not absorbed systemically when taken orally and in very low quantities dermally. IV nystatin is not recommended or used clinically because it can interfere with sterol formation and is nephrotoxic. Side effects of nystatin include diarrhea, abdominal pain, tachycardia, swelling, and muscle pain. Rarely, skin issues (rashes, burning, and itching), Stevens-Johnson Syndrome, and hypersensitive allergic reactions can occur. I believe most side effects occur from the body's response to the toxins yeast release when they lysis, not a reaction to the medication itself.

Proton Pump Inhibitors

Used mainly in people with: GERD, LERD, gastritis, *H. pylori* infection, ulcers, heartburn

SHORT TERM RANK: 4 POSSIBLY SAFE, LONG TERM RANK: 8 INCREASED CAUTION

PPIs are a group of drugs that are used to reduce stomach acid for long-term use. PPIs work by blocking the hydrogen/potassium adenosine triphosphate enzyme system of the gastric parietal cells. This enzyme system, or proton pump, is directly responsible for secreting hydrogen ions into the gastric lumen that produces stomach acid. The blocking of the hydrogen/potassium adenosine triphosphate enzyme system leads to a long-term (2-3 days) mechanism of action that is reversed when the drug is stopped, and the stomach produces new enzymes. PPIs work longer and are stronger acting compared to H2 antagonists.

Short-term (less than two weeks) use of PPIs are well tolerated and most side effects are short term. Common side effects include a headache, nausea, diarrhea, abdominal pain, fatigue, and dizziness.

Long-term use of PPIs, on the other hand, causes an increased risk of side effects, and they should only be used when all other options have been exhausted. After long term use, PPIs cause low magnesium, zinc deficiency, low B12 (from the lack of the stomach's intrinsic factor), SIBO, increased risk of *C. diff*, increased skin aging, bone fractures, increased risk of community-acquired pneumonia, development of food allergies, chronic interstitial nephritis (leads to kidney failure), and even heart arrhythmias.

The risk of SIBO is increased while taking PPIs because the opportunistic bacteria that would usually be destroyed by stomach acid when food is ingested survive and colonize the small intestine. The lack of stomach acid is also the reason for the increased risk of community-acquired pneumonia and increased risk of developing *C. diff* in people who have taken PPIs. The risk of bone fractures and osteoporosis are increased because of the interference of acid production on osteoclasts during the rebuilding of the bone. I theorize that the increase of heart palpitations is related to a decrease of magnesium caused in people who take PPIs for too long.

If I were going to take a PPI for the long-term, I would take a digestive enzyme with every meal. I would also take a good B12 supplement and take magnesium transdermally. I would also take the needed supplements to stave off osteoporosis including vitamin D, vitamin K, boron, and calcium citrate. Finally, I would take a low-dose probiotic supplement daily and follow my SIBO protocol (Ch. 9) every six months for protection.

If I were going to take a PPI, I would take some of the originally developed PPIs first including omeprazole, and lansoprazole. There is a theory that some of the newer PPIs that are "Active" forms of the originals (esomeprazole and dexlansoprazole) might have an increased side effect profile.

Ondansetron

Used mainly in people with: nausea, vomiting, IBS-D

SHORT TERM RANK: 3 SAFE, LONG TERM RANK: 7 INCREASED CAUTION, LARGE DOSE RANK (30+mg): 9 EXTREME CAUTION

Ondansetron is a serotonin 5-HT3 antagonist used in the prevention of nausea and vomiting. It works by reducing the activity of the vagus nerve, which deactivates the vomiting center in the medulla oblongata. Also, in people with IBS, it has been shown to reduce colonic contractions and motility.

Ondansetron is a well-tolerated drug with few systemic side effects. The most common side effects are constipation, dizziness, and headaches. Ondansetron has recently been discovered to cause long QT syndrome and heart arrhythmias in high doses.

Sucralfate

Used mainly in people with: ulcers

SHORT TERM RANK: 2 SAFE / LONG TERM RANK (GREATER THAN TWO WEEKS): 8 INCREASED CAUTION DUE TO ALUMINUM

Sucralfate is a cytoprotective agent and a sucrose sulfate-aluminum complex. Sucralfate binds to the stomach mucosa when ingested creating a physical barrier that protects the stomach lining from hydrochloric acid and pepsin. It stimulates bicarbonate production in the small intestine that buffers the small intestine from excess acid. It also binds with the hydrochloric acid in the stomach to form an acid buffer.

The most common side effects of sucralfate are constipation, flatulence, headache, hypophosphatemia, dry mouth, and bezoar formation. Rarely, systemic allergic reactions occur. It should not be used long-term, or kidney damage will occur due to the excess aluminum concentration in the body.

Chapter 21

Common Diagnostic Tests and Procedures for Gastrointestinal Problems

Anoscopy

An anoscopy is an examination using a rigid, tubular instrument inserted a few inches into the anus so that problems of the anal canal can be diagnosed. The width of the average bowel movement is the width of the anoscopy, so it is not too uncomfortable when it is placed inside the rectum. The doctor usually coats the anoscopy in lubricant and before insertion of the scope, you will be asked to bear down as if you had a bowel movement, and then you will be asked to relax. A doctor might shine a light into the tube so that they will have a clear view of the anus and lower rectum. Some pressure might be felt when you are receiving an anoscopy, but usually, no pain is felt.

Barium Swallow Test

Barium swallow tests are used to examine the esophagus to determine whether peristalsis and swallowing are functioning normally. Barium sulfate is usually mixed with a liquid, then a semi-solid, and then a solid food, and is individually swallowed by the person taking the test. While it is swallowed, X-rays are taken of the esophagus (two to three frames a second) so that typical swallowing technique is observed in the average person and aspiration into the lungs does not occur during swallowing. Complications of a barium swallow test are the aspiration of barium sulfate, which is an irritant outside the gastrointestinal tract, and low amounts of radiation absorbed by the body during the test.

Blood Tests

A blood test occurs when blood is extracted from a vein in the arm using a hypodermic needle, or when blood is extracted from a finger prick. Vein puncture and fingers ticking is relatively safe, and few side effects are observed like bruising and extremely rare nerve damage.

Many blood tests are given to diagnose gastrointestinal problems including:

- Antibody Tests (IGA, IGG)
- Bacterial Tests (*H. pylori*)
- Blood Glucose Tests
- Metabolic Panels
- Parasitical Tests
- RBC Tests

Colonoscopy

A colonoscopy is an endoscopic examination of the entire intestinal system using a fiber optic camera attached to a flexible tube passed through the anus. During a colonoscopy, a recording is made of the colon and polyps can be removed. Colonoscopies are used in the diagnosis of gastrointestinal hemorrhage, colon cancer, IBD, and diverticulosis. If you are over fifty, colonoscopies should be performed every ten years, as well.

To prepare for a colonoscopy the person is usually put on a low-fiber diet for one to three days before, or given at the very least area clear liquid diet. You might be given a laxative the day before the procedure to clean out the colon. Finally, you might be asked to skip NSAIDs for ten days before the procedure to reduce the risk of bleeding.

During a colonoscopy, you will be placed on a bed or operating table and will be told to lie on your side. You are then given an IV sedative. During the procedure, the doctor passes an endoscope through the intestines and looks at a monitor during the procedure to observe and to guide the scope. Air might be sent through the scope to enlarge the area and increase visibility. Lesions and polyps found in the colon can be cauterized, and biopsies can be made if needed. In most cases, a complete colonoscopy can be performed in less than fifteen minutes.

After the procedure, you will recover in a hospital bed for about an hour. You will not be able to drive home, so you will need an available ride afterward. The common side effects of a colonoscopy include post-procedural pain that is usually treated with painkillers and bleeding. Rare, but serious side effects include bowel perforation and infection.

CT Scan

CT scans were introduced to the medical diagnostic world in the 1970s. Since then, they have become one of the most common scanning procedures done today. CT scans should only be used when needed and when an MRI, x-ray, or ultrasound cannot be used for diagnosis. This precaution should be noted because of the increased ionizing radiation, which occurs during the CT scan.

During a CT scan, you will be placed on a mobile platform that goes into a rotating machine and uses ionizing radiation and cameras to take pictures of your body during the scan. As far as its diagnostic potential, CT Scans produce a 3D x-ray picture and produce better quality pictures of your organs than all other scans.

The problems with using a CT scan for diagnostics are the excess ionizing radiation and contrast dye. The excess ionizing radiation, depending on the exposed area, magnifies the amount absorbed by the body. For example, the average amount of background radiation your average person absorbs is 2.4 mSv a year. When you receive an abdomen CT, you get at least four years of background radiation at one time concentrated on a specific location on the body. This increases your risk of cancer by about a percent each time it is performed. It does not seem like a lot, but some people have multiple CT Scans over a period of time. The radiation exposure from a CT scan and contrast dyes are cumulative.

The contrast dye used for CT scans is known to cause allergic reactions in some people (radioactive iodine more than barium). Radioactive iodine should only be used in people with properly functioning kidneys. Barium use is ok for most people, but it should be used cautiously in if you have elevated blood pressure.

Endoscopy

An endoscopy is a procedure in which a flexible tube is inserted into the esophagus and stomach to evaluate its function. The tube has a light and a camera on the end of it that shows video and can take pictures during the procedure. The doctor views the video on a monitor to help guide the tube and to make observations. Biopsies could be performed during this procedure if needed.

You will be restricted from eating anything for eight hours before the procedure, and no liquids for four hours prior. You will also be sedated during the procedure. The common complications of the procedure are bleeding, aspiration, esophageal scarring, and sometimes esophageal rupture. Endoscopies are important in determining the condition of the esophagus (evaluating damage from GERD, diagnosing cancer), functionality of the LES, and conditions of the stomach (ulcers, perforations, cancer).

Endoscopic Retrograde Cholangiopancreatography

Endoscopic retrograde cholangiopancreatography is a complex diagnostic procedure that combines the use of endoscopy and fluoroscopy to diagnose and even treat gallbladder and pancreatic duct issues.

ERC can be helpful in the diagnosis of bile duct issues, tumors, pancreatic dysfunction, and pancreatitis. ERC is a very invasive procedure and has major risks including pancreatitis (occurs in up to 5% of procedures), injury to the bile ducts, gut perforation, infection, and issues that arise from surgical sedation.

Magnetic resource cholangiopancreatography has replaced ERC as the diagnostic gold standard of bile duct health. ERC can still be used to remove stones blocking the bile duct as needed and might be safer than other methods and surgeries to remove them.

Esophageal pH Monitoring Test

During an esophageal pH-monitoring test, a flexible catheter is inserted into the nose and is placed 5 cm above the upper border of the LES. A bravo pH capsule is placed on the catheter and monitors the pH of the esophagus. The catheter will be kept in place inside you for twenty-four hours. You may return to your normal activities (except for a few things like exercise, or anything heavily physical) during the test. You should only feel mild discomfort as a side effect during the test. After a twenty-four hour period, the catheter is removed, and the results are recorded. This is one of the best diagnostic tests for GERD.

Esophagogastroduodenoscopy

An esophagogastroduodenoscopy is a diagnostic, endoscopic procedure of the upper gastrointestinal tract. It is slightly more invasive than an endoscopy, which stops at the stomach. This procedure continues past the stomach and into the duodenum. It is useful in diagnosing the function of the pylorus of the stomach and the condition of the duodenum.

You will be restricted from eating anything for eight hours before the procedure, and no liquids for four hours before the procedure. You will also be sedated during the procedure. The common complications of the procedure include bleeding, esophageal scarring, aspiration, and rarely esophageal rupture, stomach perforation, and duodenal rupture.

Gastric Emptying Test (Barium Meal)

A gastric emptying test is a procedure in which radiographs of the esophagus, stomach, and duodenum are taken after barium sulfate is ingested. The radiographs taken of the gastrointestinal tract show the condition of the esophagus, LES, and stomach emptying into the duodenum. Liquid suspensions of barium sulfate are relatively non-toxic, but sometimes it can cause systemic allergic reactions and increased blood pressure. You might have to ingest gas pellets, or citric acid to help expand the stomach during the procedure.

HIDA Scan

HIDA scan is a diagnostic scan used to determine the total functionality of your gallbladder. During the exam, a radioactive tracer is injected into your body. Your body handles the tracer like bile and sends the tracer through your biliary cycle. A gamma camera takes pictures and tracks the flow of the tracer throughout your digestive system. A HIDA scan can be useful in estimating gallbladder and liver health, bile duct health, and diagnosing bile duct obstructions, abnormalities, and leaks. The test takes about an hour to perform.

The rate at which bile is released from your gallbladder is your gallbladder ejection fraction. Normal gallbladder ejection fraction ranges from 35 – 75% and may fluctuate depending on when the test was performed. Your ejection fraction score should not be the only diagnostic method used for the final decision of gallbladder removal. If you have gallstones, and they are removed, your gallbladder ejection fraction percentage and health might improve if they were causing issues. Treating gallbladder or bile duct infections can also improve your score. Finally, improving liver and pancreatic function if you are having issues with those organs might improve a low score as well.

Risks associated with a HIDA scan are low but include allergic reactions to the tracer element, bruising at the injection site, anxiety from the injected CCK, and rash development. A small amount of radiation is dosed to you through the radioactive tracer, but it should be low enough not to warrant much concern. The gamma camera gives off no radiation during the study.

Lower Gastrointestinal Series (Barium Enema)

A lower intestinal series is a medical procedure used to diagnose problems with the colon. During this procedure, an enema of barium sulfate is injected into the rectum, and radiographs are taken. During the procedure, an enema tube is inserted into you while you are lying on your side in a hospital bed. The tube releases barium sulfate into the colon while an expanding balloon keeps the barium in place. Air may be released into the colon making it easier for the imaging. The health care provider monitors the flow of the barium sulfate on an x-ray fluoroscope screen.

If you have a suspected bowel perforation, a water-soluble contrast will be given, so the barium is not absorbed into the bloodstream. Before the procedure, the large intestine must be cleaned. Usually, magnesium citrate is used to evacuate the bowel, but a saline enema may be used instead to clean the bowel. You will be put on a clear liquid diet the day before, and you will not be allowed food or liquids six hours beforehand. Liquid suspensions of barium sulfate are fairly non-toxic, but systemic allergic reactions and increased blood pressure may occur. Perforations of the intestines rarely result from the insertion of the tube.

Manometry (Esophageal)

An esophageal manometry is a test performed to assess the function of the upper esophageal sphincter, esophagus, and the lower esophageal sphincter. During the manometry, a catheter is placed into the nose, and the technician guides it into the stomach. Once the catheter is put into place, it is slowly withdrawn recording direct pressure changes and function of the sphincters. You might be asked to swallow air or water to help record the pressure changes. There is some discomfort during the procedure and sometimes causes esophageal scarring and rupture. Overall, the procedure usually takes up to an hour.

MRI

MRI is an imaging technology this is used to visualize internal structures of the body in great detail. An MRI does not use ionizing radiation when imaging but instead uses magnetic fields. Even though MRI use has been associated with RF radiation exposure, I still believe that it is a safer alternative to CT scan ionizing radiation. During an MRI, a person lies on a moveable platform that moves the person into a tunnel. A powerful magnet and imaging equipment is housed within the chassis. Contrast dyes are occasionally given during the MRI to improve imaging quality (some are radioactive).

An MRI provides good contrast images between different soft tissues of the body, and it does not use ionizing radiation like CT scans and X-rays. There are some complications of using an MRI, however. MRI machines are not as widely available as CT scans, are slower and cost more than other scans. In addition, if you have any ferromagnetic material in your body, an MRI is contraindicated because the magnetic field might pull the metal out of your body severely injuring you. Some people become claustrophobic in the MRI machine because they are placed into a confined space. Finally, there have been some reports of people dying from metal (oxygen tanks) being placed in the room when MRI has taken place, so make sure your technician spot checks that all magnetic metal is removed from the room before your MRI starts.

Sigmoidoscopy

A sigmoidoscopy is a minimally invasive medical examination of the large intestine from the rectum through the last part of the colon. There are flexible and rigid sigmoidoscopes. The flexible scope is used the most. The colon and rectum are emptied before the procedure using laxatives or enemas. A clear liquid diet is followed by the person a day before the procedure. A rigid sigmoidoscopy is seldom used and is usually only used in the area around the rectum to diagnose bleeding or inflammatory rectal disease.

During the procedure, you will be asked to lie on your left side on the examination table. The doctor then inserts a short, flexible, lighted tube into the rectum and slowly glides it through the colon. The scope transmits recorded images of inside the rectum and colon to the monitor while the doctor observes. Air is sometimes blown into the scope to inflate organs for a better view. The doctor may also take a biopsy with the scope if needed. Common complications of the procedure are bleeding and puncture of the colon. A sigmoidoscopy usually takes up to twenty minutes. You might feel some pressure in the intestines before and after the procedure.

Sitz Marker Study

During a sitz marker study, you will be asked to swallow a capsule with radiopaque rings. The capsule is digested in the gastrointestinal systems and leaves trace radiological material behind. An x-ray is taken five days later to see if, and where markers are left in the system. This test is used for people who suffer from chronic constipation. Finally, the test is performed to see total gastrointestinal functioning and emptying of the stomach and the intestines.

Stool Test

A stool test involves the collection and analysis of feces. They are used to diagnose gastrointestinal tract bleeding, SIBO, parasites, toxins from opportunistic infections like *C. diff*, virus antibodies, lactose intolerance, and fat accumulation in stools.

Ultrasound

Ultrasound is one of the safest diagnostic imaging techniques that is both noninvasive to the body itself most of the time and uses no ionizing radiation. An ultrasound machine uses sound waves to penetrate tissues to a desired depth and send back images. Ultrasounds do expose the body to an excess of RF radiation, but I still believe that the amount the body would absorb from the ultrasound is safer than using ionizing radiation scans.

Ultrasound is great for imaging muscle, soft tissue, and organs. It can also render "live" images, which can be more useful than X-rays or CT scans that must be developed for later viewing. Ultrasounds are a lot less expensive to perform compared to MRI's or CT scans.

The main limitation of ultrasounds is that bone provides too much resistance to the RF radiation; this makes ultrasound imagery of organs like the brain limited because of the skull. Gas in the gastrointestinal tract also might cause some distortions and can make organs like the pancreas hard to see. Body fat may also distort the image. Finally, the ultrasound technician must be highly qualified so that the quality images are assured. Accurate images will help physicians recommend the best treatment.

During an ultrasound, you will be instructed to lie on an examination table. The ultrasound probe is coated in conductive lubrication and placed near the area that needs to be examined. Images are then taken of the area. Ultrasounds usually run ten to twenty minutes.

Upper GI Series

An upper GI series is similar to a barium swallow test. During an upper GI test, you will be instructed to drink two liquids to help the production of the images. The first drink is usually baking soda that expands the stomach and causes gas to form. The second drink is usually barium. Barium is used to outline the esophagus and the stomach. X-rays are then taken to capture different views of the upper gastrointestinal tract.

Before the test, you will be instructed not to eat anything solid eight hours prior to the procedure. You are also instructed not to drink water three hours prior to the procedure. Nausea is common during the test because of the barium and may last up to three days afterward. An upper GI is usually used to diagnose ulcers, GERD, uncontrollable vomiting, or unexplained dark blood in stools. Although rare, systemic allergic reaction to the barium may occur.

X-ray

Standard X-rays expose the average person to a minimal amount of radiation. During an X-ray, a radiograph is taken when you are placed in front of an X-ray detector. An X-ray pulse then illuminates the targeted area. During the procedure, you might want to wear lead shielding if possible that protects the areas of the body not needed to be diagnosed from the radiation. Always ask for the thyroid guard addition to your lead vest, to protect your sensitive thyroid gland from ionizing radiation.

X-rays are commonly used in identifying skeletal problems because calcium in the bones absorbs X-rays providing contrast to the soft tissue which does not. The problem with using X-rays is that unless a person is given contrast, the X-ray does not show soft tissues or organs.

Chapter 22

The Difference in Supplement Companies

The average American purchases many of their supplements from Walmart or the local pharmacy. Most people then wonder why the supplement that they purchased made no difference in their health. Sadly, when it comes to the average person's health, most people will always go for the least expensive option. When it comes to buying the newest television, people will always spend the extra money for the best one. There is a huge difference in supplement companies and the quality of the supplements that they produce.

There is even a difference between generic medicine and patented medicine that is sold in this country, even though the FDA monitors both. The generic formula for Wellbutrin XL has been known to have increased side effect profile and was found to have decreased efficiency in the people who used it. It took FIVE years for the FDA to admit that there was a difference between the two medications and that the generic will finally be brought up to the patented standard.

You should always check the country of origin where your medicine / supplements are produced. You want it to be produced in the USA, Australia, New Zealand, Russia, Japan, Taiwan, Korea, EU, Israel, or Canada. If a product is listed as being produced anywhere else, you might want to pay more for the non-generic medicine or a different supplement made in one of these listed countries. Most of the countries listed have strict laws that regulate the production of medication and supplements, which may lead to a higher quality that you can trust.

A decent indication of an honest supplement company is if they follow at the very least GMP practices. Good manufacturing practices are a specific set of protocols that the FDA determined that were needed for the safety of producing supplements. GMP ensures that supplements you purchase are not contaminated and are of both the right dosage and potency. It is also always good to purchase a supplement that is pharmaceutical grade if possible along with it having a GMP seal. If a supplement is made from pharmaceutical grade materials, it means that the supplement could have been used in common medications or that the materials are of very high quality.

Top Five Supplement Companies

Number 5 Company: NOW

NOW produces high-quality supplements, they rarely use fillers, and their supplements reasonably priced. NOW is based out of Illinois and is a great American company! Their supplement production facility follows GMP practices in the manufacturing of their supplements and also offers body care products and sports supplements. NOW has a free online university through their website that helps consumers learn more about the supplements they are taking.

Number 4 Company: Life Extension

Life Extension is one of the oldest US-based supplement companies and manufactures their products in Florida. They are a great supplement company offering a lot of niche supplements, as well as great proprietary supplements. Life Extension does a lot of research when it comes to their supplements - more than any other supplement company in the United States does! They occasionally put fillers in their products, but they maintain a high standard of excellence. I recommend that everyone sign up for the Life Extension free magazine. It is full of great information and studies. Their production facility also follows GMP practices.

Number 3 Company: Jarrow Formulas

Even though Jarrow Formulas is more prone to put fillers in their products like magnesium stearate, they are still one of the best supplement companies. Jarrow Formulas is located in California and falls under the GMP for their facilities and supplements. They also tend to use pharmaceutical grade resources, which are the highest-grade materials you can get. For Jarrow, I highly recommend their probiotics, amino acids, and ubiquinol.

Number 2 Company: Thorne Research

I trust Thorne Research almost as much as the number one company, but they occasionally add fillers to their products. The fillers they add to their products are usually beneficial to the body (magnesium citrate, magnesium laurate). Nevertheless, they are a great American based company out of Idaho. They also practice GMPs as well as in-house laboratory testing publicizing the results afterward. Thorne Research also makes one of the only multivitamins that I can recommend, and I take their B vitamin complex daily.

Number 1 Company: Pure Encapsulations

Pure Encapsulations will always be my favorite company, but usually their supplements are the most expensive. They are located in Massachusetts, and they are a reputable American company. Their capsules are made from hypoallergenic cellulose. The best thing about them is that most of their products have no fillers in them as opposed to their cheaper competitors. These fillers can be very bad for you to ingest and include polypropylene glycol (antifreeze), magnesium stearate (rancid fat source), soy lecithin (GMO), etc. Their products are also GMP certified, and they have an "open plant" policy, which means anyone can come visit their plant. If you go to their website, they list all ingredients in their supplements and even their country of origin. Pure Encapsulations are truly the best supplement company!

Niche Companies That I Trust

These supplement companies tend to specialize in a small market or only make one type of supplement.

These are the companies I highly recommend:

- Sun Warrior
- Enzymedica: Make the best Digestive Enzymes
- Nordic Naturals: Make the some of the best fish oils!
- Sun Chlorella ✓
- Georges Aloe Vera
- North American Herb and Spice
- Clean Chlorella
- Gaia Herbs: Great NC Based Herb Company. I live in NC and have been to their farms. Top Notch!

Other Supplement Companies I Trust:

- Megafood
- Nature's Plus
- Pharmax
- Enzymatic Therapy ✓
- Renew Life ✓

- Xymogen
- Carlson
- Wakunaga
- Reserveage Organics
- Klaire Labs
- Solgar
- Source Naturals
- Carnivora

Supplement Company Tier System (Non-Niche Companies)

Top Tier:

- Pure Encapsulations
- Thorne Research
- Designs for Health
- Seeking Health
- Xymogen / NuMedica

Upper Tier:

- Jarrow Formulas
- Gaia Herbs
- Metagenics
- Pharmax
- Douglas Labs
- Klaire Labs
- Healthforce Nutritionals
- Reserveage Organics
- Life Extension

Mid Tier:

- Now
- Wakunaga
- Doctor's Best
- Renew Life
- Enzymatic Therapy
- Solgar
- Source Naturals
- Megafood
- Nature’s Plus
- Carlson

Low - Mid Tier:

- Swanson
- Vitamin Shoppe Brand
- Nature's Way
- Sundown

Low Tier:

- GNC Brand
- Vitamin World Brand

Chapter 23

Buying Locally: Local Health Food Stores and Corporations

Most people purchase their supplements online nowadays because of the ease of use. They buy their supplements from online retailers and receive their purchase on their doorstep the next day. I order my supplements online on occasion because sometimes, specialized supplements are hard to find in my area. If possible, I buy my supplements at the local health food store to help the local economy. It might cost a few more dollars for my supplements monthly, but I feel that, in the end, it is a better way that I can give back to the businesses in my local community.

When you buy online, you also might not know the quality of the supplement ordered. Buying locally is important because your sales help maintain your local economy by supplying jobs, revenue, and tax revenue for your local municipality / state. When you buy supplements locally, you can see the condition of the supplement bottle and expiration date of the supplement before purchasing. You can also ask the store employees for advice on supplements. I believe buying local at all times is one of the best things you can do personally to give back to your community.

Local health food store

Pros:

- Specialized selection.
- Offer local food, products, and supplements.
- Most workers at the local store are usually very knowledgeable about supplements.
- Very passionate workers.
- One can truly support the local economy by shopping at a local health food store.

Cons:

- Specialized selection can mean less choice.

- Sometimes workers may be the least knowledgeable due to limited training on supplements.
- Local supplement stores may be more expensive.

I love shopping at The Apple Crate, my local health store. The Apple Crate is a very nice store that sells specialized supplements from different brands and health food products, as well. Most people that work at the store are very knowledgeable, which is very important to me. One of the biggest things I despise in the natural health industry is misinformation. They also have a loyalty program where I can earn $10 back for every $100 I spend at the store, which is a great concept.

Most local health food stores have a wide selection of brands, supplements, and foods. This specialized selection of supplements can be a double-edged sword because the store can either carry the best brands for a supplement or off brands of particular supplements that are not worth purchasing. Shopping at a local health store can be a gamble sometimes. Sometimes a supplement will be top tier, and other times you must go somewhere else for the brands you might like. Most local health food store employees are very knowledgeable because they are very passionate about health. Most store owners work regular store hours and have a personal investment in being both knowledgeable and passionate about natural health.

Sometimes, you will encounter an employee who might only have basic knowledge at your local health food store because there is no systematic training program like at the bigger chains. Finally, local health food stores can be more expensive than large franchises and online companies, but I believe in paying slightly higher prices to help my local economy directly.

Vitamin Shoppe

Pros:

- Great overall selections.
- Most employees at the store usually have average knowledge of supplements.
- Some employees may have a passion for healthy living.
- You can support the local economy by shopping here.
- Competitive pricing.
- All employees receive training on supplements.
- Employees do not make a commission (therefore less pressure to make sales).

Cons:

- Less specialized selection of supplements.
- Some stores have less knowledgeable employees than others.
- Employee's passion for health usually is not as high as local health food stores.
- The Vitamin Shoppe house brand has spotty quality.

I will be honest with you, I have great respect for the Vitamin Shoppe, which is my prior employer. The Vitamin Shoppe, for the most part, respects their employees, which is rare for a corporation, and is a great place to work.

The Vitamin Shoppe does have a few advantages over the local health food stores and other corporate supplement stores. Vitamin Shoppe carries the best overall selection of supplements compared to all other supplement retailers. The only problem with this generalized selection is that niche supplements and high-tier supplements might not be found at the Vitamin Shoppe. Employees at the Vitamin Shoppe do receive education and information on supplements. This knowledge can help increase their ability to help customers. Sadly, this education can only go so far for some employees if they lack passion and treat their employment as "just another job." Employees are not paid by commission so they are not pressured to make sales pitches recommending supplements that might not be needed to improve your health.

Finally, Vitamin Shoppe does not produce its house brand of supplements. Other supplement companies do the supplement manufacturing, so the quality of an individual Vitamin Shoppe brand supplement depends on the individual supplement and can be spotty at times.

GNC

Pros:

- Most employees at GNC have average knowledge of supplements.
- Some employees can have a passion for healthy living.
- Can support the local economy by shopping here.
- Competitive pricing.
- All employees receive training on supplements.
- More locations than any supplement store.
- GNC offers the gold card discount.

Cons:

- Small selection of supplements.
- Some stores have less knowledgeable employees than others.
- Passion for health usually is not as high as local health food stores.
- GNC house brand has spotty quality.
- GNC employees are paid a commission.

Most small cities will at least have a GNC store and sometimes it is the only supplement store in town. GNC usually has a small assortment of supplements, and in the past, used to carry only their house brand of supplements. GNC currently carries supplements from more nationally recognized brands (Nordic Naturals, Nature's Way, and Now). Most employees working for GNC are educated in supplement use, knowledge and can make general supplement recommendations to improve your health. GNC has a frequent buyer's gold card discount that costs $15 a year and can help you save up to 50% on supplement purchases at GNC.

When a consumer goes into a GNC store, it is better for them to be self-informed before entering the store. GNC pays their employees sales commissions on supplements. Some employee's at GNC might use your supplement naivety to their advantage and convince you to purchase expensive supplements that you do not need.

Vitamin World

Pros:

- Most employees at Vitamin World have average knowledge of supplements.
- Some employees can have a passion for healthy living.
- Can support the local economy by shopping here.
- Lowest pricing on supplements for brick and mortar supplement stores.
- All employees receive training on supplements.

Cons:

- Small selection of supplements.
- Some stores have less knowledgeable employees than others.
- Passion for health usually is not as high as local health food stores.
- Vitamin World house brand is the least expensive: but lower quality can also come at a lower price.
- Vitamin World employees are paid a commission.

Vitamin World is the third largest supplement retailer in the United States. Vitamin World usually has a very small assortment of supplements in their stores and mostly carries its house brand of supplements. They offer a few nationally recognized brands (Source Naturals, USP Labs, and Now).

Most employees working for Vitamin World are educated in supplement use and knowledge and make general recommendations to improve your health. When a customer visits a Vitamin World, like GNC, it is good for them to be self-informed. Vitamin World pays their employees sales commissions on supplement purchases. Some employees of Vitamin World might use your supplement naivety to their advantage and convince you to purchase expensive supplements that you would not normally use or purchase.

Whole Foods

Pros:

- Wide selection of supplements and natural food products.
- Most employees at Whole Foods have average knowledge of supplements.
- Passion for healthy living is usually higher than most corporate supplement stores.
- You can support the local economy by shopping here.
- Employees that work in the supplement section receive training on supplements.

Cons:

- Whole Foods does not have a lot of stores in the U.S.
- Some stores have less knowledgeable employees than others.
- Whole Foods house supplement brand is average tier at best.
- Supplements can be almost as expensive as local health food stores.

Who does not love shopping at Whole Foods? You can purchase your grass-fed beef, MCT oil, cleaning supplies, and supplements, all in one convenient store!

Whole Foods has a good selection of supplements for a grocery store. In some Whole Foods stores, the supplement area of the store is larger than GNC, or Vitamin World stores. Most of the employees who work for Whole Foods have more passion for healthy living. This might have to do with the majority of Whole Foods stores being in college towns and affluent cities in the country where natural medicine might be more accepted.

The only cons for getting your supplements at Whole Foods is that there are not a lot of Whole Food stores in the country, so it might be hard to find one in your area. In addition, most supplements at Whole Foods are more expensive than your local health food store.

Big Box Pharmacy Stores (CVS, Walgreens, Rite Aid)

Pros:

- Big box pharmacy locations are everywhere.
- Price of supplements is lower.
- Pharmacies can carry well-known brands like Nordic Naturals and Renew Life, and Rite Aid carries GNC.

Cons:

- Pharmacists have very little knowledge of supplements.
- House brands of big box supplements are garbage.
- Big box pharmacies have very limited supplement selection.

I do not recommend that you buy your supplements from big box pharmacy stores if all possible. The supplement selection at a big box pharmacy usually is very small. Supplement quality is spotty at best unless the supplement is made from a well-known national brand. Most pharmacists are not knowledgeable about supplements and usually give inaccurate information by accident. The only advantage of shopping at a big box pharmacy store is that they are located almost everywhere in the country.

Local Compounding Pharmacy

Pros:

- Supplements are usually of high quality.
- Pharmacists usually have a knowledge of supplements and can provide decent recommendations.
- Can compound lesser known supplements and hormones.
- Compound pharmacies can make supplements for g-tubes.

Cons:

- Supplements may be expensive.
- Compounding pharmacies may have very limited supplement selection.

Your local compounding pharmacy is a lot better place to buy supplements than a big box pharmacy. Most local compounding pharmacies either will have an average assortment of different supplements or instead stock locally made compounded supplements. Compounding pharmacies also compound rare supplements, bio-identical hormonal creams, and supplements that can be used for people fed through gastrostomy tubes. Most pharmacists that work for your local compounding pharmacy have average supplement knowledge and make recommendations to improve your health. The only disadvantages of a local compounding pharmacy are that the supplements can be expensive, and the pharmacy can have limited selection depending on the size of the pharmacy.

Big Box Store (Walmart, Sam’s Club, Costco, BJ's Warehouse Club)

Pros:

- Everywhere

Cons:

- Everything

Do not buy your supplements at any big box store ever, unless they are trusted brands, and you have no other alternative to buy it elsewhere.

Chapter 24

Buying your Supplements Online: Risk vs. Reward

I do not order my supplements online unless necessary. Even though ordering your supplements online might be less expensive, most of the time you never know the quality of the supplement you might be receiving. If you buy online, you are also not supporting your local economy.

One of the main problems with ordering online is that you do not know that the supplement you are receiving is truly safe; it could be tampered with, so make sure you only use products that remain sealed. If you order an unlabeled supplement on online, the source of the supplement might be from China. Some supplements from China might be fine for use if they are produced with GMP practices, but others do not have quality control standards and often contain contaminants like heavy metals. Most unlabeled supplements online might have a low-price tag, but when you order an unlabeled supplement from the Internet, you do not know if you are getting the true supplement, a placebo, or a product that might be harmful to your health.

Another problem with ordering supplements online is that without seeing the expiration date of the supplement before ordering, you might receive a supplement from time to time that has expired. Most retailers will let you return an expired product, but unlike returning an expired supplement to a brick and mortar store quickly with a receipt, online returns can be time-consuming and it can take weeks to receive a new supplement from an online retailer.

Even though ordering supplements online might be cheaper, I only recommend ordering supplements online that you cannot find locally if all possible. If you do choose to order supplements online, use this quick reference guide to balancing the pros and cons, and choose which website is best for your needs.

Amazon.com

Pros:

- Buying your supplements on Amazon can save you a lot of money.
- Amazon carries an excellent selection of supplements.
- Amazon carries a lot of hard to find supplements.
- Competitive pricing.

- Free two-day shipping with Amazon Prime membership.
- Free three – five day shipping offered on most orders.
- Possible one-day shipping for most orders.
- Free order tracking.
- Amazon itself has a great return policy on expired supplements.
- Amazon and some of their suppliers offer a refund policy on unopened supplements.
- Amazon offers above average customer service.
- Amazon offers a good selection of organic food and products.
- Amazon has multiple reviews and an established rating system for most supplements.

Cons:

- Some supplements may be more expensive than other websites due to market demand and distributors.
- If you buy from other distributors that sell supplements on Amazon and are not the parent company, it might be more likely to receive an expired supplement.
- Different distributors have different return policies, which may cause issues with returns.
- Limited international shipping.
- Amazon does not carry as many high-tier supplements as pureformulas.com.
- If Amazon has a warehouse in the state you live in, you will be charged sales tax on every order.

If I have to order a supplement online, I use Amazon.com or PureFormulas.com to order most of my supplements. I have an Amazon Prime membership and use it to get my supplements within two days of ordering. Amazon offers many different supplements that can be hard to find on other websites, and they offer a large organic food selection and green cleaning products.

My main concerns with ordering from Amazon is that occasionally you will receive an expired supplement, and depending on what state you live in and if you have an Amazon warehouse in that state you might be charged sales tax on every purchase. If you use Amazon to purchase your supplements, try to buy them from the parent company and not other distributors unless they have a high rating. If you order your supplements from Amazon's warehouse directly, you have less of a chance to receive an expired supplement.

PureFormulas.com

Pros:

- Carries more top tier quality and hard to find supplements than any other e-commerce site.
- PureFormulas carries a near perfect selection of supplements.
- PureFormulas has a customer loyalty program.
- Excellent customer service and return policy.
- Free order tracking.
- Very low chance of receiving an expired supplement.
- They do not charge sales tax.
- PureFormulas offers coupon codes online.
- They send out coupons with every supplement shipment.
- Can pay with PayPal, which may add some extra purchase protection and enhanced refund policy.

Cons:

- Tends to be the most expensive supplement e-commerce site.
- Amazon.com offers lower shipping costs and options on most products.
- PureFormulas does not offer organic food.
- No international shipping.
- Even though PureFormulas might have the highest tier quality supplement selection, they often do not offer some mid-range supplements that are fine to use for most circumstances.

PureFormulas is a great website and Internet company from Florida that carries many top tier supplements which are hard to find even on Amazon occasionally. They carry all the top tier companies: Pure Encapsulations, Thorne Research, Designs for Health, Xymogen / NuMedica, Life Extension, Jarrow Formulas, Gaia Herbs, Metagenics, Pharmax, Douglas Labs, Klaire Labs, Healthforce Nutritionals, and Reserveage Organics.

PureFormulas also carries an excellent free frequent buyer points club, send coupons with every order, and also have excellent customer service and return policy. They also do not charge sales tax and they do not charge a lot for shipping.

The only main issue with ordering from PureFormulas is that it is the most expensive supplement e-commerce site around. Even though they tend to be more expensive, all the perks that come with ordering from them make it well worth it to use them for hard to find supplements. I still highly recommend them!

Iherb.com

Pros:

- Iherb carries a great selection of supplements.
- The website does carry some high-tier supplements.
- International shipping for most supplement orders.
- Iherb offers a reward program.
- Offers coupon codes.
- Free expedited one to five day shipping on orders over $20 in the U.S.
- Iherb does not charge sales tax for orders.
- Low chance of receiving out of date supplements.
- Iherb offers a good selection of organic food and products.
- Iherb has a good sixty-day return policy.

Cons:

- Iherb does not carry supplements from all the high-tier supplement companies.
- They do not offer an unopened refund policy.
- There are some reviews of Iherb on the Internet about occasional shoddy international shipping (long delays, losing orders).

If you are an international customer, Iherb is probably your best bet in purchasing the supplements that you need at a decent cost. For shoppers in America, I usually recommend Amazon or PureFormulas for the ordering of supplements, but Iherb is almost just as good in most circumstances. Iherb has a great selection of supplements to choose from, great customer service, they do not charge sales tax, and they offer free shipping on orders over $20. Finally, Iherb offers a reward program and offers coupon codes to help you save money on your order.

There are a few issues with ordering from Iherb in getting your supplements if you are an international customer. Some people have complained of long delays in receiving shipments (three - four weeks) and in some cases, the supplements shipped out did not even arrive! Iherb does not carry supplements from all the high-tier companies, and they also don't offer a refund policy if you are dissatisfied with the supplement.

Swansonvitamins.com

Pros:

- Swanson carries a decent selection of supplements.
- Swanson offers a large quantity of their house brand of supplements.
- Great customer service and return policy.
- Low chance of receiving an expired supplement.
- Swanson offers coupon codes online to save money.
- Swanson also offers "free" shipping.
- One-year refund policy for supplements.

Cons:

- Swanson carries a limited amount of high-tier supplements.
- The "free" shipping they offer is only for an order over $50.
- Their house brand of supplements is mid-tier.
- You have to ship the supplement back to Swanson for the refund.

Swanson offers one of the best selections of a house brand of products that I have ever seen for an e-commerce site. Some of the supplements in the house brand can range from being top tier to sadly low tier. Even though some of their supplements are questionable, I applaud them for trying to be very ambitious with having their house brand of supplements. Swanson offers a decent selection of other name brand supplements and has great customer service and return policy. Finally, Swanson offers coupon codes to help you save money, and they offer a one-year refund policy on supplements.

Swanson does offer one of the worse "free" shipping total amounts out of the e-commerce companies, which is $50. They also only carry a very limited amount of high-tier supplements. Other than that, I would trust them to purchase supplements from them online.

eBay.com

Pros:

- eBay can be the cheapest site to order your supplements. It is also the easiest way to buy supplements in bulk.
- You can pay with PayPal or a credit card for your orders.

- No sales tax.
- Sometimes free shipping is offered.
- Orders protected by PayPal.
- Largest selection of supplements on any website.
- eBay has a review system for individual sellers to help you buy with confidence.
- Offers international shipping occasionally.

Cons:

- Supplements you purchase from eBay may be from unreliable sources like China.
- Supplements have the greatest chance of being expired compared to other Internet ordering options.
- One of the easiest Internet ordering options where you can be scammed.
- PayPal protection does not always work when ordering from eBay like an Internet corporation or brick and mortar store.

If you do not have a lot of money, eBay could be the least expensive e-commerce site to purchase your supplements. ebay is also the easiest way to buy supplements in bulk; both powders that you can cap yourself, or supplements themselves. You also can pay with PayPal, which can offer you a greater sense of purchase protection than using any other form of payment, and refunds if needed. Finally, depending on the supplier, you might be able to order supplements internationally.

Ordering your supplements from eBay does come with many concerns. If you buy your supplements in bulk, you may not know the source and quality of the supplements and the country of their manufacture. Also, depending on the honesty of the supplier, you might not be sent the correct supplement that you thought you purchased, or the supplements you ordered might be out of date. PayPal's protection policy is not perfect; there are some issues were refunds for faulty products were never received, even when the purchaser was scammed!

Brick and Mortar Supplement Company Websites (Vitamin Shoppe, GNC, Vitamin World)

Pros:

- Carries an average all-around selection of supplements.
- Average customer return policy.
- Average customer service.
- Offers free shipping on differencing amounts depending on the company.
- Most items can be returned to the store easily.
- Email membership saving clubs.
- No sales tax.
- Refunds are available for unopened items.

Cons:

- Does not carry many high-tier supplements.
- Can be more expensive than the other online options.
- Does not carry organic food options.
- No international shipping.

I prefer that instead of ordering from a brick and mortar supplement company online, you get your supplements from a local brick and mortar supplement company store. Support your local economy whenever possible!

Big Box Brick and Mortar Supplement Companies Websites (Pharmacies, Walmart, Target, Warehouse Clubs)

Pros:

- None

Cons:

- Plenty

Do not buy your supplements at any big box store website ever unless they are trusted brands, and you have no other alternative to buy them elsewhere.

Appendix / Sources

General Source Information

- Balch, Phyllis. *Prescription for Nutritional Healing,* Avery Publishing, 2010.
- Balch, Phyllis. *Prescription for Herbal Healing*, Avery Publishing, 2012.
- Barron, Jon. *Lessons from the Miracle Doctors Finally*, Basic Health Publications, 2008.
- Balch, James, Stengler, Mark. *Prescription for Natural Cures,* John Wiley & Sons, 2004.
- Murray, Michael. *Encyclopedia of Nutritional Supplements,* Harmony, 1996.
- MacWilliam, Lyle. *NurtiSearch Compartive Guide to Nutritional Supplements*, Northern Dimensions Publishing, March 28, 2007.
- Gaby, Alan. *A-Z Guide to Drug-Herb-Vitamin Interactions,* Harmony, 2006.
- Gaeddert, Andrew. *Healing Digestive Disorders*, North Atlantic Books, 2004.
- Rubin, Jordan /Brasco, Joesph. *Restoring Your Digestive Health,* Twin Streams Publishing, 2003.
- Feingold, Ellen. *The Complete Self-Care Guide to Homeopathy, Herbal Remedies & Nutritional Supplements*, Homeopathy Center of Delaware, March 1, 2008.
- Dr. Brownstein, David. *Drugs That Don't Work and Natural Therapies that Do!*, Medical Alternative Press, 2007.
- Pagrana, Kathleen, Pagana, Timothy. *Mosby's Diagnostic and Laboratory Test Reference*, Mosby, October 5, 2012.
- Jane B. Reece, Lisa A. Urry, Michael L. Cain, Steven A. Wasserman, Peter Minorsky, Robert Jackson. *Campbell Biology*, Benjamin Cummings, October 7, 2010.
- Patton, Kevin, Thibodeau, Gary, Douglas, Matthew. *Essentials of Anatomy and Physiology*, Mosby, March 16, 2011.
- Bauman, Robert. *Microbiology with Diseases by Body System*, Benjamin Cummins, September 12, 2012.
- Black, Jacquelyn. *Microbiology: Principles and Explorations*, Wiley, May 1, 2012.
- Davis, William. *Wheat Belly: Loose the Wheat, Lose the Weight*, Rodale, August 30, 2011.
- Beers, Mark. *The Merck Manual*, Merck Research Laboratories, 2006.
- Tamparo, Carol, Lewis, Marcia. *Diseases of the Human Body*, F. A. Davis Company, Feb. 11, 2011.
- Sears, William, Sears, James. *The Omega-3 Effect*, Little, Brown and Company, Aug 28, 2012.
- Smith, Margaret, Morton, Dion. *The Digestive System: Systems of the Body Series*, Churchill Livingstone, November 18, 2011.
- Enders, Giulia, Gut: The Inside Story Of Our Body's Most Underrated Organ, Greystone Books, 2015.
- Axe, Josh, *Eat Dirt*, Harper Weave, 2016.
- Perlmutter, David, *Brain Maker*, Little, Brown and Company, 2015.

Difference in Supplement Companies

- Jarrow - http://www.jarrow.com/
- Pure Encapsulations - http://www.pureencapsulations.com/
- Thorne Research - http://thorne.com/
- NOW - http://www.nowfoods.com/
- Life Extension - http://www.lef.org/index.htm

How the Digestive System Works

- Beers, Mark. *The Merck Manual*, Merck Research Laboratories, 2006.
- Jane B. Reece, Lisa A. Urry, Michael L. Cain, Steven A. Wasserman, Peter Minorsky, Robert Jackson. *Campbell Biology*, Benjamin Cummings, October 7, 2010.
- Patton, Kevin, Thibodeau, Gary, Douglas, Matthew. *Essentials of Anatomy and Physiology*, Mosby, March 16, 2011.
- Smith, Margaret, Morton, Dion. *The Digestive System: Systems of the Body Series*, Churchill Livingstone, November 18, 2011.
- https://www.jackkruse.com/brain-gut-11-is-technology-your-achilles-heel/, Accessed June 16, 2016.
- http://jpp.krakow.pl/journal/archive/10_09_s3/pdf/67_10_09_s3_article.pdf, Accessed June 16, 2016.
- Ríos-lugo MJ, Cano P, Jiménez-ortega V, et al. Melatonin effect on plasma adiponectin, leptin, insulin, glucose, triglycerides and cholesterol in normal and high fat-fed rats. J Pineal Res. 2010;49(4):342-8. http://www.ncbi.nlm.nih.gov/pubmed/20663045
- Kandil TS, Mousa AA, El-gendy AA, Abbas AM. The potential therapeutic effect of melatonin in Gastro-Esophageal Reflux Disease. BMC Gastroenterol. 2010;10(1):7. http://bmcgastroenterol.biomedcentral.com/articles/10.1186/1471-230X-10-7
- Bubenik GA. Thirty four years since the discovery of gastrointestinal melatonin. J Physiol Pharmacol. 2008;59 Suppl 2:33-51. http://www.ncbi.nlm.nih.gov/pubmed/18812627
- Laurin M, Everett ML, Parker W. The cecal appendix: one more immune component with a function disturbed by post-industrial culture. Anat Rec (Hoboken). 2011;294(4):567-79. http://onlinelibrary.wiley.com/doi/10.1002/ar.21357/abstract
- Zahid A. The vermiform appendix: not a useless organ. J Coll Physicians Surg Pak. 2004;14(4):256-8. https://www.ncbi.nlm.nih.gov/pubmed/15228837
- Smith HF, Fisher RE, Everett ML, Thomas AD, Bollinger RR, Parker W. Comparative anatomy and phylogenetic distribution of the mammalian cecal appendix. J Evol Biol.

2009;22(10):1984-99.\\\ http://onlinelibrary.wiley.com/doi/10.1111/j.1420-9101.2009.01809.x/abstract;jsessionid=6B4A668B57EB425300659266E3CF943C.f04t03

Zinc

- Halpern, Georges. *Zinc Carnosine Nature's Safe and Effective Remedy For Ulcers*, Square One Publishers, May 1, 2005.

Studies

- Agren MS. Studies on zinc in wound healing. Acta Derm Venereol Suppl (Stockh). 1990;154:1-36. http://www.ncbi.nlm.nih.gov/pubmed/2275309
- Macdonald RS. The role of zinc in growth and cell proliferation. J Nutr. 2000;130(5S Suppl):1500S-8S. http://www.ncbi.nlm.nih.gov/pubmed/10801966
- Peppa M, Uribarri J, Vlassara H. Glucose, Advanced Glycation End Products, and Diabetes Complications: What Is New and What Works. Clinical Diabetes. 2003;21(4):186-187. http://clinical.diabetesjournals.org/content/21/4/186.full
- Peppa M, Raptis SA. Advanced glycation end products and cardiovascular disease. Curr Diabetes Rev. 2008;4(2):92-100. http://www.ncbi.nlm.nih.gov/pubmed/18473756

Articles

- http://www.lef.org/magazine/mag2006/dec2006_report_stomach_01.htm, Accessed April 25, 2014.
- http://www.lef.org/magazine/mag2008/jan2008_report_agingStomachs_01.htm) , Accessed April 25, 2014.
- http://lpi.oregonstate.edu/infocenter/minerals/zinc, Accessed April 25, 2014.
- http://www.lifeextension.com/magazine/2006/6/report_sod/Page-01, Accessed April 25, 2014.
- http://www.nowloss.com/ways-to-increase-testosterone-levels-naturally-without-using-steroids.htm, Accessed April 25, 2014.
- http://www.lef.org/magazine/mag2011/jan2011_Carnosine-Exceeding-Scientific-Expectations_01.htm, Accessed April 25, 2014.
- http://www.sciencedirect.com/science/article/pii/S0165017396000161, Accessed April 25, 2014.
- http://ods.od.nih.gov/factsheets/Zinc-HealthProfessional, Accessed April 25, 2014.

Magnesium

- Dean, Carolyn. *The Magnesium Miracle,* Ballantine Books, December 26, 2006.
- Seelig, Mildred / Rosanoff, Andrea. *The Magnesium Factor,* Avery Trade, August 25, 2003.
- Sircus, Mark / Reid, Daniel. *Transdermal Magnesium Therapy*, Phaelos Books & Mediawerks, January 1, 2007.

Studies

- Coudray C, Rambeau M, Feillet-coudray C, et al. Study of magnesium bioavailability from ten organic and inorganic Mg salts in Mg-depleted rats using a stable isotope approach. Magnes Res. 2005;18(4):215-23. http://www.ncbi.nlm.nih.gov/pubmed/16548135
- Mckee JA, Brewer RP, Macy GE, et al. Analysis of the brain bioavailability of peripherally administered magnesium sulfate: A study in humans with acute brain injury undergoing prolonged induced hypermagnesemia. Crit Care Med. 2005;33(3):661-6. http://www.ncbi.nlm.nih.gov/pubmed/15753761
- Ikarashi N, Mochiduki T, Takasaki A, et al. A mechanism by which the osmotic laxative magnesium sulphate increases the intestinal aquaporin 3 expression in HT-29 cells. Life Sci. 2011;88(3-4):194-200. http://www.ncbi.nlm.nih.gov/pubmed/21094173
- Seelig MS. THE REQUIREMENT OF MAGNESIUM BY THE NORMAL ADULT. SUMMARY AND ANALYSIS OF PUBLISHED DATA. Am J Clin Nutr. 1964;14(6):242-90. http://ajcn.nutrition.org/content/14/6/342.short
- Magnesium in chronic kidney disease Stages 3 and 4 and in dialysis patients. Clinical Kidney Journal. 2012;5(Suppl 1):i39. http://ckj.oxfordjournals.org/content/5/Suppl_1/i39.full
- Kaye P. The role of magnesium in the emergency department. Emergency Medicine Journal. 2002;19(4):288-291. http://emj.bmj.com/content/19/4/288.full
- Part 10.1: Life-Threatening Electrolyte Abnormalities. Circulation. 2005;112(24_suppl):IV-121-IV-125. http://circ.ahajournals.org/content/112/24_suppl/IV-121.full

Sites

- http://articles.mercola.com/sites/articles/archive/2012/12/17/magnesium-benefits.aspx, Accessed April 25, 2014.
- http://drsircus.com/medicine/magnesium/magnesium-chloride-benefits, Accessed April 25, 2014.

- http://www.globalhealingcenter.com/calcium-orotate/orotates-mineral-transporters, Accessed April 25, 2014.
- https://www.ncbi.nlm.nih.gov/pubmed/12892384, Accessed April 25, 2014.
- http://www.lef.org/magazine/mag2012/abstracts/feb2012_Magnesium-L-Threonate_01.htm, Accessed April 25, 2014.
- http://www.annualreviews.org/doi/abs/10.1146/annurev.nu.06.070186.002053, Accessed April 25, 2014.
- http://www.kidney.org/atoz/content/phosphorus.cfm, Accessed April 25, 2014.
- http://www.westonaprice.org/health-topics/dietary-supplements-what-the-industry-does-not-want-you-to-know/Accessed April 25, 2014.
- http://www.whfoods.com/genpage.php?tname=nutrient&dbid=75, Accessed April 25, 2014.
- http://chriskresser.com/another-reason-you-shouldnt-go-nuts-on-nuts, Accessed April 25, 2014.
- http://articles.mercola.com/sites/articles/archive/2012/12/17/magnesium-benefits.aspx, Accessed April 25, 2014.
- http://www.whfoods.com/genpage.php?tname=nutrient&dbid=75, Accessed April 25, 2014.
- http://ods.od.nih.gov/factsheets/Magnesium-HealthProfessional/ , Accessed April 25, 2014.
- http://emedicine.medscape.com/article/246489-overview, Accessed April 25, 2014.
- http://www.uptodate.com/contents/symptoms-of-hypermagnesemia, Accessed April 25, 2014.
- http://www.medscape.com/viewarticle/775050, Accessed April 25, 2014.
- http://www.drsircus.com/medicine/magnesium/magnesium-the-ultimate-heart-medicine, Accessed April 25, 2014.
- http://www.naturalnews.com/023511_magnesium_body_deficiency.html, Accessed April 25, 2014.
- http://www.drsircus.com/medicine/magnesium/the-insulin-magnesium-story-2, Accessed April 25, 2014.
- http://www.afibbers.org/resources/magnesiumabsorption.pdf, Accessed April 25, 2014.
- http://www.huffingtonpost.com/christiane-northrup/magnesium-calcium_b_509115.html, Accessed April 25, 2014.
- http://umm.edu/health/medical/altmed/supplement/magnesium, Accessed April 25, 2014.
- http://www.lef.org/news/LefDailyNews.htm?NewsID=17659, Accessed April 25, 2014.
- http://www.healthline.com/health/serum-magnesium-test, Accessed April 25, 2014.
- http://drcarolyndean.com/2010/06/gauging-magnesium-deficiency-symptoms, Accessed April 25, 2014.
- http://otiswoodardmd.typepad.com/my_weblog/2009/04/magnesium-do-you-have-enough.html, Accessed April 25, 2014.
- http://www.exatest.com, Accessed April 25, 2014.

Increase Stomach Acid

- Wright, Jonathan. *Why Stomach Acid Is Good For You,* M. Evans & Company, August 20, 2001.

Probiotics

- Adams, Casey. *Probiotics Protection Against Infection,* Logical Books, April 5, 2012.
- Patton, Kevin, Thibodeau, Gary, Douglas, Matthew. *Essentials of Anatomy and Physiology*, Mosby, March 16, 2011.
- Bauman, Robert. *Microbiology with Diseases by Body System*, Benjamin Cummins, September 12, 2012.
- Motarjemi, Yasmine. *Encyclopedia of Food Safety*, Academic Press, December 12, 2013.
- Lee, Yuan, Salminen, Seppo. *Handbook of Probiotics and Prebiotics*, Wiley, December 2008.

Probiotic.Org Website

- http://probiotic.org/index.htm, Accessed April 25, 2014.

Non HSO Probiotics

B. animalis

- Roselli, M. / Finamore, A. / Britti, M. / Mengheri. E / Probiotic bacteria *Bifidobacterium animalis* MB5 and *Lactobacillus rhamnosus* GG protect intestinal Caco-2 cells from the inflammation-associated response induced by enterotoxigenic *Escherichia coli* K88, British Journal of Nutrition / Volume 95 / Issue 06 / June 2006, pp 1177-1184 http://journals.cambridge.org/action/displayAbstract?fromPage=online&aid=920784

B. bifidum

- Kirjavainen, P. V. / et al. / Aberrant composition of gut microbiota of allergic infants: a target of bifidobacterial therapy at weaning? Gut 2002;51:51-55 doi:10.1136/gut.51.1.51 http://gut.bmj.com/content/51/1/51.abstract

B. longum

- Schell MA, Karmirantzou M, Snel B, et al. The genome sequence of *Bifidobacterium longum* reflects its adaptation to the human gastrointestinal tract. Proc Natl Acad Sci USA. 2002;99(22):14422-7. http://www.ncbi.nlm.nih.gov/pubmed/12381787
- Yuan J, Zhu L, Liu X, et al. A proteome reference map and proteomic analysis of *Bifidobacterium longum* NCC2705. Mol Cell Proteomics. 2006;5(6):1105-18. http://www.ncbi.nlm.nih.gov/pubmed/16549425
- Garrido D, Ruiz-moyano S, Jimenez-espinoza R, Eom HJ, Block DE, Mills DA. Utilization of galactooligosaccharides by *Bifidobacterium longum subsp. infantis* isolates. Food Microbiol. 2013;33(2):262-70. http://www.ncbi.nlm.nih.gov/pubmed/23200660
- Tanaka H, Hashiba H, Kok J, Mierau I. Bile salt hydrolase of *Bifidobacterium longum*-biochemical and genetic characterization. Appl Environ Microbiol. 2000;66(6):2502-12. http://www.ncbi.nlm.nih.gov/pubmed/10831430
- Lin MY, Chang FJ. Antioxidative effect of intestinal bacteria *Bifidobacterium longum* ATCC 15708 and *Lactobacillus acidophilus* ATCC 4356. Dig Dis Sci. 2000;45(8):1617-22. http://www.ncbi.nlm.nih.gov/pubmed/11007114
- Benno Y, Mitsuoka T. Impact of *Bifidobacterium longum* on human fecal microflora. Microbiol Immunol. 1992;36(7):683-94. http://www.ncbi.nlm.nih.gov/pubmed/1406371

E. coli Nissle

- http://www.mutaflor.com/index.html
- Kruis W, Fric P, Pokrotnieks J, et al. Maintaining remission of ulcerative colitis with the probiotic *Escherichia coli Nissle* 1917 is as effective as with standard mesalazine. Gut. 2004;53(11):1617-23. http://www.ncbi.nlm.nih.gov/pmc/articles/PMC1774300/
- Bruckschen E et al. Chronic Constipation. Comparison of Microbiological and Lactulose Treatment. [German] MMW 1994, 16: 241-245.
- Goerg KJ et al. Probiotic therapy of pseudomembranous colitis. Combination of intestinal lavage and oral administration of *Escherichia coli*. [German] DMW 1998;123:1274-1278.
- Kruis W et al. Maintaining remission of ulcerative colitis with the probiotic *Escherichia coli Nissle* 1917 is as effective as with standard mesalazine.Gut 2004, 53:1617-1623.
- Kruis W et al. Double-blind comparison of an oral *Escherichia coli* preparation and mesalazine in maintaining remission of ulcerative colitis. Aliment Pharmacol Ther 1997; 11: 853-858.
- Kuzela L et al. Induction and maintenance of remission with nonpathogenic *Escherichia coli* in patients with pouchitis. Am J Gastroenterol 2001;96:3218-3219.
- Malchow HA. Crohn's Disease and *Escherichia coli*. J Clin Gastroenterol 1997; 25: 653-658.

- Malchow H et al. Colonization of adults by an apathogenic *E. coli* strain administered after gut decontamination. Gastroenterology 1995; Suppl. 108: 869.
- Möllenbrink M et al. Treatment of chronic constipation with physiologic *Escherichia coli* bacteria. Results of a clinical study of the effectiveness and tolerance of microbiological therapy with the *E. coli* Nissle 1917 strain (Mutaflor) [German] Med Klin 1994, 89: 587-93.
- Rembacken BJ et al. Non-pathogenic *Escherichia coli* versus mesalazine for the treatment of ulcerative colitis: a randomised trial. Lancet 1999; 354:635-639.
- Schütz E. The treatment of intestinal diseases with Mutaflor. A multicenter retrospective study. [German] Fortschr Med 1989; 107: 599-602
- Tromm A et al. The probiotic *E. coli* strain *Nissle* 1917 for the treatment of collagenous colitis: First results of an open-labelled trial Z. Gastroenterol, 2004, 365-369.

Lactobacilus acidophilus

- Kim JY, Kwon JH, Ahn SH, et al. Effect of probiotic mix (*Bifidobacterium bifidum, Bifidobacterium lactis, Lactobacillus acidophilus*) in the primary prevention of eczema: a double-blind, randomized, placebo-controlled trial. Pediatr Allergy Immunol. 2010;21(2 Pt 2):e386-93. http://onlinelibrary.wiley.com/doi/10.1111/j.1399-3038.2009.00958.x/full

Lactobacilus brevis

- Linsalata M, Russo F, Berloco P, et al. The influence of *Lactobacillus brevis* on ornithine decarboxylase activity and polyamine profiles in *Helicobacter pylori*-infected gastric mucosa. Helicobacter. 2004;9(2):165-72. http://onlinelibrary.wiley.com/doi/10.1111/j.1083-4389.2004.00214.x/abstract;jsessionid=8B870943E70A8BBE77993641B40693A9.d04t02?deniedAccessCustomisedMessage=&userIsAuthenticated=false

Lactobacilus bulgaricus

- Wollowski I, Rechkemmer G, Pool-zobel BL. Protective role of probiotics and prebiotics in colon cancer. Am J Clin Nutr. 2001;73(2 Suppl):451S-455S. https://www.ncbi.nlm.nih.gov/pubmed/17200238

Lactobacilus helveticus

- http://www.sciencedirect.com/science/article/pii/S0022030294770260, Accessed April 25, 2014.

Lactobacillus reuteri

- http://journals.lww.com/pidj/Abstract/1997/12000/Bacteriotherapy_with_Lactobacillus_reuteri_in.2.aspx, Accessed April 25, 2014.
- Savino F, Pelle E, Palumeri E, Oggero R, Miniero R. *Lactobacillus reuteri* (American Type Culture Collection Strain 55730) versus simethicone in the treatment of infantile colic: a prospective randomized study. Pediatrics. 2007;119(1):e124-30. https://www.ncbi.nlm.nih.gov/pubmed/17200238

Lactobacillus plantarum

- Niedzielin K, Kordecki H, Birkenfeld B. A controlled, double-blind, randomized study on the efficacy of *Lactobacillus plantarum* 299V in patients with irritable bowel syndrome. Eur J Gastroenterol Hepatol. 2001;13(10):1143-7. http://www.ncbi.nlm.nih.gov/pubmed/11711768

S. boulardii

- Kelesidis T, Pothoulakis C. Efficacy and safety of the probiotic *Saccharomyces boulardii* for the prevention and therapy of gastrointestinal disorders. Therap Adv Gastroenterol. 2012;5(2):111-25. http://www.ncbi.nlm.nih.gov/pmc/articles/PMC3296087/
- Surawicz CM, Elmer GW, Speelman P, Mcfarland LV, Chinn J, Van belle G. Prevention of antibiotic-associated diarrhea by *Saccharomyces boulardii*: a prospective study. Gastroenterology. 1989;96(4):981-8. http://www.ncbi.nlm.nih.gov/pubmed/2494098

- Kelesidis T, Pothoulakis C. Efficacy and safety of the probiotic *Saccharomyces boulardii for* the prevention and therapy of gastrointestinal disorders. Therap Adv Gastroenterol. 2012;5(2):111-25. http://www.ncbi.nlm.nih.gov/pmc/articles/PMC3296087/

S. salivarius

- Burton JP, Chilcott CN, Moore CJ, Speiser G, Tagg JR. A preliminary study of the effect of probiotic *Streptococcus salivarius* K12 on oral malodour parameters. J Appl Microbiol. 2006;100(4):754-64. http://www.ncbi.nlm.nih.gov/pubmed/16553730

HSO'S

Acinetobacter Genus

- Glew RH, Moellering RC, Kunz LJ. Infections with *Acinetobacter calcoaceticus (Herellea vaginicola)*: clinical and laboratory studies. Medicine (Baltimore). 1977;56(2):79-97. http://www.ncbi.nlm.nih.gov/pubmed/846390
- http://journals.lww.com/infectdis/Fulltext/2008/01000/Drug_Resistant_Acinetobacter.1.aspx, Accessed April 25, 2014.

Arthobacter Genus

- Bernasconi E, Valsangiacomo C, Peduzzi R, Carota A, Moccetti T, Funke G. *Arthrobacter woluwensis* subacute infective endocarditis: case report and review of the literature. Clin Infect Dis. 2004;38(4):e27-31. http://www.ncbi.nlm.nih.gov/pubmed/14765360
- Funke G, Hutson RA, Bernard KA, Pfyffer GE, Wauters G, Collins MD. Isolation of *Arthrobacter* spp. from clinical specimens and description of *Arthrobacter cumminsii* sp. nov. and Arthrobacter woluwensis sp. nov. J Clin Microbiol. 1996;34(10):2356-63. http://www.ncbi.nlm.nih.gov/pmc/articles/PMC229268/
- http://cid.oxfordjournals.org/content/38/4/e27.full.pdf, Accessed April 25, 2014.
- Funke G, Hutson RA, Bernard KA, Pfyffer GE, Wauters G, Collins MD. Isolation of *Arthrobacter* spp. from clinical specimens and description of *Arthrobacter cumminsii* sp. nov. and Arthrobacter woluwensis sp. nov. J Clin Microbiol. 1996;34(10):2356-63. http://jcm.asm.org/content/34/10/2356

Azotobacter Genus

- http://commtechlab.msu.edu/sites/dlc-me/zoo/zdrs0309.html, Accessed April 25, 2014.

B. subtilis

Studies

- Goossens D, Jonkers D, Russel M, et al. Survival of the probiotic, *L. plantarum* 299v and its effects on the faecal bacterial flora, with and without gastric acid inhibition. Dig Liver Dis. 2005;37(1):44-50. http://www.ncbi.nlm.nih.gov/pubmed/15702859
- Rigaux P, Daniel C, Hisbergues M, et al. Immunomodulatory properties of *Lactobacillus plantarum* and its use as a recombinant vaccine against mite allergy. Allergy. 2009;64(3):406-14. http://www.ncbi.nlm.nih.gov/pubmed/19120072
- Grangette C, Nutten S, Palumbo E, et al. Enhanced antiinflammatory capacity of a *Lactobacillus plantarum* mutant synthesizing modified teichoic acids. Proc Natl Acad Sci USA. 2005;102(29):10321-6. http://www.ncbi.nlm.nih.gov/pubmed/15985548
- Nicholson WL, Munakata N, Horneck G, Melosh HJ, Setlow P. Resistance of *Bacillus* endospores to extreme terrestrial and extraterrestrial environments. Microbiol Mol Biol Rev. 2000;64(3):548-72. http://www.ncbi.nlm.nih.gov/pubmed/10974126
- Oggioni MR, Pozzi G, Valensin PE, Galieni P, Bigazzi C. Recurrent septicemia in an immunocompromised patient due to probiotic strains of *Bacillus subtilis*. J Clin Microbiol. 1998;36(1):325-6. http://jcm.asm.org/content/36/1/325.full?ijkey=1903da10e5f13b43cfe75e8ae3b2de7e0ee01a92&keytype2=tf_ipsecsha
- Richard V, Van der auwera P, Snoeck R, Daneau D, Meunier F. Nosocomial bacteremia caused by Bacillus species. Eur J Clin Microbiol Infect Dis. 1988;7(6):783-5. http://www.ncbi.nlm.nih.gov/pubmed/3145864
- Jeon YL, Yang JJ, Kim MJ, et al. Combined *Bacillus licheniformis* and *Bacillus subtilis* infection in a patient with oesophageal perforation. J Med Microbiol. 2012;61(Pt 12):1766-9. http://www.ncbi.nlm.nih.gov/pubmed/22918867
- Chen GC, Ramanathan VS, Law D, et al. Acute liver injury induced by weight-loss herbal supplements. World J Hepatol. 2010;2(11):410-5. http://www.ncbi.nlm.nih.gov/pmc/articles/PMC3004035/

Websites

- http://link.springer.com/article/10.1007%2Fs12602-013-9136-0, Accessed April 25, 2014.
- http://web.mst.edu/~microbio/BIO221_2009/B_subtilis.html, Accessed April 25, 2014.
- http://www.cdc.gov/anthrax/, Accessed April 25, 2014.
- http://www.avianbiotech.com/diseases/clostridium.htm, Accessed April 25, 2014.
- http://sporegen.com/uploads/publications/Hong2009.pdf, Accessed April 25, 2014.

- http://informahealthcare.com/doi/abs/10.1080/089106000435491, Accessed April 25, 2014.
- http://micro.cornell.edu/research/epulopiscium/bacterial-endospores, Accessed April 25, 2014.
- http://www.protexin.com/attachments/Probiotic%20News%20Issue%201.pdf, Accessed April 25, 2014.
- http://www.fda.gov/ohrms/dockets/dockets/95s0316/95s-0316-rpt0277-Attachment-F-Sonenshein-vol214.pdf, Accessed April 25, 2014.
- http://www.epa.gov/oppt/biotech/pubs/fra/fra009.htm, Accessed April 25, 2014.
- http://www.bulletproofexec.com/the-red-meat-scapegoat-the-new-york-times-carnitine-heart-disease-and-science/, Accessed April 25, 2014.
- http://chriskresser.com/treating-sibo-cold-thermogenisis-and-when-to-take-probiotics, Accessed April 25, 2014.
- http://www.marksdailyapple.com/eating-earth-exploring-the-mysterious-world-of-geophagy/#axzz2kgVmG8lD, Accessed April 25, 2014.
- https://files.nyu.edu/jmm257/public/querencias/natto.html, Accessed April 25, 2014.
- http://sporegen.com/uploads/publications/Hong2009.pdf, Accessed April 25, 2014.
- http://blog.listentoyourgut.com/bacterial-soil-organisms-hsos-sos-sbos-etc/, Accessed April 25, 2014.
- http://www.bulletproofexec.com/the-red-meat-scapegoat-the-new-york-times-carnitine-heart-disease-and-science/, Accessed April 25, 2014.

Brevibacteria Genus

- Gruner E, Pfyffer GE, Von graevenitz A. Characterization of *Brevibacterium* spp. from clinical specimens. J Clin Microbiol. 1993;31(6):1408-12. http://jcm.asm.org/content/31/6/1408.full.pdf
- https://bioweb.uwlax.edu/bio203/s2012/fischer_jaco/, Accessed April 25, 2014.

Enterococcus faecalis

- Molander A, Reit C, Dahlen G, Kvist T: Microbiological status of root-filled teeth with apical periodontitis, Int Endod J 31:1, 1998 http://www.nejm.org/doi/full/10.1056/NEJM199501053320105
- Murray BE. The life and times of the *Enterococcus.* Clin Microbiol Rev. 1990;3(1):46-65. http://www.ncbi.nlm.nih.gov/pmc/articles/PMC358140/
- Nallapareddy SR, Singh KV, Sillanpää J, et al. Endocarditis and biofilm-associated pili of *Enterococcus faecalis*. J Clin Invest. 2006;116(10):2799-807. http://www.jci.org/articles/view/29021

- http://www.ijaaonline.com/article/S0924-8579(07)72177-5/abstract, Accessed April 25, 2014.
- http://www.life.umd.edu/classroom/bsci424/PathogenDescriptions/Enterococcus.htm, Accessed April 25, 2014.

Prebiotics

Arabinogalactans

- http://www.altmedrev.com/publications/4/2/96.pdf, Accessed June 16, 2016.
- http://www.dadamo.com/txt/index.pl?3004, Accessed June 16, 2016.
- https://www.researchgate.net/publication/11839126_Effects_of_Dietary_Arabinogalactan_on_Gastrointestinal_and_Blood_Parameters_in_Healthy_Human_Subjects, Accessed June 16, 2016.
- http://foodandnutritionresearch.net/index.php/fnr/article/viewFile/1801/1708, Accessed June 16, 2016.
- Bodera P. Influence of prebiotics on the human immune system (GALT). Recent Pat Inflamm Allergy Drug Discov. 2008;2(2):149-53. http://www.ingentaconnect.com/content/ben/iad/2008/00000002/00000002/art00010?crawler=true
- Fonseca C, Romão R, Rodrigues de sousa H, Hahn-hägerdal B, Spencer-martins I. L-Arabinose transport and catabolism in yeast. FEBS J. 2007;274(14):3589-600. http://www.ncbi.nlm.nih.gov/pubmed/17627668

Inulin / FOS

- http://www.marksdailyapple.com/prebiotics/. Accessed April 27, 2014
- http://www.breakingtheviciouscycle.info/knowledge_base/detail/inulin/. Accessed April 27, 2014

Lactulose

- Beers, Mark. *The Merck Manual*, Merck Research Laboratories, 2006.

- Shukla S, Shukla A, Mehboob S, Guha S. Meta-analysis: the effects of gut flora modulation using prebiotics, probiotics and synbiotics on minimal hepatic encephalopathy. Aliment Pharmacol Ther. 2011;33(6):662-71. http://www.ncbi.nlm.nih.gov/pubmed/21251030

XOS

- http://www.marksdailyapple.com/prebiotics/. Accessed April 27, 2014
- Xylooligosaccharides (XOS) as an Emerging Prebiotic: Microbial Synthesis, Utilization, Structural Characterization, Bioactive Properties, and Applications. Comprehensive Reviews in Food Science and Food Safety. 10(1):2. http://onlinelibrary.wiley.com/doi/10.1111/j.1541-4337.2010.00135.x/abstract

IOS

- http://www.efsa.europa.eu/en/efsajournal/pub/1801. Accessed April 27, 2014.
- http://www.fda.gov/downloads/Food/IngredientsPackagingLabeling/GRAS/NoticeInventory/ucm268863.pdf. Accessed April 27, 2014.
- Rycroft CE, Jones MR, Gibson GR, Rastall RA. A comparative in vitro evaluation of the fermentation properties of prebiotic oligosaccharides. J Appl Microbiol. 2001;91(5):878-87. http://www.ncbi.nlm.nih.gov/pubmed/11722666
- Harmsen HJ, Wildeboer-veloo AC, Raangs GC, et al. Analysis of intestinal flora development in breastfed and formula-fed infants by using molecular identification and detection methods. J Pediatr Gastroenterol Nutr. 2000;30(1):61-7. http://www.ncbi.nlm.nih.gov/pubmed/10630441

MOS

- Oyofo BA, Deloach JR, Corrier DE, Norman JO, Ziprin RL, Mollenhauer HH. Prevention of *Salmonella typhimurium* colonization of broilers with D-mannose. Poult Sci. 1989;68(10):1357-60. http://www.ncbi.nlm.nih.gov/pubmed/2685797

GOS

- Bouhnik Y, Raskine L, Simoneau G, et al. The capacity of nondigestible carbohydrates to stimulate fecal *Bifidobacteria* in healthy humans: a double-blind, randomized, placebo-controlled, parallel-group, dose-response relation study. Am J Clin Nutr. 2004;80(6):1658-64. http://www.ncbi.nlm.nih.gov/pubmed/15585783
- Shoaf K, Mulvey GL, Armstrong GD, Hutkins RW. Prebiotic galactooligosaccharides reduce adherence of enteropathogenic *Escherichia coli* to tissue culture cells. Infect Immun. 2006;74(12):6920-8. http://www.ncbi.nlm.nih.gov/pubmed/16982832
- Searle LE, Best A, Nunez A, et al. A mixture containing galactooligosaccharide, produced by the enzymic activity of *Bifidobacterium bifidum*, reduces *Salmonella enterica serovar Typhimurium* infection in mice. J Med Microbiol. 2009;58(Pt 1):37-48. http://www.ncbi.nlm.nih.gov/pubmed/19074651
- Depeint F, Tzortzis G, Vulevic J, I'anson K, Gibson GR. Prebiotic evaluation of a novel galactooligosaccharide mixture produced by the enzymatic activity of *Bifidobacterium bifidum* NCIMB 41171, in healthy humans: a randomized, double-blind, crossover, placebo-controlled intervention study. Am J Clin Nutr. 2008;87(3):785-91. http://ajcn.nutrition.org/content/87/3/785.abstract
- Whisner CM, Martin BR, Schoterman MH, et al. Galacto-oligosaccharides increase calcium absorption and gut *Bifidobacteria* in young girls: a double-blind cross-over trial. Br J Nutr. 2013;110(7):1292-303. http://www.ncbi.nlm.nih.gov/pubmed/23507173
- Hughes C, Davoodi-semiromi Y, Colee JC, et al. Galactooligosaccharide supplementation reduces stress-induced gastrointestinal dysfunction and days of cold or flu: a randomized, double-blind, controlled trial in healthy university students. Am J Clin Nutr. 2011;93(6):1305-11. http://www.ncbi.nlm.nih.gov/pubmed/21525194
- Weaver CM, Martin BR, Nakatsu CH, et al. Galactooligosaccharides improve mineral absorption and bone properties in growing rats through gut fermentation. J Agric Food Chem. 2011;59(12):6501-10. http://www.ncbi.nlm.nih.gov/pubmed/21553845
- Rycroft CE, Jones MR, Gibson GR, Rastall RA. A comparative in vitro evaluation of the fermentation properties of prebiotic oligosaccharides. J Appl Microbiol. 2001;91(5):878-87. http://www.ncbi.nlm.nih.gov/pubmed/11722666
- Niittynene Lenna / et al. Galacto-oligosaccharides and Bowel Function Scand J Food Nutrition. June 2007. http://www.ncbi.nlm.nih.gov/pmc/articles/PMC2607002/

Histamine

- Preedy, Victor. *Processing and Impact on Active Components in Food*, Academic Press, 2014.
- http://sepa.duq.edu/regmed/immune/histamine.html, Accessed June 16, 2016.
- http://www.scielo.br/pdf/abd/v85n2/en_10, Accessed June 16, 2016.
- http://www.allergynutrition.com/wp-content/uploads/2014/05/Histamine-DAO-and-Probiotics-Revised.pdf, Accessed June 16, 2016.
- https://www.bulletproofexec.com/why-yogurt-and-probiotics-make-you-fat-and-foggy/, Accessed June 16, 2016.

- http://arbl.cvmbs.colostate.edu/hbooks/pathphys/endocrine/otherendo/histamine.html, Accessed June 16, 2016.
- Clemetson CA. Histamine and ascorbic acid in human blood. J Nutr. 1980;110(4):662-8. http://jn.nutrition.org/content/110/4/662.extract
- Capozzi V, Russo P, Ladero V, et al. Biogenic Amines Degradation by Lactobacillus plantarum: Toward a Potential Application in Wine. Front Microbiol. 2012;3:122. http://www.ncbi.nlm.nih.gov/pmc/articles/PMC3316997

Opportunistic / Infectious Bacteria

- Black, Jacquelyn. *Microbiology: Principles and Explorations*, Wiley, May 1, 2012.
- Bauman, Robert. *Microbiology with Diseases by Body System*, Benjamin Cummins, September 12, 2012.
- Beers, Mark. The *Merck Manual*, Merck Research Laboratories, 2006.
- Tamparo, Carol, Lewis, Marcia. *Diseases of the Human Body*, F. A. Davis Company, Feb. 11, 2011.
- http://www.uib.es/depart/dba/microbiologia/ADSenfcoml/material_archivos/infeccion%20gastrointestinal.pdf, Accessed April 25, 2014.

Supplements

- Balch, James, Stengler, Mark. *Prescription for Natural Cures,* John Wiley & Sons, 2004.
- Balch, Phyllis. *Prescription for Nutritional Healing,* Avery Publishing, 2010.
- Bowden, Jonny. *Zinc Carnosine: The Most Effective Natural Cures on Earth*, Fair Winds Press, August 1, 2011.
- Feingold, Ellen. *The Complete Self-Care Guide to Homeopathy, Herbal Remedies & Nutritional Supplements*, Homeopathy Center of Delaware, March 1, 2008.
- Halpern, Georges. *Zinc Carnosine Nature's Safe and Effective Remedy For Ulcers*, Square One Publishers, May 1, 2005.
- MacWilliam, Lyle. *NurtiSearch Compartive Guide to Nutritional Supplements*, Northern Dimensions Publishing, March 28, 2007.
- Murray, Michael. *Encyclopedia of Nutritional Supplements,* Harmony, 1996.

5-HTP

- http://www.naturalmedicinejournal.com/journal/2011-10/many-uses-5-htp, Accessed April 28, 2014
- https://www.scribd.com/document/80455343/5HTP-as-Precursor, Accessed April 28, 2014
- Saegusa Y, Takeda H, Muto S, et al. Decreased motility of the lower esophageal sphincter in a rat model of gastroesophageal reflux disease may be mediated by reductions of serotonin and acetylcholine signaling. Biol Pharm Bull. 2011;34(5):704-11. http://www.ncbi.nlm.nih.gov/pubmed/21532161
- Rattan S, Goyal RK. Effects of 5-hydroxytryptamine on the lower esophageal sphincter in vivo: evidence for multiple sites of action. J Clin Invest. 1977;59(1):125-33. http://www.ncbi.nlm.nih.gov/pmc/articles/PMC333339/

Allicin C

- Cutler RR, Wilson P. Antibacterial activity of a new, stable, aqueous extract of allicin against methicillin-resistant *Staphylococcus aureus.* Br J Biomed Sci. 2004;61(2):71-4. http://www.ncbi.nlm.nih.gov/pubmed/15250668

Collagen

- https://www.jstage.jst.go.jp/article/jnsv/52/3/52_3_211/_article, Accessed April 28, 2014
- http://wellnessmama.com/3380/why-ive-been-drinking-green-jello-well-almost/, Accessed April 28, 2014
- Schauss AG, Stenehjem J, Park J, Endres JR, Clewell A. Effect of the novel low molecular weight hydrolyzed chicken sternal cartilage extract, BioCell Collagen, on improving osteoarthritis-related symptoms: a randomized, double-blind, placebo-controlled trial. J Agric Food Chem. 2012;60(16):4096-101. http://www.ncbi.nlm.nih.gov/pubmed/22486722?dopt=Abstract

Chlorella

- http://articles.mercola.com/sites/articles/archive/2012/02/01/is-this-one-of-natures-most-powerful-detoxification-tools.aspx, Accessed April 28, 2014
- http://robbwolf.com/2012/01/19/trojan-horses-of-chlorella-superfood/. Accessed September 19, 2016.
- http://www.sciencedirect.com/science/article/pii/S1364032114002342. Accessed September 19, 2016.

- Rai UN, Singh NK, Upadhyay AK, Verma S. Chromate tolerance and accumulation in Chlorella vulgaris L.: role of antioxidant enzymes and biochemical changes in detoxification of metals. Bioresour Technol. 2013;136:604-9. http://www.ncbi.nlm.nih.gov/pubmed/23567737
- Armstrong PB, Armstrong MT, Pardy RL, Child A, Wainwright N. Immunohistochemical demonstration of a lipopolysaccharide in the cell wall of a eukaryote, the green alga, Chlorella. Biol Bull. 2002;203(2):203-4. http://www.ncbi.nlm.nih.gov/pubmed/12414578
- Erratum for PMID 21180585. Therap Adv Gastroenterol. 2012;5(5):371. http://ini.sagepub.com/content/3/6/437.abstract

Colloidal Silver

- http://www.scientificamerican.com/article/silver-makes-antibiotics-thousands-of-times-more-effective/, Accessed April 28, 2014
- http://news.rice.edu/2012/07/11/ions-not-particles-make-silver-toxic-to-bacteria-2/, Accessed April 28, 2014

Diatomaceous Earth

- http://wolfcreekranch1.tripod.com/defaq.html, Accessed April 28, 2014
- http://npic.orst.edu/factsheets/degen.html, Accessed April 28, 2015
- http://healthwyze.org/index.php/component/content/article/243-eliminating-the-parasites-that-you-almost-certainly-have-and-curing-lupus.html, Accessed April 28, 2014
- http://www.richsoil.com/diatomaceous-earth.jsp, Accessed April 28, 2014
- http://wellnessmama.com/1969/are-there-bugs-in-your-belly/, Accessed April 28, 2014

Digestive Enzyme

- http://www.lef.org/magazine/mag2009/jan2009_Optimize-Digestive-Health_01.htm, Accessed April 28, 2014
- http://www.lef.org/magazine/mag2013/jan2013_Are-You-Obtaining-the-Proper-Enzymes_01.htm, Accessed April 28, 2014
- http://www.globalhealingcenter.com/natural-health/glucoamylase/, Accessed April 28, 2014
- http://www.globalhealingcenter.com/natural-health/beta-glucanase/, Accessed April 28, 2014
- http://www.eng.umd.edu/~nsw/ench485/lab14.htm, Accessed April 28, 2014

- http://www.gmo-compass.org/eng/database/enzymes/92.pectinase.html, Accessed April 28, 2014
- http://www.globalhealingcenter.com/natural-health/health-benefits-of-hemicellulase, Accessed April 28, 2014
- http://www.globalhealingcenter.com/natural-health/xylanase/, Accessed April 28, 2014
- http://www.klaire.com/images/dppiv_update_article.pdf, Accessed April 28, 2014
- http://www.lef.org/magazine/mag2008/may2008_Powerful-Relief-from-Inflammatory-Pain-And-Other-Age-Related-Disorders_01.htm, Accessed April 28, 2014
- http://www.lef.org/magazine/mag2009/jan2009_Optimize-Digestive-Health_01.htm, Accessed April 28, 2014
- http://www.bio.davidson.edu/Courses/Molbio/MolStudents/spring2010/Gonzalez_Stewart/pepsin.html, Accessed April 28, 2014
- http://www.naturaldigestivehealing.com/blog/2011/10/03/why-i-don%E2%80%99t-recommend-HCL-and-digestive-enzymes/Accessed April 28, 2014

Fish Oil

- Sears, William, Sears, James. *The Omega-3 Effect*, Little, Brown and Company, Aug 28, 2012.

Lactoferrin

- http://robbwolf.com/2011/03/15/the-paleo-solution-episode-71/, Accessed April 28, 2014
- http://www.stanford.edu/group/virus/reo/2005/drug_profile.htm, Accessed April 28, 2014
- https://www.researchgate.net/publication/231583765_Lactoferrin_-_A_multifunctional_protein_with_antimicrobial_properties, Accessed April 28, 2014
- http://www.hnmama.com/html/2013/shike/2.pdf, Accessed April 28, 2014
- https://www.cabdirect.org/cabdirect/abstract/20003015397, Accessed April 28, 2014
- http://aac.asm.org/content/48/4/1242, Accessed April 28, 2014
- http://www.stritch.luc.edu/depts/indii/spec/2009/5-20-2009.pdf, Accessed April 28, 2014
- Manev V, Maneva A, Sirakov L. Effect of lactoferrin on the phagocytic activity of polymorphonuclear leucocytes isolated from blood of patients with autoimmune diseases and *Staphylococcus aureus* allergy. Adv Exp Med Biol. 1998;443:321-30. http://www.ncbi.nlm.nih.gov/pubmed/9781376
- Di mario F, Aragona G, Dal bò N, et al. Use of bovine lactoferrin for *Helicobacter pylori* eradication. Dig Liver Dis. 2003;35(10):706-10. http://www.ncbi.nlm.nih.gov/pubmed/14620619

- Tanaka K, Ikeda M, Nozaki A, et al. Lactoferrin inhibits hepatitis C virus viremia in patients with chronic hepatitis C: a pilot study. Jpn J Cancer Res. 1999;90(4):367-71. http://www.ncbi.nlm.nih.gov/pubmed/10363572
- Nozaki A, Ikeda M, Naganuma A, et al. Identification of a lactoferrin-derived peptide possessing binding activity to hepatitis C virus E2 envelope protein. J Biol Chem. 2003;278(12):10162-73. http://www.ncbi.nlm.nih.gov/pubmed/12522210
- Troost FJ, Steijns J, Saris WH, Brummer RJ. Gastric digestion of bovine lactoferrin in vivo in adults. J Nutr. 2001;131(8):2101-4. http://jn.nutrition.org/content/131/8/2101.long
- Lönnerdal B, Iyer S. Lactoferrin: molecular structure and biological function. Annu Rev Nutr. 1995;15:93-110. http://www.ncbi.nlm.nih.gov/pubmed/8527233
- Bharadwaj S, Naidu AG, Betageri GV, Prasadarao NV, Naidu AS. Milk ribonuclease-enriched lactoferrin induces positive effects on bone turnover markers in postmenopausal women. Osteoporos Int. 2009;20(9):1603-11. http://www.ncbi.nlm.nih.gov/pubmed/19172341
- Karns K, Herr AE. Human tear protein analysis enabled by an alkaline microfluidic homogeneous immunoassay. Anal Chem. 2011;83(21):8115-22. http://pubs.acs.org/doi/abs/10.1021/ac202061v
- Lönnerdal B, Bryant A. Absorption of iron from recombinant human lactoferrin in young US women. Am J Clin Nutr. 2006;83(2):305-9. http://ajcn.nutrition.org/content/83/2/305.full
- Lupetti A, Paulusma-annema A, Welling MM, et al. Synergistic activity of the N-terminal peptide of human lactoferrin and fluconazole against *Candida* species. Antimicrob Agents Chemother. 2003;47(1):262-7. http://www.ncbi.nlm.nih.gov/pmc/articles/PMC149030/
- Takakura N, Wakabayashi H, Ishibashi H, et al. Oral lactoferrin treatment of experimental oral candidiasis in mice. Antimicrob Agents Chemother. 2003;47(8):2619-23. http://www.ncbi.nlm.nih.gov/pmc/articles/PMC166093/

L-Glutamine

- http://umm.edu/health/medical/altmed/supplement/glutamine, Accessed April 28, 2014
- http://www.researchgate.net/publication/5743856_Rapid_healing_of_peptic_ulcers_in_patients_receiving_fresh_cabbage_juice, Accessed April 28, 2014

Lauricidin

- http://www.wellnessresources.com/tips/articles/monolaurin_a_natural_immune_boosting_powerhouse/, Accessed April 28, 2014
- http://www.ppt-health.com/candida-yeast-infections-overview/how-monolaurin-helps-candida-big-time/, Accessed April 28, 2014
- http://www.westonaprice.org/ask-the-doctor/herpes, Accessed April 28, 2014

- Strandberg KL, Peterson ML, Lin YC, Pack MC, Chase DJ, Schlievert PM. Glycerol monolaurate inhibits *Candida* and *Gardnerella vaginalis* in vitro and in vivo but not *Lactobacillus*. Antimicrob Agents Chemother. 2010;54(2):597-601. http://www.ncbi.nlm.nih.gov/pubmed/20008774

Manuka Honey

- http://www.plosone.org/article/info%3Adoi%2F10.1371%2Fjournal.pone.0057679, Accessed April 28, 2014

Melatonin

- http://www.biomedcentral.com/1471-230X/10/7, Accessed April 28, 2014
- Kandil TS, Mousa AA, El-gendy AA, Abbas AM. The potential therapeutic effect of melatonin in Gastro-Esophageal Reflux Disease. BMC Gastroenterol. 2010;10:7. http://www.ncbi.nlm.nih.gov/pmc/articles/PMC2821302/

R-Lipoic Acid

- http://www.lef.org/magazine/mag2005/feb2005_report_lipoic_01.htm, Accessed April 28, 2014
- http://www.lef.org/magazine/mag2007/oct2007_nu_lipoic_acid_01.htm, Accessed April 28, 2014
- Ranieri M, Sciuscio M, Cortese A, et al. Possible role of alpha-lipoic acid in the treatment of peripheral nerve injuries. J Brachial Plex Peripher Nerve Inj. 2010;5:15. http://www.ncbi.nlm.nih.gov/pmc/articles/PMC2939615/
- Ziegler D, Reljanovic M, Mehnert H, Gries FA. Alpha-lipoic acid in the treatment of diabetic polyneuropathy in Germany: current evidence from clinical trials. Exp Clin Endocrinol Diabetes. 1999;107(7):421-30. http://www.ncbi.nlm.nih.gov/pubmed/10595592

Ox Bile

- http://www.drdavidwilliams.com/importance-of-bile-acid#axzz2aAqxl28f, Accessed April 28, 2014

Oxaloacetate

- https://selfhacked.com/2016/08/06/16-scientifically-proven-benefits-oxaloacetate/,Accessed September 09, 2016
- https://blog.bulletproof.com/alan-cash-upgraded-aging-living-longer-with-oxaloacetate-183/,Accessed September 09, 2016
- Wilkins HM, Harris JL, Carl SM, et al. Oxaloacetate activates brain mitochondrial biogenesis, enhances the insulin pathway, reduces inflammation and stimulates neurogenesis. Hum Mol Genet. 2014;23(24):6528-41. http://www.ncbi.nlm.nih.gov/pmc/articles/PMC4271074

Seacure

- http://www.optimumchoices.com/Seacure_research.htm, Accessed April 28, 2014

Undecylenic Acid

- http://www.altmedrev.com/publications/7/1/68.pdf
- http://www.altmedrev.com/publications/7/1/68.pdf. Accessed September 19, 2016.
- Mclain N, Ascanio R, Baker C, Strohaver RA, Dolan JW. Undecylenic acid inhibits morphogenesis of Candida albicans. Antimicrob Agents Chemother. 2000;44(10):2873-5. http://www.ncbi.nlm.nih.gov/pubmed/10991877

Zeaxanthin

- https://www.macular.org/zeaxanthin, Accessed April 28, 2014

Zinc Carnosine

- http://www.lef.org/magazine/mag2008/jan2008_report_agingStomachs_01.htm, Accessed April 28, 2014

- http://lpi.oregonstate.edu/infocenter/minerals/zinc, Accessed April 28, 2014
- http://www.lef.org/magazine/mag2007/jan2007_report_sod_01.htm, Accessed April 28, 2014
- http://www.nowloss.com/ways-to-increase-testosterone-levels-naturally-without-using-steroids.htm, Accessed April 28, 2014
- http://www.lef.org/magazine/mag2011/jan2011_Carnosine-Exceeding-Scientific-Expectations_01.htm, Accessed April 28, 2014
- http://clinical.diabetesjournals.org/content/21/4/186.full, Accessed April 28, 2014
- http://www.sciencedirect.com/science/article/pii/S0165017396000161, Accessed April 28, 2014
- http://ods.od.nih.gov/factsheets/Zinc-HealthProfessional, Accessed April 28, 2014
- Agren MS. Studies on zinc in wound healing. Acta Derm Venereol Suppl (Stockh). 1990;154:1-36. http://www.ncbi.nlm.nih.gov/pubmed/2275309
- Macdonald RS. The role of zinc in growth and cell proliferation. J Nutr. 2000;130(5S Suppl):1500S-8S. http://www.ncbi.nlm.nih.gov/pubmed/10801966
- Peppa M, Raptis SA. Advanced glycation end products and cardiovascular disease. Curr Diabetes Rev. 2008;4(2):92-100. http://www.ncbi.nlm.nih.gov/pubmed/18473756

Herbs

- Balch, Phyllis. *Prescription for Nutritional Healing,* Avery Publishing, 2010.
- Balch, Phyllis. *Prescription for Herbal Healing*, Avery Publishing, 2012.
- Feingold, Ellen. *The Complete Self-Care Guide to Homeopathy, Herbal Remedies & Nutritional Supplements*, Homeopathy Center of Delaware, March 1, 2008.

Aloe Vera

- http://blog.samlennon.net/blog/wp-content/uploads/2012/08/AloeVeraCure.pdf, Accessed April 28, 2014

Astragulus

- http://umm.edu/health/medical/altmed/herb-interaction/possible-interactions-with-astragalus, Accessed April 28, 2014

- Wang DQ, Ding BG, Ma YQ, et al. [Studies on protective effect of total flavonoids of Astragalus on liver damage induced by paracetamol]. Zhongguo Zhong Yao Za Zhi. 2001;26(7):483-6. http://www.ncbi.nlm.nih.gov/pubmed/12776364

Black Raspberries

- Wang DQ, Ding BG, Ma YQ, et al. [Studies on protective effect of total flavonoids of Astragalus on liver damage induced by paracetamol]. Zhongguo Zhong Yao Za Zhi. 2001;26(7):483-6. http://www.ncbi.nlm.nih.gov/pubmed/16800781

Black Walnut Hulls

- http://wellnessmama.com/257/herb-profile-black-walnut-hull/, Accessed April 28, 2014

Boswellia

- https://www.ncbi.nlm.nih.gov/pmc/articles/PMC3309643/, Accessed April 28, 2014
- http://naturalingredient.org/wp/wp-content/uploads/Boswellia_serrata_Monograph.pdf, Accessed April 28, 2014
- Gupta I, Parihar A, Malhotra P, et al. Effects of Boswellia serrata gum resin in patients with ulcerative colitis. Eur J Med Res. 1997;2(1):37-43. http://www.ncbi.nlm.nih.gov/pubmed/9049593

Butchers Broom

- Kathy Abascal and Eric Yarnell. Alternative and Complementary Therapies. December 2005, 11(6): 285-289. doi:10.1089/act.2005.11.285.

Caradmom

- https://www.hdg.muohio.edu/EatingAtMiami/NutritionResources/index.php?fact=Cardamom, Accessed April 28, 2014

Chamomile

- Srivastava JK, Shankar E, Gupta S. Chamomile: A herbal medicine of the past with bright future. Mol Med Rep. 2010;3(6):895-901. http://www.ncbi.nlm.nih.gov/pmc/articles/PMC2995283/

Echinacea

- Mir-rashed N, Cruz I, Jessulat M, et al. Disruption of fungal cell wall by antifungal Echinacea extracts. Med Mycol. 2010;48(7):949-58. http://www.ncbi.nlm.nih.gov/pubmed/20429770

Fennel

- http://www.doctoroz.com/videos/natural-cures-your-most-embarrassing-problems, Accessed April 28, 2014

Ginger

- Gupta S, Ravishankar S. A comparison of the antimicrobial activity of garlic, ginger, carrot, and turmeric pastes against *Escherichia coli O157:H7* in laboratory buffer and ground beef. Foodborne Pathog Dis. 2005;2(4):330-40. http://www.ncbi.nlm.nih.gov/pubmed/16366855
- Ernst E, Pittler MH. Efficacy of ginger for nausea and vomiting: a systematic review of randomized clinical trials. Br J Anaesth. 2000;84(3):367-71. http://www.ncbi.nlm.nih.gov/pubmed/10793599

Goldenseal

- http://www.journalofnaturalproducts.com/Volume3/8_Res_paper-7.pdf, Accessed April 28, 2014
- http://www.anaturalhealingcenter.com/documents/Thorne/articles/Berberine.pdf, Accessed April 28, 2014
- Yu HH, Kim KJ, Cha JD, et al. Antimicrobial activity of berberine alone and in combination with ampicillin or oxacillin against methicillin-resistant *Staphylococcus aureus*. J Med Food. 2005;8(4):454-61. http://www.ncbi.nlm.nih.gov/pubmed/16379555
- Cernáková M, Kostálová D. Antimicrobial activity of berberine--a constituent of Mahonia aquifolium. Folia Microbiol (Praha). 2002;47(4):375-8. http://www.ncbi.nlm.nih.gov/pubmed/12422513

Horse Chestnut

- http://www.drweil.com/vitamins-supplements-herbs/herbs/horse-chestnut/, Accessed April 28, 2014

Licorice

- http://www.naturalmedicinejournal.com/journal/2009-11/deglycyrrhizinated-licorice-gastrointestinal-ulcers, Accessed April 28, 2014
- Das SK, Das V, Gulati AK, Singh VP. Deglycyrrhizinated liquorice in aphthous ulcers. J Assoc Physicians India. 1989;37(10):647. https://www.ncbi.nlm.nih.gov/pubmed/2632514

Marshmallow Root

- http://umm.edu/health/medical/altmed/herb/marshmallow, Accessed April 28, 2014

Mastic Gum

- http://www.nejm.org/doi/full/10.1056/NEJM199812243392618, Accessed April 28, 2014
- Dabos KJ, Sfika E, Vlatta LJ, Giannikopoulos G. The effect of mastic gum on *Helicobacter pylori*: a randomized pilot study. Phytomedicine. 2010;17(3-4):296-9. http://www.ncbi.nlm.nih.gov/pubmed/19879118

Peppermint Oil

- http://bioweb.uwlax.edu/bio203/s2009/johnson_nic4/Classification.htm, Accessed April 28, 2014
- http://ag.arizona.edu/yavapai/publications/yavcobulletins/Growing%20Herbs.pdf, Accessed April 28, 2014
- http://www.greenmedinfo.com/blog/power-peppermint-15-health-benefits-revealed, Accessed April 28, 2014
- http://umm.edu/health/medical/altmed/herb/peppermint, Accessed April 28, 2014
- http://www.painresearchforum.org/news/8488-kappa-opioid-receptors-rekindling-flame, Accessed April 28, 2014
- http://journals.cambridge.org/action/displayAbstract?fromPage=online&aid=464364, Accessed April 28, 2014
- http://www.karger.com/Article/FullText/89139, Accessed April 28, 2014
- http://onlinelibrary.wiley.com/doi/10.1111/j.2042-7158.1994.tb03871.x/pdf, Accessed April 28, 2014
- http://cancerres.aacrjournals.org/content/64/22/8365, Accessed April 28, 2014
- http://www.findaphd.com/search/ProjectDetails.aspx?PJID=47927, Accessed April 28, 2014
- http://www.sciencedirect.com/science/article/pii/S1878535211000232, Accessed April 28, 2014
- http://www.aafp.org/afp/2007/0401/p1027.html, Accessed April 28, 2014
- http://www.altmedrev.com/publications/7/5/410.pdf, Accessed April 28, 2014
- http://www.patient.co.uk/medicine/peppermint-oil-capsules-colpermin-mintec-apercap, Accessed April 28, 2014
- http://umm.edu/health/medical/altmed/herb/peppermint, Accessed April 28, 2014
- http://www.sciencedirect.com/science/article/pii/S1590865807000618, Accessed April 28, 2014
- http://www.sciencedaily.com/releases/2012/05/120525103354.htm, Accessed April 28, 2014
- Quigley EM. Bacterial flora in irritable bowel syndrome: role in pathophysiology, implications for management. J Dig Dis. 2007;8(1):2-7. http://www.ncbi.nlm.nih.gov/pubmed/17261128
- Dukowicz AC, Lacy BE, Levine GM. Small intestinal bacterial overgrowth: a comprehensive review. Gastroenterol Hepatol (N Y). 2007;3(2):112-22. http://www.ncbi.nlm.nih.gov/pmc/articles/PMC3099351/

Sangre de Drago

- http://www.webmd.com/vitamins-supplements/ingredientmono-755-sangre%20de%20grado.aspx?activeingredientid=755&, Accessed April 28, 2014
- http://www.naturalnews.com/026764_Sangre_de_Drago_medicinal_power.html, Accessed April 28, 2014
- Tradtrantip L, Namkung W, Verkman AS. Crofelemer, an antisecretory antidiarrheal proanthocyanidin oligomer extracted from Croton lechleri, targets two distinct intestinal chloride channels. Mol Pharmacol. 2010;77(1):69-78. http://www.ncbi.nlm.nih.gov/pmc/articles/PMC2802429/
- Miller MJ, Macnaughton WK, Zhang XJ, et al. Treatment of gastric ulcers and diarrhea with the Amazonian herbal medicine Sangre de Grado. Am J Physiol Gastrointest Liver Physiol. 2000;279(1):G192-200. http://www.ncbi.nlm.nih.gov/pubmed/10898763

Slippery Elm Bark

- http://umm.edu/health/medical/altmed/herb/slippery-elm, Accessed April 28, 2014

Triphala

- http://www.mapi.com/ayurvedic-knowledge/plants-spices-and-oils/triphala-a-powerhouse-ayurvedic-herb.html#gsc.tab=0, Accessed April 28, 2014
- Biradar YS, Jagatap S, Khandelwal KR, Singhania SS. Exploring of Antimicrobial Activity of Triphala Mashi-an Ayurvedic Formulation. Evid Based Complement Alternat Med. 2008;5(1):107-13. http://www.ncbi.nlm.nih.gov/pmc/articles/PMC2249739/

Antibiotic and Medicine Guide

- Beers, Mark. *The Merck Manual*, Merck Research Laboratories, 2006.
- *Physicians' Desk Reference*, PDR Network LLC, 2011.
- http://www.fda.gov/drugs/drugsafety/postmarketdrugsafetyinformationforpatientsandproviders/ucm111085.htm, Accessed April 28, 2014

Common Diagnostic Tests

- Beers, Mark. *The Merck Manual*, Merck Research Laboratories, 2006.
- Pagrana, Kathleen, Pagana, Timothy. *Mosby's Diagnostic and Laboratory Test Reference*, Mosby, October 5, 2012.
- http://owndoc.com/candida-albicans/candida-facts/
- https://www.cedars-sinai.edu/Patients/Programs-and-Services/Imaging-Center/For-Patients/Exams-by-Procedure/X-ray-and-Fluoroscopy/Sitz-Marker-Study.aspx
- http://my.clevelandclinic.org/services/Esophageal_pH_Test/hic_24-Hour_Esophageal_pH_Test.aspx

GERD

- Beers, Mark. *The Merck Manual*, Merck Research Laboratories, 2006.
- Wright, Jonathan. *Why Stomach Acid Is Good For You,* M. Evans & Company, August 20, 2001.
- Rodriguez, Jorge / Wyler, Susan. *The Acid Reflux Solution*, Ten Speed Press, March 27, 2012.
- Brownstein, David. *Drugs That Don't Work and Natural Therapies That Do!*, Medical Alternative Press, 2007.
- Rubin, Jordan /Brasco, Joseph. *Restoring Your Digestive Health*, Twin Streams Publishing, 2003.

Sites

- http://chriskresser.com/the-hidden-causes-of-heartburn-and-gerd, Accessed April 28, 2014.
- http://www.siboinfo.com/symptoms.html, Accessed April 28, 2014.
- http://gut.bmj.com/content/54/suppl_1/i13.full, Accessed April 28, 2014.
- http://chriskresser.com/fodmaps-could-common-foods-be-harming-your-digestive-health, Accessed April 28, 2014.
- http://chriskresser.com/are-gmos-safe, Accessed April 28, 2014.
- http://www.webmd.com/heartburn-gerd/guide/lifestyle-changes-heartburn, Accessed April 28, 2014.
- http://www.ucdmc.ucdavis.edu/welcome/features/20081204_heartburn/index.html, Accessed April 28, 2014.
- http://www.ecaware.org/what-is-esophageal-cancer/risk-factors/acid-reflux-gerd/, Accessed April 28, 2014.
- http://www.drlwilson.com/articles/candida.htm, Accessed April 28, 2014.
- http://www.bobcotton.com/gerdsalt.htm, Accessed April 28, 2014.
- http://www.westonaprice.org/digestive-disorders/acid-reflux-a-red-flag, Accessed April 28, 2014.

- http://www.slate.com/articles/health_and_science/science/2010/08/dont_just_sit_there.html, Accessed April 28, 2014.
- http://www.fda.gov/drugs/drugsafety/ucm245011.htm, Accessed April 28, 2014.
- http://www.preventionandhealing.com/articles/Acid_Reflux_and_Rebellious_Stomach-NEW.pdf, Accessed April 28, 2014.
- http://www.gastro.theclinics.com/article/S0889-8553%2805%2970102-3/abstract, Accessed April 28, 2014.
- http://www.hon.ch/OESO/books/Vol_6_Barrett_s_Esophagus/Articles/vol2/art023.html, Accessed April 28, 2014.

Studies

- Pali-schöll I, Jensen-jarolim E. Anti-acid medication as a risk factor for food allergy. Allergy. 2011;66(4):469-77. http://www.ncbi.nlm.nih.gov/pubmed/21121928
- Compare D, Pica L, Rocco A, et al. Effects of long-term PPI treatment on producing bowel symptoms and SIBO. Eur J Clin Invest. 2011;41(4):380-6 http//www.ncbi.nlm.nih.gov/pubmed/21128930

SIBO

- Dr. Brownsetin, David. *Drugs That Don't Work and Natural Therapies that Do!*, Medical Alternative Press, 2007.

Leaky Gut

- http://www.optimumchoices.com/Seacure_research.htm, Accessed April 28, 2014.

Peppermint Oil

- http://www.altmedrev...ons/7/5/410.pdf, Accessed April 28, 2014.

Biofilms

- https://selfhacked.com/2016/03/01/44-science-backed-ways-to-inhibit-biofilms-naturally-with-references/, Accessed April 28, 2014.
- http://chriskresser.com/treating-sibo-cold-thermogenisis-and-when-to-take-probiotics, Accessed April 28, 2014.
- http://www.advancedhealing.com/dr-ettingers-biofilm-protocol-for-lyme-and-gut-pathogens/, Accessed April 28, 2014.
- Barrett JS, Canale KE, Gearry RB, Irving PM, Gibson PR. Probiotic effects on intestinal fermentation patterns in patients with irritable bowel syndrome. World J Gastroenterol. 2008;14(32):5020-4. http://www.ncbi.nlm.nih.gov/pmc/articles/PMC2742929/
- Kite P, Eastwood K, Sugden S, Percival SL. Use of in vivo-generated biofilms from hemodialysis catheters to test the efficacy of a novel antimicrobial catheter lock for biofilm eradication in vitro. J Clin Microbiol. 2004;42(7):3073-6. http://jcm.asm.org/content/42/7/3073.full.pdf
- Wakabayashi H, Yamauchi K, Kobayashi T, Yaeshima T, Iwatsuki K, Yoshie H. Inhibitory effects of lactoferrin on growth and biofilm formation of *Porphyromonas gingivalis* and *Prevotella intermedia*. Antimicrob Agents Chemother. 2009;53(8):3308-16. http://www.ncbi.nlm.nih.gov/pmc/articles/PMC2715627/

SIYO

- http://owndoc.com/candida-albicans/candida-facts/, Accessed April 28, 2014.
- http://www.yeastinfection.org/functional-candida-testing-elisa-blood-and-saliva-tests/, Accessed April 28, 2014.
- http://owndoc.com/candida-albicans/spit-test-candida-diagnosis-unreliable/, Accessed April 28, 2014.
- http://www.drlwilson.com/articles/candida.htm, Accessed April 28, 2014.
- Parodi A, Paolino S, Greco A, et al. Small intestinal bacterial overgrowth in rosacea: clinical effectiveness of its eradication. Clin Gastroenterol Hepatol. 2008;6(7):759-6 http://www.ncbi.nlm.nih.gov/pubmed/18456568
- Muñoz P, Bouza E, Cuenca-estrella M, et al. *Saccharomyces cerevisiae* fungemia: an emerging infectious disease. Clin Infect Dis. 2005;40(11):1625-34. http://www.ncbi.nlm.nih.gov/pubmed/15889360

General SIBO Information

- http://www.siboinfo.com/overview.html, Accessed April 28, 2014.
- http://www.siboinfo.com/testing1.html, Accessed April 28, 2014.
- http://www.siboinfo.com/overview.html, Accessed April 28, 2014.
- http://chriskresser.com/treating-sibo-cold-thermogenisis-and-when-to-take-probiotics, Accessed April 28, 2014.
- http://ndnr.com/web-articles/gastrointestinal/small-intestine-bacterial-overgrowth-2/, Accessed April 28, 2014.
- http://www.siboinfo.com/prevention.html, Accessed April 28, 2014.
- Bures J, Cyrany J, Kohoutova D, et al. Small intestinal bacterial overgrowth syndrome. World J Gastroenterol. 2010;16(24):2978-90. http://www.ncbi.nlm.nih.gov/pmc/articles/PMC2890937/
- Rhoads JM, Argenzio RA, Chen W, et al. L-glutamine stimulates intestinal cell proliferation and activates mitogen-activated protein kinases. Am J Physiol. 1997;272(5 Pt 1):G943-53. http://www.ncbi.nlm.nih.gov/pubmed/9176200

Curcumin

- http://lpi.oregonstate.edu/infocenter/phytochemicals/curcumin/, Accessed April 28, 2014.
- Auricchio S, De ritis G, De vincenzi M, et al. Mannan and oligomers of N-acetylglucosamine protect intestinal mucosa of celiac patients with active disease from in vitro toxicity of gliadin peptides. Gastroenterology. 1990;99(4):973-8. http://www.ncbi.nlm.nih.gov/pubmed/2394351

H. pylori and Gastritis

H. pylori General Info

- http://chriskresser.com/more-evidence-to-support-the-theory-that-gerd-is-caused-by-bacterial-overgrowth, Accessed April 28, 2014.
- http://digestive.niddk.nih.gov/ddiseases/pubs/hpylori/, Accessed April 28, 2014.
- http://www.cancer.gov/cancertopics/factsheet/Risk/h-pylori-cancer, Accessed April 28, 2014.
- http://www.mayoclinic.com/health/h-pylori/DS00958/DSECTION=symptoms, Accessed April 28, 2014.
- http://www.med.nyu.edu/medicine/labs/blaserlab/, Accessed April 28, 2014.
- http://www.nytimes.com/2011/11/01/health/scientist-examines-possible-link-between-antibiotics-and-obesity.html?_r=0, Accessed April 28, 2014.

- http://www.sciencedaily.com/releases/2008/10/081006092511.htm, Accessed April 28, 2014.
- Blaser MJ. *Helicobacter pylori* and gastric diseases. BMJ. 1998;316(7143):1507-10. http://www.ncbi.nlm.nih.gov/pmc/articles/PMC1113159/

H. pylori Supplements

- Balch, Phyllis. Prescription for Herbal Healing, Avery Publishing, 2012.
- http://www.anaturalhealingcenter.com/documents/Thorne/articles/helicobacter_pylori.pdf , Accessed April 28, 2014.
- http://www.meschinohealth.com/ArticleDirectory/Oil_Of_Oregano_Natures_Antibiotic_And_Anti-Fungal_Supplement, Accessed April 28, 2014.
- Dabos KJ, Sfika E, Vlatta LJ, Giannikopoulos G. The effect of mastic gum on *Helicobacter pylori*: a randomized pilot study. Phytomedicine. 2010;17(3-4):296-9. http://www.ncbi.nlm.nih.gov/pubmed/19879118
- Zhang L, Ma J, Pan K, Go VL, Chen J, You WC. Efficacy of cranberry juice on *Helicobacter pylori* infection: a double-blind, randomized placebo-controlled trial. *Helicobacter*. 2005;10(2):139-45. http://www.ncbi.nlm.nih.gov/pubmed/15810945
- Nzeako BC, Al-namaani F. The antibacterial activity of honey on *Helicobacter pylori*. Sultan Qaboos Univ Med J. 2006;6(2):71-6. http://www.ncbi.nlm.nih.gov/pmc/articles/PMC3074916/

Gastritis / Ulcers General Information

- Beers, Mark. The Merck Manual, Merck Research Laboratories, 2006.
- http://digestive.niddk.nih.gov/ddiseases/pubs/hpylori/, Accessed April 28, 2014.

Ulcer Supplements:

- http://news.harvard.edu/gazette/story/2009/05/glutamine-supplements-show-promise-in-treating-stomach-ulcers/, Accessed April 28, 2014.
- Mahmood A, Fitzgerald AJ, Marchbank T, et al. Zinc carnosine, a health food supplement that stabilises small bowel integrity and stimulates gut repair processes. Gut. 2007;56(2):168-75. http://www.ncbi.nlm.nih.gov/pmc/articles/PMC1856764/
- Das SK, Das V, Gulati AK, Singh VP. Deglycyrrhizinated liquorice in aphthous ulcers. J Assoc Physicians India. 1989;37(10):647. http://www.ncbi.nlm.nih.gov/pubmed/2632514

Zinc carnosine:

- Halpern, Georges. *Zinc Carnosine Nature's Safe and Effective Remedy For Ulcers*, Square One Publishers, May 1, 2005.
- http://www.lef.org/magazine/mag2008/jan2008_report_agingStomachs_01.htm, Accessed April 28, 2014.

DGL licorice:

- Bowden, Jonny. *The Most Effective Natural Cures on Earth*, Fair Winds Press, August 1, 2011.
- http://www.naturalmedicinejournal.com/journal/2009-11/deglycyrrhizinated-licorice-gastrointestinal-ulcers, Accessed April 28, 2014.

Activated charcoal:

- http://healthwyze.org/index.php/component/content/article/408-how-to-quickly-remedy-food-poisoning.html, Accessed April 28, 2014.

GMO Information, Posture, Clothing

GMO's and the Standard American Diet

- http://www.nongmoproject.org/learn-more/what-is-gmo/, Accessed April 28, 2014.
- http://www.nongmoshoppingguide.com/, Accessed April 28, 2014.
- http://www.mnn.com/food/healthy-eating/stories/genetic-engineering-vs-selective-breeding, Accessed April 28, 2014.
- http://www.greenmedinfo.com/blog/new-study-proves-bt-toxins-gmos-toxic-mammalian-blood, Accessed April 28, 2014.
- http://www.businessinsider.com/walmart-is-going-to-sell-monsantos-genetically-modified-corn-and-it-wont-be-labeled-2012-8, Accessed April 28, 2014.
- http://www.wheatbellyblog.com/2012/04/the-happy-wheat-free-intestine/, Accessed April 28, 2014.

- http://responsibletechnology.org/gmo-education/65-health-risks-of-gm-foods/, Accessed April 28, 2014.
- http://www.drfranklipman.com/got-tummy-troubles/, Accessed April 28, 2014.
- http://www.cornucopia.org/wp-content/uploads/2013/02/Carrageenan-Report1.pdf, Accessed April 28, 2014.
- http://digitaljournal.com/article/325050, Accessed April 28, 2014.
- http://www.responsibletechnology.org/gmo-education, Accessed April 28, 2014.
- Rao SS, Attaluri A, Anderson L, Stumbo P. Ability of the normal human small intestine to absorb fructose: evaluation by breath testing. Clin Gastroenterol Hepatol. 2007;5(8):959-63. http://www.ncbi.nlm.nih.gov/pmc/articles/PMC1994910/

LES

Calcium Citrate: Dr. Leo Galland

- http://www.huffingtonpost.com/leo-galland-md/acid-reflux-the-truth-beh_b_541649.html, Accessed April 28, 2014.

R-Lipoic Acid

- Ranieri M, Sciuscio M, Cortese A, et al. Possible role of alpha-lipoic acid in the treatment of peripheral nerve injuries. J Brachial Plex Peripher Nerve Inj. 2010;5:15 http://www.ncbi.nlm.nih.gov/pmc/articles/PMC2939615/
- Ziegler D, Reljanovic M, Mehnert H, Gries FA. Alpha-lipoic acid in the treatment of diabetic polyneuropathy in Germany: current evidence from clinical trials. Exp Clin Endocrinol Diabetes. 1999;107(7):421-30. http://www.ncbi.nlm.nih.gov/pubmed/10595592

Melatonin

- http://www.biomedcentral.com/1471-230X/10/7, Accessed April 28, 2014.
- Jentoft JE, Smith LM, Fu XD, Johnson M, Leis J. Conserved cysteine and histidine residues of the avian myeloblastosis virus nucleocapsid protein are essential for viral replication but are not "zinc-binding fingers". Proc Natl Acad Sci USA. 1988;85(19):7094-8. http://www.ncbi.nlm.nih.gov/pmc/articles/PMC2821302/

5-HTP

- http://www.naturalmedicinejournal.com/journal/2011-10/many-uses-5-htp, Accessed April 28, 2014.
- https://www.scribd.com/document/80455343/5HTP-as-Precursor, Accessed April 28, 2014.
- Saegusa Y, Takeda H, Muto S, et al. Decreased motility of the lower esophageal sphincter in a rat model of gastroesophageal reflux disease may be mediated by reductions of serotonin and acetylcholine signaling. Biol Pharm Bull. 2011;34(5):704-11. http://www.ncbi.nlm.nih.gov/pubmed/21532161
- Rattan S, Goyal RK. Effects of 5-hydroxytryptamine on the lower esophageal sphincter in vivo: evidence for multiple sites of action. J Clin Invest. 1977;59(1):125-33. http://www.ncbi.nlm.nih.gov/pmc/articles/PMC333339/

Candida albicans

- Boroch, Ann. *The Candida Cure*, Quintessential Healing Publishing, Inc., 2009.

Candida General Information

- http://emedicine.medscape.com/article/781215-clinical, Accessed April 28, 2014.
- http://onlinelibrary.wiley.com/doi/10.1002/cbf.1533/pdf, Accessed April 28, 2014
- http://www.marksdailyapple.com/candida/#axzz2gFRgEAgw, Accessed April 28, 2014
- http://www.medicinenet.com/white_tongue/symptoms.htm, Accessed April 28, 2014
- http://www.drlwilson.com/articles/candida.htm, Accessed April 28, 2014
- http://www.healingnaturallybybee.com/articles/heal2.php, Accessed April 28, 2014
- Bernhardt H, Wellmer A, Zimmermann K, Knoke M. Growth of *Candida albicans* in normal and altered faecal flora in the model of continuous flow culture. Mycoses. 1995;38(7-8):265-70. http://www.ncbi.nlm.nih.gov/pubmed/8559187
- Cat TB, Charash W, Hebert J, et al. Potential influence of antisecretory therapy on the development of *Candida*-associated intraabdominal infection. Ann Pharmacother. 2008;42(2):185-91. http://www.ncbi.nlm.nih.gov/pubmed/18212256

Herx Information and Protocols

- http://candidapage.com/aldehyde.shtml, Accessed April 28, 2014
- http://www.drsusanmarra.com/sites/default/files/resources/forms/HerxheimerReaction110811.pdf, Accessed April 28, 2014

Candida Protocol Supplements

- http://www.newswithviews.com/Howenstine/james49.htm, Accessed April 28, 2014
- http://onlinelibrary.wiley.com/doi/10.1111/j.1574-6968.2010.02037.x/abstract, Accessed April 28, 2014
- http://www.biomedcentral.com/content/pdf/1472-6831-10-18.pdf, Accessed April 28, 2014
- http://www.thecandidadiet.com/oreganooil.htm, Accessed April 28, 2014
- http://www.wellnessresources.com/health/articles/niacinamide_turns_out_to_be_a_potent_candida-killing_nutrient/, Accessed April 28, 2014
- http://www.wellnessresources.com/tips/articles/monolaurin_a_natural_immune_boosting_powerhouse/, Accessed April 28, 2014
- http://www.allicinfacts.com/about-allicin/medical-uses/allicin-medical-uses-c/, Accessed April 28, 2014
- http://www.thecandidadiet.com/olive-leaf-extract.htm, Accessed April 28, 2014

Monolaurin

- http://www.touroinstitute.com/natural%20bactericidal.pdf, Accessed April 28, 2014
- Carpo BG, Verallo-rowell VM, Kabara J. Novel antibacterial activity of monolaurin compared with conventional antibiotics against organisms from skin infections: an in vitro study. J Drugs Dermatol. 2007;6(10):991-8. http://www.ncbi.nlm.nih.gov/pubmed/17966176

Oregano Oil

- http://jmm.sgmjournals.org/content/56/4/519.full, Accessed April 28, 2014

Molybdenum

- http://www.arthritistrust.org/Articles/Molybdenum%20for%20Candida%20albicans%20Patients.pdf, Accessed April 28, 2014

Coconut Oil

- http://www.naturalnews.com/025199_oil_coconut.html, Accessed April 28, 2014
- Ogbolu DO, Oni AA, Daini OA, Oloko AP. In vitro antimicrobial properties of coconut oil on *Candida* species in Ibadan, Nigeria. J Med Food. 2007;10(2):384-7. http://www.ncbi.nlm.nih.gov/pubmed/17651080

Constipation and Chloride

Constipation Information

- Beers, Mark. *The Merck Manual*, Merck Research Laboratories, 2006.
- Jones, Wes. *Cure Constipation Now*, Berkley Trade, July 7, 2009.

Constipation Protocols

- http://www.huffingtonpost.com/2012/10/01/squatty-potty-wants-to-en_n_1929747.html, Accessed April 28, 2014
- http://steveclarknd.com/?page_id=201, Accessed April 28, 2014
- http://www.lef.org/protocols/gastrointestinal/constipation_01.html, Accessed April 28, 2014
- http://www.lef.org/protocols/gastrointestinal/constipation_05.htm#supplements, Accessed April 28, 2014
- http://lpi.oregonstate.edu/infocenter/phytochemicals/curcumin/, Accessed April 28, 2014
- Rhoads JM, Argenzio RA, Chen W, et al. L-glutamine stimulates intestinal cell proliferation and activates mitogen-activated protein kinases. Am J Physiol. 1997;272(5 Pt 1):G943-53. http://www.ncbi.nlm.nih.gov/pubmed/9176200

- Auricchio S, De ritis G, De vincenzi M, et al. Mannan and oligomers of N-acetylglucosamine protect intestinal mucosa of celiac patients with active disease from in vitro toxicity of gliadin peptides. Gastroenterology. 1990;99(4):973-8. http://www.ncbi.nlm.nih.gov/pubmed/2394351

Importance of Chloride

- http://www.bobcotton.com/gerdsalt.htm, Accessed April 28, 2014

Gallbladder, Liver, and Pancreas

- Beers, Mark. *The Merck Manual*, Merck Research Laboratories, 2006.
- Jane B. Reece, Lisa A. Urry, Michael L. Cain, Steven A. Wasserman, Peter Minorsky, Robert Jackson. *Campbell Biology*, Benjamin Cummings, October 7, 2010.
- Patton, Kevin, Thibodeau, Gary, Douglas, Matthew. *Essentials of Anatomy and Physiology*, Mosby, March 16, 2011.

Gallbladder, Liver, and Pancreas General Information

- http://www.jackkruse.com/cpc-3-do-you-need-a-gallbladder/, Accessed April 28, 2014

Gallbladder, Liver, and Pancreas Protocols

R-Lipoic Acid

- http://www.lef.org/magazine/mag2005/feb2005_report_lipoic_01.htm, Accessed April 28, 2014
- http://www.lef.org/magazine/mag2007/oct2007_nu_lipoic_acid_01.htm, Accessed April 28, 2014

- Bustamante J, Lodge JK, Marcocci L, Tritschler HJ, Packer L, Rihn BH. Alpha-lipoic acid in liver metabolism and disease. Free Radic Biol Med. 1998;24(6):1023-39. http://www.ncbi.nlm.nih.gov/pubmed/9607614
- Jacob S, Ruus P, Hermann R, et al. Oral administration of RAC-alpha-lipoic acid modulates insulin sensitivity in patients with type-2 diabetes mellitus: a placebo-controlled pilot trial. Free Radic Biol Med. 1999;27(3-4):309-14. http://www.ncbi.nlm.nih.gov/pubmed/10468203

Milk Thistle

- http://www.umm.edu/altmed/articles/milk-thistle-000266.htm, Accessed April 28, 2014

Liver Protocols

- http://onlinelibrary.wiley.com/doi/10.1111/liv.12025/full, Accessed April 28, 2014
- http://www.healthyimmunity.com/pdfs/Schisandra_Strengthens_Liver.pdf, Accessed April 28, 2014
- http://www.lef.org/magazine/mag2010/may2010_N-Acetyl-Cysteine_01.htm, Accessed April 28, 2014
- http://ajcn.nutrition.org/content/58/1/103.abstract, Accessed April 28, 2014
- http://www.bulletproofexec.com/calcium-d-glucarate/, Accessed April 28, 2014
- Pradhan SC, Girish C. Hepatoprotective herbal drug, silymarin from experimental pharmacology to clinical medicine. Indian J Med Res. 2006;124(5):491-504. http://www.ncbi.nlm.nih.gov/pubmed/17213517
- Wang DQ, Ding BG, Ma YQ, et al. [Studies on protective effect of total flavonoids of Astragalus on liver damage induced by paracetamol]. Zhongguo Zhong Yao Za Zhi. 2001;26(7):483-6. http://www.ncbi.nlm.nih.gov/pubmed/12776364
- Kent KD, Harper WJ, Bomser JA. Effect of whey protein isolate on intracellular glutathione and oxidant-induced cell death in human prostate epithelial cells. Toxicol In Vitro. 2003;17(1):27-33. http://www.ncbi.nlm.nih.gov/pubmed/12537959

Gallbladder Protocols

- http://www.drdavidwilliams.com/importance-of-bile-acid#axzz2ifPBvwr9, Accessed April 28, 2014
- http://www.mayoclinic.com/health/gallbladder-cleanse/AN01283, Accessed April 28, 2014

- http://www.motilitysociety.org/patient/pdf/Dumping%20Diet%205%204b%202006.pdf, Accessed April 28, 2014
- Ko CW. Magnesium: does a mineral prevent gallstones?. Am J Gastroenterol. 2008;103(2):383-5. http://www.ncbi.nlm.nih.gov/pubmed/18289201

Pancreas

- http://drsircus.com/medicine/magnesium/the-insulin-magnesium-story-2, Accessed April 28, 2014
- http://www.nlm.nih.gov/medlineplus/ency/article/003135.htm, Accessed April 28, 2014
- Jones K. Review of sangre de drago (Croton lechleri)--a South American tree sap in the treatment of diarrhea, inflammation, insect bites, viral infections, and wounds: traditional uses to clinical research. J Altern Complement Med. 2003;9(6):877-96. http://www.ncbi.nlm.nih.gov/pubmed/14736360
- Iodice S, Gandini S, Maisonneuve P, Lowenfels AB. Tobacco and the risk of pancreatic cancer: a review and meta-analysis. Langenbecks Arch Surg. 2008;393(4):535-45. http://www.ncbi.nlm.nih.gov/pubmed/18193270

Parasites

Parasite General Information

- Beers, Mark. *The Merck Manual*, Merck Research Laboratories, 2006.
- http://www.cdc.gov/parasites/water.html, Accessed April 28, 2014
- http://www.cdc.gov/parasites/trichinellosis/gen_info/faqs.html, Accessed April 28, 2014
- http://www.nbcnews.com/health/cat-poop-parasites-may-pose-public-health-hazard-study-suggests-6C10574506, Accessed April 28, 2014
- http://www.cdc.gov/parasites/hookworm/, Accessed April 28, 2014
- http://www.who.int/bulletin/volumes/87/2/07-047308/en/, Accessed April 28, 2014
- https://fri.wisc.edu/files/Briefs_File/parasites.pdf, Accessed April 28, 2014
- http://www.totalityofbeing.com/FramelessPages/Articles/organic_vs_nonorganic.html, Accessed April 28, 2014
- http://www.huffingtonpost.com/2012/07/05/toxoplasma-gondii-brain-parasite-suicide-cats_n_1651523.html, Accessed April 28, 2014

Piperine

- http://apps.who.int/medicinedocs/en/d/Jwhozip48e/6.5.html, Accessed April 28, 2014
- http://www.ingentaconnect.com/content/govi/pharmaz/2008/00000063/00000005/art00005?crawler=true, Accessed April 28, 2014
- http://www.sciencedaily.com/releases/2009/03/090311085151.htm, Accessed April 28, 2014
- http://www.sciencedirect.com/science/article/pii/0005273695000558, Accessed April 28, 2014
- http://www.sciencedirect.com/science/article/pii/S0960894X04005177, Accessed April 28, 2014
- https://www.ncbi.nlm.nih.gov/pmc/articles/PMC3588050/, Accessed April 28, 2014
- Veerareddy PR, Vobalaboina V, Nahid A. Formulation and evaluation of oil-in-water emulsions of piperine in visceral leishmaniasis. Pharmazie. 2004;59(3):194-7. http://www.ncbi.nlm.nih.gov/pubmed/15074591
- Atal N, Bedi KL. Bioenhancers: Revolutionary concept to market. J Ayurveda Integr Med. 2010;1(2):96-9. http://www.ncbi.nlm.nih.gov/pmc/articles/PMC3151395/
- Li S, Lei Y, Jia Y, Li N, Wink M, Ma Y. Piperine, a piperidine alkaloid from Piper nigrum re-sensitizes P-gp, MRP1 and BCRP dependent multidrug resistant cancer cells. Phytomedicine. 2011;19(1):83-7. http://www.ncbi.nlm.nih.gov/pubmed/21802927
- Ferreira C, Soares DC, Barreto-junior CB, et al. Leishmanicidal effects of piperine, its derivatives, and analogues on Leishmania amazonensis. Phytochemistry. 2011;72(17):2155-64. http://www.ncbi.nlm.nih.gov/pubmed/21885074
- Singh TU, Kumar D, Tandan SK. Paralytic effect of alcoholic extract of Allium sativum and Piper longum on liver amphistome, Gigantocotyle explanatum. Indian J Pharmacol. 2008;40(2):64-8. http://www.ncbi.nlm.nih.gov/pmc/articles/PMC3025128/

Diatomaceous Earth

- http://wolfcreekranch1.tripod.com/defaq.html, Accessed April 28, 2014
- http://npic.orst.edu/factsheets/degen.html, Accessed April 28, 2014
- http://healthwyze.org/index.php/component/content/article/243-eliminating-the-parasites-that-you-almost-certainly-have-and-curing-lupus.html, Accessed April 28, 2014
- http://www.richsoil.com/diatomaceous-earth.jsp, Accessed April 28, 2014
- http://wellnessmama.com/1969/are-there-bugs-in-your-belly/, Accessed April 28, 2014

Black Walnut / Wormwood

- http://www.janethull.com/newsletter/0709/getting_the_bugs_out.php, Accessed April 28, 2014

D-Limonene

- https://www.lef.org/magazine/mag2007/apr2007_atd_01.htm, Accessed April 28, 2014
- http://www.anaturalhealingcenter.com/documents/Thorne/articles/Limonene12-3.pdf, Accessed April 28, 2014
- http://www.lef.org/magazine/mag2006/sep2006_cover_heartburn_01.htm, Accessed April 28, 2014
- http://www.epa.gov/iris/subst/0682.htm, Accessed April 28, 2014
- http://www.biochemcorp.com/dlimonene2.htm, Accessed April 28, 2014
- http://www.anaturalhealingcenter.com/documents/Thorne/articles/Limonene12-3.pdf, Accessed April 28, 2014
- Sun J. D-Limonene: safety and clinical applications. Altern Med Rev. 2007;12(3):259-64. http://www.ncbi.nlm.nih.gov/pubmed/18072821
- Vigushin DM, Poon GK, Boddy A, et al. Phase I and pharmacokinetic study of D-limonene in patients with advanced cancer. Cancer Research Campaign Phase I/II Clinical Trials Committee. Cancer Chemother Pharmacol. 1998;42(2):111-7. http://www.ncbi.nlm.nih.gov/pubmed/9654110
- Jia SS, Xi GP, Zhang M, et al. Induction of apoptosis by D-limonene is mediated by inactivation of Akt in LS174T human colon cancer cells. Oncol Rep. 2013;29(1):349-54. http://www.ncbi.nlm.nih.gov/pubmed/23117412
- Chidambara murthy KN, Jayaprakasha GK, Patil BS. D-limonene rich volatile oil from blood oranges inhibits angiogenesis, metastasis and cell death in human colon cancer cells. Life Sci. 2012;91(11-12):429-39. http://www.ncbi.nlm.nih.gov/pubmed/22935404

LERD

- Bauer, Marc / Koufman, Jamie / Stern, Jordan. *Dropping Acid: The Reflux Diet Cookbook & Cure*, Reflux Cookbooks, September 16, 2010.
- http://www.voiceinstituteofnewyork.com/articles-and-publications/acid-reflux-15-groundbreaking-articles/, Accessed April 25, 2014.

Gastroparesis

Gastroparesis Caused by Nerve Damage

- http://my.clevelandclinic.org/disorders/gastroparesis/dd_overview.aspx, Accessed April 28, 2014

Ginger

- Wu KL, Rayner CK, Chuah SK, et al. Effects of ginger on gastric emptying and motility in healthy humans. Eur J Gastroenterol Hepatol. 2008;20(5):436-40. http://www.ncbi.nlm.nih.gov/pubmed/18403946
- Hu ML, Rayner CK, Wu KL, et al. Effect of ginger on gastric motility and symptoms of functional dyspepsia. World J Gastroenterol. 2011;17(1):105-10. http://www.ncbi.nlm.nih.gov/pmc/articles/PMC3016669/

Low Residue Diet

- http://www.colemangastro.com/patient-education/gastroparesis-diet, Accessed April 28, 2014

Cyclic Vomiting Syndrome

Cause of Cyclic Vomiting Syndrome is Mitochondrial Disturbance

- http://ghr.nlm.nih.gov/condition/cyclic-vomiting-syndrome, Accessed April 28, 2014
- Boles RG, Williams JC. Mitochondrial disease and cyclic vomiting syndrome. Dig Dis Sci. 1999;44(8 Suppl):103S-107S. http://www.ncbi.nlm.nih.gov/pubmed/10490048

L-Carnosine

- http://www.biomedcentral.com/1471-2377/11/102, Accessed April 28, 2014
- Van calcar SC, Harding CO, Wolff JA. L-carnitine administration reduces number of episodes in cyclic vomiting syndrome. Clin Pediatr (Phila). 2002;41(3):171-4. http://www.ncbi.nlm.nih.gov/pubmed/11999680

CoQ10

- http://articles.mercola.com/sites/articles/archive/2012/06/07/dr-robert-barry-on-coq10.aspx, Accessed April 28, 2014
- http://www.lef.org/magazine/mag2008/feb2008_Alleviating-Congestive-Heart-Failure-With-Coenzyme-Q10_01.htm, Accessed April 28, 2014
- http://www.lef.org/magazine/mag2007/jan2007_report_coq10_01.htm, Accessed April 28, 2014
- http://www.marksdailyapple.com/managing-your-mitochondria-nutrients-and-supplements/#axzz2hICMvYjy, Accessed April 28, 2014
- http://www.sciencemag.org/content/336/6086/1241, Accessed April 28, 2014
- http://www.lef.org/protocols/dental/gingivitis_05.htm, Accessed April 28, 2014
- http://www.coconutresearchcenter.com/hwnl_4-2.htm, Accessed April 28, 2014
- http://www.westonaprice.org/cardiovascular-disease/coenzyme-q10-for-healthy-hearts, Accessed April 28, 2014

PQQ

- http://www.lef.org/magazine/mag2011/feb2011_Generate-Fresh-Mitochondria-with-PQQ_01.htm, Accessed April 28, 2014

Barrett's Esophagus

- http://www.naturalnews.com/034863_licorice_Barretts_esophagus_remedies.html, Accessed April 28, 2014
- http://www.lef.org/magazine/mag2007/apr2007_atd_01.htm, Accessed April 28, 2014

- http://cancer.osu.edu/mediaroom/releases/Pages/Black-Raspberries-May-Prevent-Esophageal-Cancer.aspx, Accessed April 28, 2014
- Kresty LA, Frankel WL, Hammond CD, et al. Transitioning from preclinical to clinical chemopreventive assessments of lyophilized black raspberries: interim results show berries modulate markers of oxidative stress in Barrett's esophagus patients. Nutr Cancer. 2006;54(1):148-56. http://www.ncbi.nlm.nih.gov/pubmed/16800781

Esophageal Spasms

Cayenne

- https://www.caymanchem.com/article/2116, Accessed April 28, 2014
- http://cdn.intechopen.com/pdfs/32237/InTech-Neural_regulatory_mechanisms_of_esophageal_motility_and_its_implication_for_gerd.pdf, Accessed April 28, 2014

Peppermint Oil

- Pimentel M, Bonorris GG, Chow EJ, Lin HC. Peppermint oil improves the manometric findings in diffuse esophageal spasm. J Clin Gastroenterol. 2001;33(1):27-31. http://www.ncbi.nlm.nih.gov/pubmed/11418786

Nutcracker Esophagus

Peppermint Oil

- http://www.umm.edu/altmed/articles/peppermint-000269.htm, Accessed April 28, 2014

Abdominal Hernia

- http://www.shouldice.com/the_shouldice_repair.htm, Accessed April 28, 2014

SIBO

- Dr. Brownsetin, David. *Drugs That Don't Work and Natural Therapies that Do!*, Medical Alternative Press, 2007.

Leaky Gut

- http://www.optimumchoices.com/Seacure_research.htm, Accessed April 28, 2014

Peppermint Oil

- http://www.altmedrev...ons/7/5/410.pdf, Accessed April 28, 2014
- Grigoleit HG, Grigoleit P. Peppermint oil in irritable bowel syndrome. Phytomedicine. 2005;12(8):601-6. https://www.ncbi.nlm.nih.gov/pubmed/16121521

Biofilms

- https://selfhacked.com/2016/03/01/44-science-backed-ways-to-inhibit-biofilms-naturally-with-references/, Accessed April 28, 2014
- http://chriskresser.com/treating-sibo-cold-thermogenisis-and-when-to-take-probiotics, Accessed April 28, 2014
- http://www.advancedhealing.com/dr-ettingers-biofilm-protocol-for-lyme-and-gut-pathogens/, Accessed April 28, 2014
- Kite P, Eastwood K, Sugden S, Percival SL. Use of in vivo-generated biofilms from hemodialysis catheters to test the efficacy of a novel antimicrobial catheter lock for biofilm eradication in vitro. J Clin Microbiol. 2004;42(7):3073-6. http://jcm.asm.org/content/42/7/3073.full.pdf
- Barrett JS, Canale KE, Gearry RB, Irving PM, Gibson PR. Probiotic effects on intestinal fermentation patterns in patients with irritable bowel syndrome. World J Gastroenterol. 2008;14(32):5020-4. http://www.ncbi.nlm.nih.gov/pmc/articles/PMC2742929/

- Wakabayashi H, Yamauchi K, Kobayashi T, Yaeshima T, Iwatsuki K, Yoshie H. Inhibitory effects of lactoferrin on growth and biofilm formation of Porphyromonas gingivalis and *Prevotella* intermedia. Antimicrob Agents Chemother. 2009;53(8):3308-16. http://www.ncbi.nlm.nih.gov/pmc/articles/PMC2715627/

SIYO

- http://owndoc.com/candida-albicans/candida-facts/, Accessed April 28, 2014
- http://www.yeastinfection.org/functional-candida-testing-elisa-blood-and-saliva-tests/, Accessed April 28, 2014
- http://owndoc.com/candida-albicans/spit-test-candida-diagnosis-unreliable/, Accessed April 28, 2014
- http://www.drlwilson.com/articles/candida.htm, Accessed April 28, 2014
- Parodi A, Paolino S, Greco A, et al. Small intestinal bacterial overgrowth in rosacea: clinical effectiveness of its eradication. Clin Gastroenterol Hepatol. 2008;6(7):759-64. http://www.ncbi.nlm.nih.gov/pubmed/18456568
- Muñoz P, Bouza E, Cuenca-estrella M, et al. *Saccharomyces cerevisiae* fungemia: an emerging infectious disease. Clin Infect Dis. 2005;40(11):1625-34. http://www.ncbi.nlm.nih.gov/pubmed/15889360

General SIBO Information

- http://www.siboinfo.com/overview.html, Accessed April 28, 2014
- http://chriskresser.com/treating-sibo-cold-thermogenisis-and-when-to-take-probiotics, Accessed April 28, 2014
- http://ndnr.com/web-articles/gastrointestinal/small-intestine-bacterial-overgrowth-2/, Accessed April 28, 2014
- http://www.siboinfo.com/testing1.html, Accessed April 28, 2014
- http://www.siboinfo.com/overview.html, Accessed April 28, 2014
- Bures J, Cyrany J, Kohoutova D, et al. Small intestinal bacterial overgrowth syndrome. World J Gastroenterol. 2010;16(24):2978-90. http://www.ncbi.nlm.nih.gov/pmc/articles/PMC2890937/
- Rhoads JM, Argenzio RA, Chen W, et al. L-glutamine stimulates intestinal cell proliferation and activates mitogen-activated protein kinases. Am J Physiol. 1997;272(5 Pt 1):G943-53. http://www.ncbi.nlm.nih.gov/pubmed/9176200
- Bures J, Cyrany J, Kohoutova D, et al. Small intestinal bacterial overgrowth syndrome. World J Gastroenterol. 2010;16(24):2978-90. http://www.ncbi.nlm.nih.gov/pmc/articles/PMC2890937/

Curcumin

- http://lpi.oregonstate.edu/infocenter/phytochemicals/curcumin/, Accessed April 28, 2014
- Auricchio S, De ritis G, De vincenzi M, et al. Mannan and oligomers of N-acetylglucosamine protect intestinal mucosa of celiac patients with active disease from in vitro toxicity of gliadin peptides. Gastroenterology. 1990;99(4):973-8. http://www.ncbi.nlm.nih.gov/pubmed/2394351

IBS

- Lacy, Brian. *Making Since of IBS*, John Hopkins University Press, 2006.

SIBO as a Cause

- Posserud I, Stotzer PO, Björnsson ES, Abrahamsson H, Simrén M. Small intestinal bacterial overgrowth in patients with irritable bowel syndrome. Gut. 2007;56(6):802-8. http://www.ncbi.nlm.nih.gov/pmc/articles/PMC1954873/
- Karantanos T, Markoutsaki T, Gazouli M, Anagnou NP, Karamanolis DG. Current insights in to the pathophysiology of Irritable Bowel Syndrome. Gut Pathog. 2010;2(1):3. http://www.gutpathogens.com/content/2/1/3

Adrenal Fatigue

- http://www.drlam.com/articles/Top_10_adrenal_fatigue_facts_made_easy.asp, Accessed April 28, 2014
- www.drlam.com, Accessed April 28, 2014

Chronic Functional Abdominal Pain

- http://www.iffgd.org/site/gi-disorders/functional-gi-disorders/functional-abdominal-pain-syndrome, Accessed April 28, 2014
- http://www.merckmanuals.com/home/digestive_disorders/symptoms_of_digestive_disorders/chronic_and_recurring_abdominal_pain.html, Accessed April 28, 2014
- Chiou E, Nurko S. Management of functional abdominal pain and irritable bowel syndrome in children and adolescents. Expert Rev Gastroenterol Hepatol. 2010;4(3):293-304. http://www.ncbi.nlm.nih.gov/pmc/articles/PMC2904303/

Intestinal Renewal

N-Acetyl Glucosamine

- Salvatore S, Heuschkel R, Tomlin S, et al. A pilot study of N-acetyl glucosamine, a nutritional substrate for glycosaminoglycan synthesis, in paediatric chronic inflammatory bowel disease. Aliment Pharmacol Ther. 2000;14(12):1567-79. http://www.ncbi.nlm.nih.gov/pubmed/11121904

L-Glutamine

- http://www.altmedrev.com/publications/4/4/239.pdf, Accessed April 28, 2014

Celiac Disease

- Beers, Mark. *The Merck Manual*, Merck Research Laboratories, 2006.
- Green, Peter / Jones, Rory. *Celiac Disease A Hidden Epidemic*, Collins Publishing, 2006.
- Davis, William. *Wheat Belly: Loose the Wheat, Lose the Weight*, Rodale, August 30, 2011.
- Tamparo, Carol, Lewis, Marcia. *Diseases of the Human Body*, F. A. Davis Company, Feb. 11, 2011.
- http://www.klaire.com/images/dppiv_update_article.pdf, Accessed April 28, 2014

IBD

- Beers, Mark. The *Merck Manual*, Merck Research Laboratories, 2006.
- Saibil, Fred. *Crohn's Disease and Ulcerative Colitis*, Firefly Books, 2011.
- Tamparo, Carol, Lewis, Marcia. *Diseases of the Human Body*, F. A. Davis Company, Feb. 11, 2011.
- http://www.drhoffman.com/page.cfm/169, Accessed April 28, 2014
- http://www.crohns.org/treatment/, Accessed April 28, 2014
- http://www.notmilk.com/drgreger.html, Accessed April 28, 2014
- http://emedicine.medscape.com/article/222664-treatment, Accessed April 28, 2014
- http://aas.bf.uni-lj.si/avgust2007/09bupesh.pdf, Accessed April 28, 2014
- Pierce ES. Ulcerative colitis and Crohn's disease: is *Mycobacterium avium subspecies paratuberculosis* the common villain?. Gut Pathog. 2010;2(1):21. http://www.gutpathogens.com/content/2/1/21
- Pierce ES. Possible transmission of *Mycobacterium avium subspecies paratuberculosis* through potable water: lessons from an urban cluster of Crohn's disease. Gut Pathog. 2009;1(1):17. http://www.gutpathogens.com/content/1/1/17
- Hermon-taylor J. *Mycobacterium avium subspecies paratuberculosis*, Crohn's disease and the Doomsday scenario. Gut Pathog. 2009;1(1):15. http://www.gutpathogens.com/content/1/1/15
- Hermon-taylor J. Gut pathogens: invaders and turncoats in a complex cosmos. Gut Pathog. 2009;1(1):3. http://www.gutpathogens.com/content/1/1/3
- Sullam PM. Rifabutin therapy for disseminated *Mycobacterium avium* complex infection. Clin Infect Dis. 1996;22 Suppl 1:S37-41. http://www.ncbi.nlm.nih.gov/pubmed/8785255\

Appendix

- http://www.sciencedaily.com/releases/2007/10/071008102334.htm, Accessed April 28, 2014
- http://www.the-scientist.com/?articles.view/articleNo/34416/title/Appendix-Not-Totally-Useless/, Accessed April 28, 2014

Hemorrhoid

- http://www.cayennepepper.info/cayenne-pepper-hemorrhoid-cure.html, Accessed April 28, 2014
- http://scialert.net/fulltext/?doi=ijp.2013.1.11, Accessed April 28, 2014
- http://www.webmd.com/vitamins-supplements/ingredientmono-227-WITCH%20HAZEL.aspx?activeIngredientId=227&activeIngredientName=WITCH%20HAZEL, Accessed April 28, 2014

Colon Cleansing

Colon Cleansing General Information

- Jones, Wes. *Cure Constipation Now*, Berkley Trade, July 7, 2009.
- Monastyrsky, Konstantin. *Fiber Menace*, Ageless Press, October 15, 2005.
- http://www.mayoclinic.com/health/colon-cleansing/AN00065, Accessed April 28, 2014
- http://www.ext.colostate.edu/pubs/foodnut/09333.html, Accessed April 28, 2014
- http://www.webmd.com/diet/fiber-health-benefits-11/insoluble-soluble-fiber, Accessed April 28, 2014
- http://chriskresser.com/myths-and-truths-about-fiber, Accessed April 28, 2014
- http://www.nlm.nih.gov/medlineplus/ency/article/002136.htm, Accessed April 28, 2014
- http://www.webmd.com/diet/fiber-health-benefits-11/insoluble-soluble-fiber, Accessed April 28, 2014
- http://www.gutsense.org/reports/myth.html, Accessed April 28, 2014

Colon Cleansing Protocols

Bentonite Clay

- http://www.californiaearthminerals.com/media/damrau-diarrhea-trials--bentonite-kills-germs-in-your-body.pdf, http://sonnes.com/store/?wpsc-product=7-detoxificant-32-oz-liquid, Accessed April 28, 2014

Chlorella

- Steinblock, David. *Chlorella: Natural Medicinal Algae*, Aging Research Inst, September 1992.

Other Supplements

- http://www.altmedrev.com/publications/7/5/410.pdf, Accessed April 28, 2014
- http://chriskresser.com/treating-sibo-cold-thermogenisis-and-when-to-take-probiotics, Accessed April 28, 2014
- https://selfhacked.com/2016/03/01/44-science-backed-ways-to-inhibit-biofilms-naturally-with-references/, Accessed April 28, 2014
- http://www.planetherbs.com/specific-herbs/the-wonders-of-triphala.html, Accessed April 28, 2014
- https://californiaearthminerals.com/media/damrau-diarrhea-trials--bentonite-kills-germs-in-your-body.pdf, http://sonnes.com/store/?wpsc-product=7-detoxificant-32-oz-liquid, Accessed April 28, 2014
- http://benthamscience.com/open/jebp/articles/V005/SI0010JEBP/47JEBP.pdf, Accessed April 28, 2014
- http://www.plosone.org/article/info%3Adoi%2F10.1371%2Fjournal.pone.0015099, Accessed April 28, 2014
- http://naturalmedicinejournal.com/article_content.asp?article=106, Accessed April 28, 2014
- Grigoleit HG, Grigoleit P. Peppermint oil in irritable bowel syndrome. Phytomedicine. 2005;12(8):601-6. http://www.ncbi.nlm.nih.gov/pubmed/16121521
- Ogbolu DO, Oni AA, Daini OA, Oloko AP. In vitro antimicrobial properties of coconut oil on *Candida* species in Ibadan, Nigeria. J Med Food. 2007;10(2):384-7. http://www.ncbi.nlm.nih.gov/pubmed/17651080

79338334R10228

Made in the USA
San Bernardino, CA
14 June 2018